Female Pelvic Imaging

Editors

NEERAJ LALWANI
THEODORE J. DUBINSKY

RADIOLOGIC CLINICS
OF NORTH AMERICA

www.radiologic.theclinics.com

Consulting Editor
FRANK H. MILLER

November 2013 • Volume 51 • Number 6

ELSEVIER

1600 John F. Kennedy Boulevard • Suite 1800 • Philadelphia, Pennsylvania, 19103-2899

http://www.theclinics.com

RADIOLOGIC CLINICS OF NORTH AMERICA Volume 51, Number 6
November 2013 ISSN 0033-8389, ISBN 13: 978-0-323-26600-0

Editor: Adrianne Brigido

Radiologic Clinics of North America (ISSN 0033-8389) is published bimonthly by Elsevier Inc., 360 Park Avenue South, New York, NY 10010-1710. Months of issue are January, March, May, July, September, and November. Periodicals postage paid at New York, NY and additional mailing offices. Subscription prices are USD 438 per year for US individuals, USD 685 per year for US institutions, USD 210 per year for US students and residents, USD 511 per year for Canadian individuals, USD 858 per year for Canadian institutions, USD 630 per year for international individuals, USD 858 per year for international institutions, and USD 302 per year for Canadian and foreign students/residents. To receive student and resident rate, orders must be accompanied by name of affiliated institution, date of term and the signature of program/residency coordinatior on institution letterhead. Orders will be billed at individual rate until proof of status is received. Foreign air speed delivery is included in all *Clinics* subscription prices. All prices are subject to change without notice. **POSTMASTER:** Send address changes to *Radiologic Clinics of North America*, Elsevier Health Sciences Division, Subscription Customer Service, 3251 Riverport Lane, Maryland Heights, MO63043. **Customer Service: Telephone: 1-800-654-2452** (U.S. and Canada); **1-314-447-8871** (outside U.S. and Canada). **Fax: 1-314-447-8029. E-mail: journalscustomerservice-usa@elsevier.com** (for print support); **journalsonlinesupport-usa@elsevier.com** (for online support).

Reprints. For copies of 100 or more of articles in this publication, please contact the Commercial Reprints Department, Elsevier Inc., 360 Park Avenue South, New York, New York 10010-1710. Tel.: +1-212-633-3874; Fax: +1-212-633-3820; E-mail: reprints@elsevier.com.

Radiologic Clinics of North America also published in Greek Paschalidis Medical Publications, Athens, Greece.

Radiologic Clinics of North America is covered in *MEDLINE/PubMed (Index Medicus), EMBASE/Excerpta Medica, Current Contents/Life Sciences, Current Contents/Clinical Medicine, RSNA Index to Imaging Literature, BIOSIS, Science Citation Index,* and *ISI/BIOMED*.

Printed in the United States of America.

Contributors

CONSULTING EDITOR

FRANK H. MILLER, MD
Professor of Radiology; Chief, Body Imaging,
Section and Fellowship Program and GI,
Radiology; Medical Director MRI, Department
of Radiology, Feinberg School of Medicine,
Northwestern University, Chicago, Illinois

EDITORS

NEERAJ LALWANI, MD
Assistant Professor, Department of Radiology,
University of Washington, School of Medicine,
Seattle, Washington

THEODORE J. DUBINSKY, MD
The Laurence A. Mack Endowed Professor of
Radiology, Obstetrics and Gynecology, and
Reproductive Health Sciences, University of
Washington, School of Medicine, Seattle,
Washington

AUTHORS

SUSAN ACKERMAN, MD
Professor of Radiology, Department of
Radiology and Radiological Sciences, Medical
University of South Carolina, Charleston,
South Carolina

BRIAN C. ALLEN, MD
Assistant Professor, Abdominal Imaging,
Department of Radiology, Wake Forest
University School of Medicine, Wake Forest
Baptist Medical Center, Winston-Salem,
North Carolina

ROCHELLE ANDREOTTI, MD
Clinical Professor of Radiology, Department
of Radiology, Vanderbilt University Medical
Center, Nashville, Tennessee

MUNAZZA ANIS, MD
Assistant Professor of Radiology, Department
of Radiology and Radiological Sciences,
Medical University of South Carolina,
Charleston, South Carolina

LINDA ARMSTRONG, DO
Women's Imaging Fellow, Department of
Radiology, Vanderbilt University Medical
Center, Nashville, Tennessee

PUNEET BHARGAVA, MD
Assistant Professor, Department of
Radiology, VA Puget Sound Health Care
System, Seattle, Washington

PRIYA R. BHOSALE, MD
Diagnostic Radiology, The University of Texas
MD Anderson Cancer Center, Houston, Texas

MANJIRI K. DIGHE, MD
Associate Professor, Department of Radiology,
University of Washington, Seattle, Washington

VIKRAM DOGRA, MD
Professor of Imaging Science, Urology, and
Biomedical Imaging, Department of Imaging
Sciences, University of Rochester Medical
Center, Rochester, New York

NAJLA FASIH, MD
Assistant Professor, Department of Medical Imaging, The Ottawa Hospital, University of Ottawa, Ottawa, Ontario, Canada

ARTHUR FLEISCHER, MD
Professor of Radiology, Department of Radiology, Vanderbilt University Medical Center, Nashville, Tennessee

ANDRES GARZA-BERLANGA, MD
Assistant Professor of Radiology, Department of Radiology, UT Health Science Center at San Antonio, San Antonio, Texas

VERGHESE GEORGE, MBBS, FRCR
Assistant Professor, Department of Diagnostic and Interventional Imaging, The University of Texas Health Science Center at Houston, Texas

ABID IRSHAD, MBBS
Professor of Radiology, Department of Radiology and Radiological Sciences, Medical University of South Carolina, Charleston, South Carolina

KATHERINE KAPROTH-JOSLIN, MD, PhD
Radiology Resident, Department of Imaging Sciences, University of Rochester Medical Center, Rochester, New York

ASHISH KHANDELWAL, MD
Department of Radiology, Brigham and Women's Hospital, Harvard Medical School, Boston, Massachusetts

ANIA KIELAR, MD
Assistant Professor, Department of Medical Imaging, The Ottawa Hospital, University of Ottawa, Ottawa, Ontario, Canada

GHAZWAN M. KROMA, MD
Assistant Professor of Radiology, Department of Radiology, UT Health Science Center at San Antonio, San Antonio, Texas

CHANDANA LALL, MD
Department of Radiology, University of California, Irvine, Orange, California

NEERAJ LALWANI, MD
Assistant Professor, Department of Radiology, University of Washington, School of Medicine, Seattle, Washington

JEAN H. LEE, MD
Assistant Professor, Department of Radiology, University of Washington, Seattle, Washington

MADELENE LEWIS, MD
Assistant Professor of Radiology, Department of Radiology and Radiological Sciences, Medical University of South Carolina, Charleston, South Carolina

JOHN R. LEYENDECKER, MD
Professor, Abdominal Imaging, Department of Radiology, Wake Forest University School of Medicine, Wake Forest Baptist Medical Center, Winston-Salem, North Carolina

JORGE LOPERA, MD
Professor of Radiology, Department of Radiology, UT Health Science Center at San Antonio, San Antonio, Texas

CHRISTINE O. MENIAS, MD
Department of Radiology, Mayo Clinic LL Radiology, Scottsdale, Arizona

MARIAM MOSHIRI, MD
Assistant Professor, Department of Radiology, University of Washington, Seattle, Washington

ARPIT NAGAR, MD
Department of Radiology, Ohio State University Medical Center, Columbus, Ohio

SRINIVASA R. PRASAD, MD
Professor of Radiology, Section of Body Imaging, The University of Texas MD Anderson Cancer Center, Houston, Texas

SHETAL N. SHAH, MD
Director, PET-MR; Co-director, Diagnostic Radiology and PET Imaging, Center for PET and Molecular Imaging, Cleveland Clinic Foundation, Cleveland, Ohio

ALAMPADY K.P. SHANBHOGUE, MD
Department of Radiology, Beth Israel Medical Center, New York, New York

CARY LYNN SIEGEL, MD
Professor of Radiology, Washington University School of Medicine; Director of Genitourinary Radiology; Director of Gastrointestinal Radiology, Abdominal Imaging Section, Mallinckrodt Institute of Radiology, St Louis, Missouri

VENKATESWAR RAO SURABHI, MD
Assistant Professor, Department of Diagnostic and Interventional Imaging, The University of Texas Health Science Center at Houston, Texas

RAJEEV SURI, MD
Associate Professor of Radiology, Department of Radiology, UT Health Science Center at San Antonio, San Antonio, Texas

JOHN THOMAS, MD
Interventional Radiologist, Methodist Hospital, San Antonio, Texas

SREE HARSHA TIRUMANI, MD
Department of Imaging, Dana-Farber Cancer Institute/Brigham and Women's Hospital, Harvard Medical School, Boston, Massachusetts

RAGHUNANDAN VIKRAM, MBBS, MRCP, FRCR
Diagnostic Radiology, The University of Texas MD Anderson Cancer Center, Houston, Texas

CHITRA VISWANATHAN, MD
Diagnostic Radiology, The University of Texas MD Anderson Cancer Center, Houston, Texas

Contents

Magnetic Resonance Imaging of Female Urethral and Periurethral Disorders   941

Venkateswar Rao Surabhi, Christine O. Menias, Verghese George, Cary Lynn Siegel, and
Srinivasa R. Prasad

> This article reviews the normal anatomy of the female urethra, magnetic resonance
> (MR) imaging techniques, and the role of MR imaging in the evaluation of diverse
> urethral and periurethral diseases. Salient MR imaging findings of common and
> uncommon cystic urethral lesions (urethral diverticulum, Skene cyst, and vaginal
> cysts), and masses (urethral carcinoma, leiomyoma, melanoma, fibroepithelial polyp,
> caruncle, and mucosal prolapse) are presented. The evolving role of dynamic MR in
> the evaluation of stress urinary incontinence is reviewed.

Placental Evaluation with Magnetic Resonance   955

Brian C. Allen and John R. Leyendecker

> Because of the high maternal morbidity and mortality of undiagnosed placental
> abnormalities, there is a need for accurate antenatal diagnosis. Important placental
> features amenable to investigation with magnetic resonance (MR) imaging include
> variant placental location and morphology, and abnormal implantation or invasion
> of placenta into the myometrium. MR imaging features permit the diagnosis of
> abnormal placentation include placental lobulation with uterine contour deformity,
> interruption of the inner low signal-intensity myometrial layer, and placental hetero-
> geneity resulting from dark intraplacental bands and abnormal vascularity.

Imaging of Female Infertility: A Pictorial Guide to the Hysterosalpingography,
Ultrasonography, and Magnetic Resonance Imaging Findings of the Congenital
and Acquired Causes of Female Infertility   967

Katherine Kaproth-Joslin and Vikram Dogra

> Hysterosalpingography is the gold standard in assessing the patency of the fallopian
> tubes, which is among the most common causes of female factor infertility, making
> this technique the most frequent first-choice imaging modality in the assessment of
> female infertility. Ultrasonography and magnetic resonance imaging are typically
> used for evaluation of indeterminate or complicated cases of female infertility and
> presurgical planning. Imaging also plays a role in the detection of the secondary
> causes of ovarian factor infertility, including endometriosis and polycystic ovarian
> syndrome.

Obstetric (Nonfetal) Complications   983

Alampady K.P. Shanbhogue, Christine O. Menias, Neeraj Lalwani, Chandana Lall,
Ashish Khandelwal, and Arpit Nagar

> Pregnancy predisposes women to a wide array of obstetric and gynecological com-
> plications which are often complex, challenging and sometimes life-threatening.
> While some of these are unique to pregnancy, a few that occur in nonpregnant
> women are more common during pregnancy. Imaging plays a crucial role in the

diagnosis and management of pregnancy-related obstetric and gynecologic complications. Ultrasonography and magnetic resonance imaging confer the least risk to the fetus and should be the preferred examinations for evaluating these complications. Multidetector computed tomography should be used after carefully weighing the risk-benefit ratio based on the clinical condition in question. Interventional radiology is emerging as a preferred, noninvasive or minimally invasive treatment option that can obviate surgery and its antecedent short term and long term complications. Knowledge of appropriateness of imaging and image guided intervention is necessary for accurate patient management.

The approach to imaging in pregnancy is unique, as it is essential to minimize radiation exposure to the fetus. Ultrasonography and magnetic resonance imaging are the chief modalities for evaluation of the pregnant patient with abdominal pain. Use of computed tomography should not be delayed when there is a need for early diagnosis. This article discusses test selection and underlying reasoning, with a description of common imaging features of different causes of acute abdominal pain in pregnancy. Also discussed are current evidence-based recommendations for the use of iodinated and gadolinium-based contrast agents and the importance of patient counseling.

Imaging plays a crucial role in diagnosis and management of gestational trophoblastic disease. Ultrasonography is the initial investigation of choice for the diagnosis. Pelvic magnetic resonance (MR) imaging is used as a problem-solving tool for assessment of degree of local invasion. Chest radiography is the recommended initial radiographic staging modality, and chest computed tomography is performed if the radiograph is negative. ^{18}F-Fluorodeoxyglucose positron emission tomography has been shown to be useful in assessing the active or viable sites of metastases, thereby determining the need for tumor resectability in chemoresistant disease.

Three-dimensional (3D) sonography can significantly improve on the diagnostic ability of two-dimensional sonography of the pelvic organs. 3D sonography has become a problem-solving technique in the evaluation of a variety of gynecologic disorders involving the uterus, adnexa, and pelvic floor. It allows an accurate depiction of the uterine cavity and outline of the uterus in the coronal plane. 3D sonography is less expensive than other modalities, is convenient, and does not have the risk of radiation or potential nephrotoxicity from contrast that other imaging modalities have. It is a cost-effective tool to assess the pelvic organs.

In uterine fibroid embolization (UFE), knowledge of the potential ovarian-uterine anastomoses is important because they provide collateral blood flow that may result in the failure of the UFE or ovarian nontarget embolization. Uterine artery embolization is an alternative treatment of postpartum hemorrhage with 80% to 90% bleeding control and in which fertility can be preserved. Diagnosis of pelvic congestion syndrome on routine sonographic or computed tomography/magnetic resonance imaging is often missed. Fallopian tube recanalization allows couples to have unlimited attempts to conceive naturally and avoids the risks (multiple pregnancies, ovarian hyperstimulation syndrome), and high cost of in vitro fertilization.

The primary imaging modality for evaluation of ovarian cystic lesions is pelvic ultrasonography. Most ovarian cysts are benign and demonstrate typical sonographic features that support benignity. However, some ovarian cystic lesions have indeterminate imaging features, and the approach to management varies. This article discusses how to recognize and diagnose different types of ovarian cystic lesions, including an approach to management. The learning objective is to recognize imaging features of ovarian cystic lesions.

Cross-sectional imaging modalities play a pivotal role in the diagnosis and multidisciplinary management of patients with endometrial and cervical carcinomas. Ultrasonography, including sonohysterography, permits evaluation of endometrial abnormalities and characterization of adnexal masses. Computed tomography, particularly in conjunction with ^{18F}-fluorodeoxyglucose positron emission tomography, is increasingly used to stage the cancers and to detect disease recurrence. Magnetic resonance imaging plays a major role in accurate locoregional staging of these cancers, and significantly influences treatment decisions and outcomes. This article discusses the role of imaging modalities in the diagnosis, management, and surveillance of these cancers.

The role of Positron Emission Tomography/Computed Tomography (PET/CT) in the evaluation of various gynecologic malignancies in light of current available data is presented and illustrated with imaging examples, pearls, and common pitfalls. 18F-fluorodeoxyglucose PET/CT is being increasingly used in management of gynecologic malignancy and has useful applications in cervical, ovarian, and endometrial carcinoma. Sensitivity and specificity are superior compared with conventional imaging. However, there are limitations of which the reporting physician should be aware. This article introduces the available evidence and discusses the role of PET/CT in various gynecologic malignancies and highlights imaging pearls and potential pitfalls.

Pelvic floor dysfunction is largely a complex problem of multiparous and postmenopausal women and is associated with pelvic floor or organ descent. Physical examination can underestimate the extent of the dysfunction and misdiagnose the disorders. Functional magnetic resonance (MR) imaging is emerging as a promising tool to evaluate the dynamics of the pelvic floor and use for surgical triage and operative planning. This article reviews the anatomy and pathology of pelvic floor dysfunction, typical imaging findings, and the current role of functional MR imaging.

PROGRAM OBJECTIVE

The objective of the Radiologic Clinics of North America is to keep practicing radiologists and radiology residents up to date with current clinical practice in radiology by providing timely articles reviewing the state of the art in patient care.

TARGET AUDIENCE

Practicing radiologists, radiology residents, and other health care professionals who provide patient care utilizing radiologic findings.

LEARNING OBJECTIVES

Upon completion of this activity, participants will be able to:
1. Discuss imaging of female urethral and periurethral disorders, pelvic floor dysfunction, and acute abdomen in pregnancy.
2. Describe the clinical applications for three dimensional volumetric sonography in gynecology.
3. Discuss obstetric (non-fetal) complications.

ACCREDITATION

The Elsevier Office of Continuing Medical Education (EOCME) is accredited by the Accreditation Council for Continuing Medical Education (ACCME) to provide continuing medical education for physicians.

The EOCME designates this enduring material for a maximum of 15 *AMA PRA Category 1 Credit*(s)™. Physicians should claim only the credit commensurate with the extent of their participation in the activity.

All other health care professionals requesting continuing education credit for this enduring material will be issued a certificate of participation.

DISCLOSURE OF CONFLICTS OF INTEREST

The EOCME assesses conflict of interest with its instructors, faculty, planners, and other individuals who are in a position to control the content of CME activities. All relevant conflicts of interest that are identified are thoroughly vetted by EOCME for fair balance, scientific objectivity, and patient care recommendations. EOCME is committed to providing its learners with CME activities that promote improvements or quality in healthcare and not a specific proprietary business or a commercial interest.

The planning committee, staff, authors and editors listed below have identified no financial relationships or relationships to products or devices they or their spouse/life partner have with commercial interest related to the content of this CME activity:
Susan Ackerman, MD; Brian C. Allen, MD; Rochelle Andreotti, MD; Munazza Anis, MD; Linda Armstrong, DO; Puneet Bhargava, MD; Priya R. Bhosale, MD; Adrianne Brigido; Nicole Congleton; Manjiri K. Dighe, MD; Vikram Dogra, MD; Theodore J. Dubinsky, MD; Najla Fasih, MD; Arthur Fleischer, MD; Andres Garza-Berlanga, MD; Verghese George, MBBS, FRCR; Brynne Hunter; Abid Irshad, MBBS; Katherine Kaproth-Joslin, MD/PhD; Ashish Khandelwal, MD; Ania Kielar, MD; Ghazwan M. Kroma, MD; Chandana Lall, MD; Neeraj Lalwani, MD; Sandy Lavery; Jean H. Lee, MD; Madelene Lewis, MD; John R. Leyendecker, MD; Jorge Lopera, MD, FSIR; Jill McNair; Christine O. Menias, MD; Frank H. Miller, MD; Mariam Moshiri, MD; Arpit Nagar, MD; Srinivasa R. Prasad, MD; Shetal N. Shah, MD; Alampady K.P. Shanbhogue, MD; Cary Lynn Siegel, MD; Karthikeyan Subramaniam; Venkateswar Rao Surabhi, MD; Rajeev Suri, MD; John Thomas, MD; Sree Harsha Tirumani, MD; Raghunandan Vikram, MBBS, MRCP, FRCR; Chitra Viswanathan, MD.

The planning committee, staff, authors and editors listed below have identified financial relationships or relationships to products or devices they or their spouse/life partner have with commercial interest related to the content of this CME activity:
John Leyendecker, MD has royalties/patents with Elsevier.
Mariam Moshiri, MD is a consultant/advisor for and recieves patents/royalties from Amirsys, Inc.

UNAPPROVED/OFF-LABEL USE DISCLOSURE

The EOCME requires CME faculty to disclose to the participants:
1. When products or procedures being discussed are off-label, unlabelled, experimental, and/or investigational (not US Food and Drug Administration (FDA) approved); and
2. Any limitations on the information presented, such as data that are preliminary or that represent ongoing research, interim analyses, and/or unsupported opinions. Faculty may discuss information about pharmaceutical agents that is outside of FDA-approved labelling. This information is intended solely for CME and is not intended to promote off-label use of these medications. If you have any questions, contact the medical affairs department of the manufacturer for the most recent prescribing information.

TO ENROLL

To enroll in the *Radiologic Clinics of North America* Continuing Medical Education program, call customer service at 1-800-654-2452 or sign up online at http://www.theclinics.com/home/cme. The CME program is available to subscribers for an additional annual fee of USD $288.

METHOD OF PARTICIPATION

In order to claim credit, participants must complete the following:
1. Complete enrolment as indicated above.
2. Read the activity.
3. Complete the CME Test and Evaluation. Participants must achieve a score of 70% on the test. All CME Tests and Evaluations must be completed online.

CME INQUIRIES/SPECIAL NEEDS

For all CME inquiries or special needs, please contact elsevierCME@elsevier.com.

RADIOLOGIC CLINICS OF NORTH AMERICA

Preface

Diagnostic imaging has undergone a rapid and intense change in the last decade. The role of a modern radiologist in diagnosing female pelvic pathologies is crucial and has significantly expanded along with the recent advances in imaging techniques. However, the complexity of these newer imaging techniques remains a challenge. Comprehensive information about these modalities and techniques is not readily available in the literature. For these reasons, this issue of the *Radiologic Clinics of North America* is dedicated to addressing current state-of-the-art applications of imaging techniques to female pelvic imaging.

We are blessed to have a team of outstanding contributors, all experts in their fields, provide state-of-the-art reviews for this issue of the *Radiologic Clinics of North America*. All the topics included in this issue have real-world application for the practicing radiologist. The articles are designed to allow the reader to organize the practical information in a meaningful fashion. We firmly believe the information encompassed within this issue will help practicing radiologists provide clinically relevant information to referring physicians and positively impact the patient management. In addition, this issue will also be beneficial to colleagues in all other medical specialties who consistently work to improve patient care and quality of life for women presenting with complex pelvic pathologies.

Topics covered in this issue include MR imaging of female urethra and periurethral disorders, MR evaluation of placenta, imaging of female infertility, obstetric (nonfetal) complications (including gestational trophoblastic disease), imaging of acute abdomen in pregnancy, 3D pelvic sonography, role of interventional procedures in ob/gyn, approach to ovarian cystic lesions, imaging of gynecologic malignancies (including PET), and MR imaging of pelvic floor dysfunction.

We would like to thank this talented group of contributors for their excellent contributions and outstanding efforts to assemble this issue of the *Radiologic Clinics of North America*; they have made editing this issue a pleasure. In addition, we wish to thank Dr Frank Miller, Elsevier, and their staff members; we particularly thank Adrianne Brigido, for the support and help she provided to us as this issue was being planned and prepared.

We hope that this issue will serve to update the practicing radiologists, clinicians, and academicians on a wide range of established and novel diagnostic methods and will be a valuable resource for the current practice of female pelvic imaging.

Neeraj Lalwani, MD
Department of Radiology
University of Washington, School of Medicine
Seattle, WA 98104-2499, USA

Theodore J. Dubinsky, MD
University of Washington, School of Medicine
Seattle, WA 98104-2499, USA

E-mail addresses:
neerajl@u.washington.edu (N. Lalwani)
tdub@u.washington.edu (T.J. Dubinsky)

Radiol Clin N Am 51 (2013) xiii
http://dx.doi.org/10.1016/j.rcl.2013.09.003
0033-8389/13/$ – see front matter © 2013 Published by Elsevier Inc.

Magnetic Resonance Imaging of Female Urethral and Periurethral Disorders

Venkateswar Rao Surabhi, MD[a],*,
Christine O. Menias, MD[b], Verghese George, MBBS, FRCR[a],
Cary Lynn Siegel, MD[c,d], Srinivasa R. Prasad, MD[e]

KEYWORDS

- Female urethra • Magnetic resonance imaging • Diverticulum • Carcinoma • Leiomyoma
- Stress urinary incontinence

KEY POINTS

- Endoluminal magnetic resonance (MR) imaging, allowing high-resolution delineation of the female urethra, assists in the diagnosis of a wide spectrum of urethral disorders.
- Diverticulum is the most common cystic lesion of the urethra that communicates with its lumen.
- MR imaging plays a seminal role in triaging urethral carcinoma patients to surgery as opposed to neoadjuvant chemoradiotherapy by identifying key prognostic factors such as location, size, and, most importantly, locoregional invasion.
- Urethral leiomyomas demonstrate T2 isointense to hyperintense signal on MR imaging in contradistinction to typical uterine leiomyomas that are dark on T2.
- Dynamic pelvic MR imaging is very helpful for establishing urethral hypermobility in the workup of stress urinary incontinence.

INTRODUCTION

Imaging of the female urethra is typically requested for assessment of a wide array of lower urinary tract symptoms. Voiding cystourethrography and ultrasonography are commonly performed tests for initial evaluation of urethral symptoms. Urethrography provides limited information about disorders that are contiguous with the urethral lumen. High-resolution transvaginal or transperineal ultrasonography with employment of Doppler techniques is a useful test in the diagnosis and characterization of urethral abnormalities. However, it is limited by operator dependence, small field of view, and limited ability to identify the neck of the diverticula. Evolving technological advances in magnetic resonance (MR) imaging software and hardware, including coils, permits high-resolution, noninvasive, cross-sectional imaging of the urethra. MR imaging can accurately diagnose a wide spectrum of urethral/periurethral abnormalities and provide a road map for surgeons. Moreover, dynamic MR imaging allows functional assessment of urethral mobility.

In this article, MR imaging techniques for the evaluation of the female urethra are described. The radiological characteristics of cystic abnormalities and "masses" involving the urethra and periurethral region are discussed.

[a] Department of Diagnostic and Interventional Imaging, The University of Texas Health Science Center at Houston, 6431 Fannin St, MSB 2.130, Houston, TX 77030, USA; [b] Department of Radiology, Mayo Clinic LL Radiology, 13400 E Shea Blvd, Scottsdale, AZ 85259, USA; [c] Department of Radiology, Mallinckrodt Institute of Radiology, 510 S Kingshighway Blvd, Saint Louis, MO 63110, USA; [d] Washington University School of Medicine, Saint Louis, MO 63105, USA; [e] Section of Body Imaging, The University of Texas MD Anderson Cancer Center, 1400 Pressler Street, Unit 1473, Houston, TX 77030, USA
* Corresponding author.
E-mail address: Venkateswar.R.Surabhi@uth.tmc.edu

Radiol Clin N Am 51 (2013) 941–953
http://dx.doi.org/10.1016/j.rcl.2013.07.001
0033-8389/13/$ – see front matter © 2013 Elsevier Inc. All rights reserved.

MR IMAGING TECHNIQUE

MR imaging, on account of its multiplanar scanning capability, superior tissue distinction, and exquisite contrast resolution, is considered the imaging modality of choice for the diagnosis, characterization, localization, and presurgical planning in patients with urethral and periurethral disorders. Imaging with a pelvic phased-array coil may involve use of a torso or cardiac coil at 1.5 or 3 T. Although high-quality images may be acquired using a pelvic phased-array coil, endovaginal, endorectal or, much less commonly, endourethral coils can be used to achieve significantly enhanced resolution and high signal-to-noise ratio (SNR).[1] Endovaginal imaging may be performed at 1.5 or 3 T using a compatible rigid cylindrical coil or a single-use inflatable coil. The endoluminal (most commonly endovaginal) approach is particularly useful in evaluating urethral diverticula, especially in the topographic localization of the diverticulum, assessment of complications, and depiction of the diverticular ostia.[2]

MR imaging involves obtaining 3-plane high-resolution images angled along and perpendicular to the plane of the urethra. The small field of view (FOV) required to image the relatively small structure of the urethra at high resolution necessitates the use of phase oversampling techniques to avoid aliasing. Small slice thickness and a high matrix are also recommended to reduce voxel volume and thus increase spatial resolution. Because the combination of a small FOV and reduced voxel volume tends to decrease SNR, increasing the number of signal averages (or number of excitations) is often required. The resulting increase in scan time does not significantly affect image quality because the lower pelvis is relatively immune to respiratory motion artifacts.

High-resolution, 3-plane, T2-weighted fast spin-echo (FSE/TSE) sequences form the mainstay of the imaging protocol; fat saturation may be applied to 1 of the planes as desired. The FOV should cover the bladder base to the urethral meatus craniocaudally, and the periurethral soft tissues laterally. Before running the FSE sequences, T2-weighted single-shot coronal images may be obtained for planning purposes; these images should be of sufficiently large FOV to include the kidneys. The use of intravenous contrast is indicated in the assessment of infectious, inflammatory, and neoplastic pathology of the urethra; precontrast and postcontrast, high-resolution, fat-saturated, FSE T1-weighted images are typically obtained. The authors' institutional MR imaging parameters are summarized in **Tables 1** and **2**.

NORMAL URETHRAL ANATOMY

The female urethra is a 4-cm long tubular structure, extending from the bladder neck to the external urethral meatus. The 3 layers of a normal urethra are an inner layer of mucosal epithelium with in-foldings, a middle submucosal layer of a rich vascular network of elastic tissue, and an outer collagen-rich muscular envelope. These 3 components contribute to the typical target-like appearance at MR imaging, particularly on T2-weighted images secondary to a low-signal mucosal layer, high-signal submucosa, and low-signal muscle layer (**Fig. 1**).[3] Whereas the proximal one-third of the female urethra is lined by transitional epithelium, the distal two-thirds is lined by stratified squamous epithelium. There are multiple small submucosal and periurethral glands that drain into the lumen of the urethra. Skene glands are a conglomeration of small glands that secrete mucus into either side of the distal urethra at the external meatus.

The periurethral space contains various ligaments that support the urethra: the pubourethral and urethropelvic (paraurethral, periurethral, and suburethral) ligaments (**Fig. 2**). The pubourethral ligaments are located superiorly between the urethra and pubic symphysis, and the urethropelvic ligaments provide lateral attachment to the arcus tendineus.[4,5]

Table 1
Pelvic phased-array coil MR urethra protocol

Sequence	FOV (cm)	Matrix	TR/TE (ms)	ST/SG (mm)	NEX
Coronal T2 SSFSE	30	256 × 128	645/85	6/7	0.5
Axial, coronal, and sagittal T2 FRFSE	20–27	512 × 256	3000/100	3/0.3	3–4
Axial T2 FRFSE FS (optional)	20	512 × 256	4500/105	3/0.3	3–4
Axial FS T1 FSE (pre- and postcontrast)	20	512 × 256	450/2.5	3/0.3	2

Abbreviations: FOV, field of view; FRFSE, fast recovery fast spin-echo; FS, fat-saturated; FSE, fast spin-echo; NEX, number of excitations; SSFSE, single-shot fast spin-echo sequence; ST/SG, slice thickness and slice gap; TR/TE, repetition time and echo time.

Table 2
Endovaginal coil MR urethra protocol

Sequence	FOV (cm)	Matrix	TR/TE (ms)	ST/SG (mm)	NEX
Coronal T2 SSFSE (body coil)	30	256 × 128	645/85	6/7	0.5
Axial, coronal, and sagittal T2 FRFSE	18–20	512 × 256	2500/100	3/0	3–4
Axial T2 FRFSE FS (optional)	18	512 × 256	4000/105	3/0	3–4
Axial FS T1 FSE (pre- and postcontrast)	20	512 × 256	450/2.5	3/0	2

These are guidelines for use on a SIGNA HD xt 1.5-T imager (GE Healthcare). The names of the sequences and parameter values may vary with other scanners.

Abbreviations: FOV, field of view; FRFSE, fast recovery fast spin-echo; FS, fat-saturated; FSE, fast spin-echo; NEX, number of excitations; SSFSE, single-shot fast spin-echo sequence; ST/SG, slice thickness and slice gap; TR/TE, repetition time and echo time.

PERIURETHRAL CYSTIC LESIONS

Cystic lesions of the urethra and periurethral location are frequently encountered in gynecologic and female urologic practices. The diverticulum is the most common cystic lesion of the urethra, which communicates with its lumen. Lesions arising from the periurethral tissues and vagina can present as cystic lesions in the region. Presenting symptoms range from mild discomfort or fullness to urinary symptoms such as incontinence or obstructive voiding symptoms. In most cases, urethral and periurethral cystic lesions can be distinguished from one another based on MR imaging findings by determining if there is a communication between the lesion and the urethra (diverticulum), organ of origin from the vaginal wall (vaginal cysts),

and distal urethral/juxtameatal location and teardrop configuration of Skene-duct cysts.[6]

URETHRAL DIVERTICULUM

Urethral diverticulum is a focal outpouching of the urethra that typically projects posteriorly into the urethrovaginal space. Urethral diverticula have been reported to occur in 1% to 5% of the general female population.[7] Although they may present at any age, urethral diverticula are most frequently diagnosed between the third and fifth decades of life.[8,9]

Urethral diverticula are frequently misdiagnosed because of the nonspecific nature of their presenting symptoms. Although classically described as the "3 Ds" (dysuria, dyspareunia, and postvoid

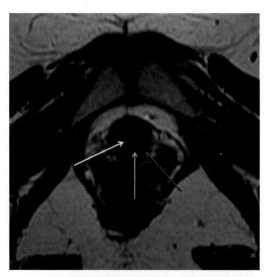

Fig. 1. Normal urethral zonal anatomy. Axial T2-weighted MR image obtained with a pelvic phased-array coil shows a target-like appearance secondary to inner hypointense mucosal layer (*yellow arrow*), middle hyperintense submucosal layer (*green arrow*), and outer hypointense muscular layer (*red arrow*).

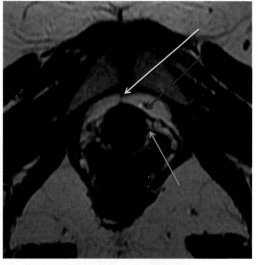

Fig. 2. Normal urethral supporting ligaments. Axial T2-weighted MR image obtained with a pelvic phased-array coil shows pubourethral ligament (*yellow arrow*), periurethral ligament (*green arrow*), and paraurethral ligament (*red arrow*).

dribbling), the presenting complaints are wide-ranging and include recurrent urinary infections, urinary frequency and urgency, stress or urge incontinence, and hematuria.[10] Rarer presentations include a tender periurethral mass, discharge of pus from the urethral meatus, and urinary retention.[11] To avoid being overlooked, the condition should be included in the differential diagnosis during the clinical workup of women with unexplained lower urinary tract symptoms.[12]

Multiple theories have been postulated to explain the etiopathogenesis of urethral diverticula. Most urethral diverticula are acquired. Congenital urethral diverticula are considered extremely rare; these are typically seen in males, and are anteriorly located.[12] Congenital female diverticula have been thought to develop from cloacogenic rests, vaginal wall cysts, and faulty union of primordial folds.[2,13] Although multiple possible acquired causes including obstetric trauma and urethrovaginal surgery[2] have been proposed, the most popular hypothesis is that of an obstructed paraurethral gland. Paraurethral glands of Skene are tubuloalveolar mucous glands that line the mid and distal urethra, and are located at the posterolateral aspect of the urethra bilaterally. It has been proposed that obstruction of paraurethral gland(s) predisposes to superimposed infection; subsequent rupture into the urethral lumen and epithelialization forms an urothelium-lined diverticulum.[14,15] In support of this theory, most urethral diverticula are located in the distal two-thirds of the urethra, and posterolaterally between 3 o'clock and 9 o'clock positions.[8] MR imaging is considered the imaging modality of choice for the diagnosis of and comprehensive presurgical planning for patients with urethral diverticula.[2,13] MR imaging has been reported to be more sensitive in the detection of diverticula than fluoroscopic urethrography or fiber-optic urethroscopy.[16]

The classic diverticulum typically appears as a round or oval cystic structure located at the posterolateral aspect of the mid to distal urethra, typically at or above the level of the pubic symphysis (Fig. 3). The diverticulum is typically hyperintense on T2-weighted and hypointense on T1-weighted images. Hemorrhagic or proteinaceous debris within the diverticulum may show high signal intensity on T1-weighted and variable signal intensity on T2-weighted imaging. The ostium of the diverticulum may be seen as a beak-like extension of the diverticula through the muscular and submucosal layers of the urethra (Figs. 4 and 5). Visualization of the ostium is significantly better on endoluminal imaging and on postcontrast imaging.[9] High-resolution, fat-saturated, postcontrast FSE T1-weighted images are extremely useful in the identification of the diverticular neck (see Figs. 4 and 5). The urethral diverticula may have complex U-shaped ("horseshoe") or circumferential ("saddlebag") configurations.[2,17] Rarely, the diverticulum may be anteriorly located or involve the proximal urethra (see Fig. 5). The latter may result in mass effect at the bladder base on urography; this has been described as the female prostate sign.[18] Urethral diverticula may be single or multiple, and their cavities may be unilocular (see Fig. 3) or multiseptated (see Fig. 5).[3] For preoperative planning purposes, it is important that the diverticula are described in terms of their number, size, location, configuration, sac contents (if any), position of the neck and ostium, and distance of the ostium from the bladder neck.[9] Resection of the diverticular neck is critical in preventing its recurrence.[19] Radiologists often use a "clock-face" template on axial MR images to convey the location of the urethral diverticulum and neck, with the 12 o'clock position representing the midline anterior aspect of the urethra (see Figs. 4 and 5B).[3]

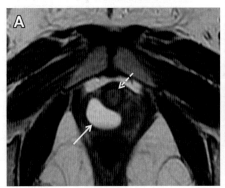
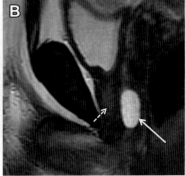

Fig. 3. Unilocular urethral diverticulum. (A) Axial and (B) sagittal T2-weighted images obtained with a pelvic phased-array coil showing a typically located unilocular urethral diverticulum (*white arrow*) involving the right posterolateral aspect of the distal urethra (*dashed white arrow*).

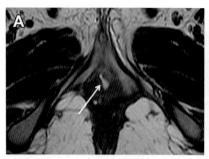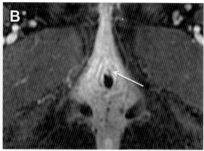

Fig. 4. Diverticular ostium on pelvic phased-array coil MR images. (*A*) T2-weighted MR image showing a tubular, very low-lying cystic lesion at the meatus (*white arrow*). (*B*) The diverticular ostium (*white arrow*) communicating with the urethral lumen at the 6 o'clock position is clearly seen.

Complications of Urethral Diverticulum

Recurrent urinary tract infections

Because of anatomic factors, urethral diverticula are prone to infections resulting in recurrent urinary tract infections (UTIs) in 30% to 50% of patients.[13] The rarer proximal urethral diverticula can cause obstruction of the bladder outlet, again predisposing to recurrent UTIs.[20] The most common pathogens involved include *Escherichia coli*, *Chlamydia* species, and gonococci. On imaging, the walls and septae of an infected diverticulum typically show irregularity, thickening, and increased enhancement. Layering debris and altered signal intensity may also be seen within the diverticular cavity (**Fig. 6**).

Rupture

A rare complication is spontaneous rupture of the diverticulum into the urethrovaginal space or fistulization into the vagina.[21] Presence of fluid within the urethrovaginal space, seen as high T2 signal or a high signal tract leading from the urethra to the vagina on fat-suppressed images, should alert the radiologist to these complications. In the subacute setting, rupture may result in extension of the inflammatory process beyond the cavity of the diverticulum (see **Fig. 6**).

Calculi

Stagnant urine within the diverticular cavity predisposes to the formation of calculi, usually calcium phosphate or calcium oxalate stones. Approximately 1.5% to 10% of patients with urethral diverticula develop calculi. On MR imaging, the calculi are seen as low-signal (T1 and T2) foci within the dependent aspect of the diverticular cavity (**Fig. 7**).[2] Urethral obstruction caused by dislodged diverticular calculi has been reported in the literature.[22]

Malignancy

Malignant transformation of a urethral diverticulum is rare, representing 5% of all urethral carcinomas. It has been postulated that repeated injury to the diverticular wall predisposes to adenomatous

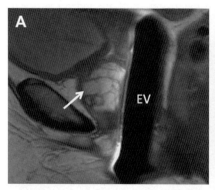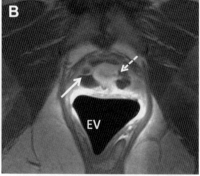

Fig. 5. Female prostate sign. (*A*) Sagittal T2 and (*B*) axial postcontrast T1-weighted endoluminal MR images showing an atypical urethral diverticulum (*white arrow*) with nearly circumferential involvement of the proximal urethra, producing the MR imaging equivalent of the female prostate sign. Multiple thin septations are noted within the diverticulum, these show minimal postcontrast enhancement. Note the subtle ostium (*dashed white arrow*) at the 3 o'clock position; visualization of diverticular ostia is significantly superior on endoluminal MR imaging. EV, endovaginal coil.

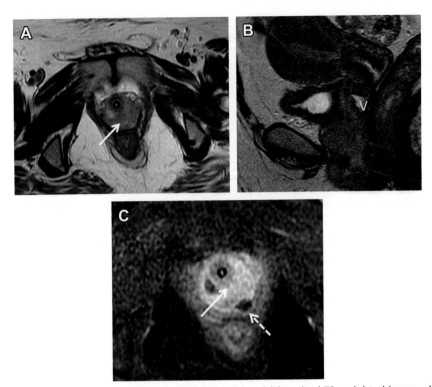

Fig. 6. Infected and ruptured urethral diverticulum. (*A*) Axial and (*B*) sagittal T2-weighted images showing heterogeneous, inflammatory soft tissue within the diverticular cavity (*white arrow*) associated with extension of inflammatory process into the urethrovaginal space (*red arrows*) indicating rupture. V, vagina. (*C*) Axial postcontrast fat-saturated T1-weighted image showing heterogeneous, enhancing inflammatory soft tissue within the diverticular cavity (*white arrow*). Note breach of the diverticular wall posteriorly on the left (*dashed white arrow*) indicating rupture of the diverticulum.

metaplasia and the development of intradiverticular neoplasia. Of diverticular cancers, 61% are adenocarcinomas, 27% transitional cell carcinomas, and 12% squamous cell carcinomas.[23,24] Carcinomas arising in a urethral diverticulum are usually late stage, with high rates of postsurgical recurrence and early metastases.[2]

Intradiverticular malignancy is best seen on postcontrast T1-weighted images as an enhancing mass within the diverticula (**Fig. 8**). Large masses may completely fill and obliterate the cystic space. The tumor may show variable signal intensity on T2-weighted imaging; extradiverticular extension is characterized by disruption of the

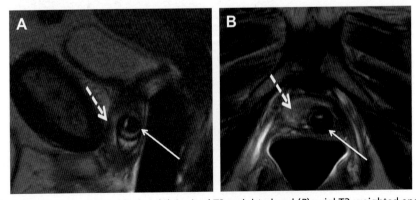

Fig. 7. Urethral diverticulum with a calculus. (*A*) Sagittal T2-weighted and (*B*) axial T2-weighted endovaginal MR images demonstrate a calculus (*white arrow*) within a urethral diverticulum. Note anterior and rightward displacement of urethra (*dashed white arrow*).

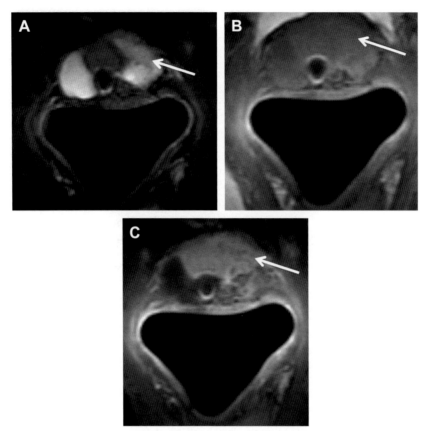

Fig. 8. Adenocarcinoma arising within the urethral diverticulum. (*A*) Axial fat-saturated T2-weighted, (*B*) axial precontrast T1-weighted, and (*C*) axial fat-saturated postcontrast T1-weighted endovaginal MR images demonstrate a complex urethral diverticulum with ill-defined, isointense T2 and T1 signal and heterogeneously enhancing soft tissue (*white arrow*) component within the anterior aspect of the diverticular cavity.

low-signal wall of the diverticulum. In the absence of contiguous invasion, it may be difficult to distinguish between malignancy and benign granulation tissue on MR imaging. Histopathologic examination after tissue sampling may be required for confirmation of the diagnosis.[24] Some benign lesions, such as nephrogenic adenomas, have also been reported to arise from within the urethral diverticula.[25]

VAGINAL CYSTS

Müllerian and mesonephric remnants tend to be located in the vagina, particularly along the anterolateral aspect of the vagina. Typically cysts of the Gartner duct (arising from mesonephric remnant) are located in the upper vagina, but these cysts can arise from the lower third of the vagina and may mimic a urethral diverticulum (**Fig. 9**). The distinction between müllerian and Gartner-duct cysts is not important and is not possible based on imaging findings. Renal anomalies have been reported in association with Gartner-duct cysts.[6]

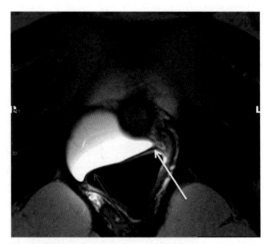

Fig. 9. Cyst of Gartner duct. Axial T2-weighted endovaginal MR image demonstrates a well-circumscribed cyst arising from the right side of anterior vaginal wall (*red arrow*). Note the normal thickness of anterior vaginal wall on the left side (*white arrow*).

SKENE-DUCT CYSTS

Skene glands are bilateral and are located in the floor of the distal urethra. Ductal obstruction secondary to infection or trauma leads to formation of Skene-duct cysts. Most of these cysts are clinically insignificant, but cysts larger than 2 cm often cause urinary symptoms such as dysuria or obstructive voiding symptoms.[6,13] A Skene-duct cyst must be distinguished from a urethral diverticulum. MR imaging findings in favor of Skene cysts are location along the lateral aspect of the distal urethra/meatus (Fig. 10), teardrop shape, and paired nature on either side of the distal urethra.

URETHRAL CARCINOMA

Carcinoma of the female urethra is a rare entity, accounting for only 0.02% of all female cancers.[26] Transitional cell carcinoma, adenocarcinoma, and squamous cell carcinoma are the most common pathologic subtypes of urethral cancer. Less common subtypes include clear-cell type of adenocarcinoma and small-cell carcinoma. Urethral carcinoma encompassing both squamous and transitional cell histologic features has been categorized as epidermoid type.[26] The proximal one-third of the female urethra is lined by transitional epithelium and the distal two-thirds by stratified squamous epithelium. Skene glands near the meatus are lined by columnar epithelium, and secrete mucus into the urethra via 2 Skene ducts. Transitional cell carcinomas and adenocarcinomas tend to arise from the proximal one-third of the urethra whereas squamous cell carcinomas tend to arise from the distal two-thirds of the urethra, in keeping with urethral epithelial lining.[27] However, there are exceptions to this rule, particularly for tumors arising from urethral diverticula and Skene glands.[27]

The primary treatment of choice is surgical resection for localized urethral tumors and chemoradiation followed by surgery for tumors with periurethral extension or metastatic inguinal lymphadenopathy. Outcome depends on the stage at initial diagnosis and location, with posterior urethral tumors carrying a poorer prognosis than anterior ones.[26]

The key role of MR imaging is in the detection of urethral tumor extension into paraurethral tissues and anterior vaginal wall, which renders the tumor a high stage (Fig. 11). MR imaging also helps in the detection of inguinal and pelvic lymphadenopathy (see Fig. 11).[27] The 3 most important prognostic features of urethral cancer, namely tumor location, size, and depth of paraurethral and anterior vaginal wall invasion, can be accurately assessed with MR imaging, thus providing vital information regarding tumor resectability and the triage of patients to primary surgery or treatment with neoadjuvant chemoradiation.[28]

URETHRAL/PERIURETHRAL LEIOMYOMA

Leiomyomas are benign mesenchymal tumors that arise from the smooth muscle. Leiomyomas of the urethra are rare, and most frequently involve the proximal segment.[29] Smaller leiomyomas are confined to the urethra, but larger leiomyomas might protrude through the urethral meatus or extend into the paraurethral region.[30] Whereas tumors arising from the posterior urethral wall present with dyspareunia, tumors arising in the lateral and anterior walls are more frequently associated with UTIs and the presence of a mass.[29] Urethral leiomyomas demonstrate T2-hyperintense or T2-isointense signal on MR imaging, as opposed to uterine leiomyomas (Fig. 12).[29] Enhancement pattern varies from mild enhancement to avid enhancement. Surgical excision is the treatment of choice.

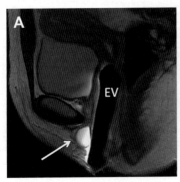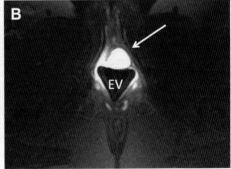

Fig. 10. Cyst of Skene duct. (A) Sagittal T2-weighted and (B) axial T2-weighted endoluminal MR images showing a "teardrop" cyst (white arrow) at the urethral meatus without any communication to the urethra. EV, endovaginal coil.

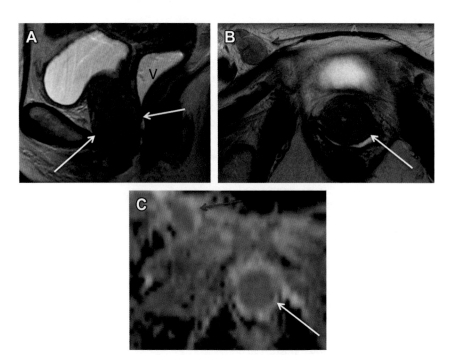

Fig. 11. Urethral squamous cell carcinoma. (*A*) Sagittal T2-weighted and (*B*) axial T2-weighted MR images obtained with a pelvic phased-array coil showing a large infiltrative mass (*white arrow*) involving the proximal and distal parts of urethra, with associated invasion of anterior wall of the vagina (*yellow arrow*) and metastatic right inguinal lymph node (*red arrow*). V, vagina distended with ultrasound gel. (*C*) Apparent diffusion coefficient (ADC) map shows hypointense signal of the urethral mass (*white arrow*) and right inguinal lymph node (*red arrow*), consistent with diffusion restriction.

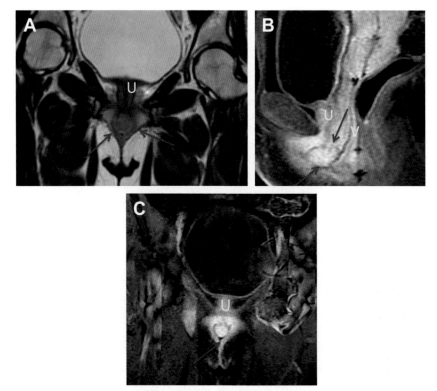

Fig. 12. Urethral leiomyoma. (*A*) Coronal T2-weighted MR image shows a mildly T2-hyperintense mass lesion (*red arrows*) at the urethral meatus. (*B*) Sagittal, fat-saturated, postcontrast T1-weighted and (*C*) coronal fat-saturated postcontrast T1-weighted MR images obtained with a pelvic phased-array coil showing homogeneous enhancement of the urethral meatus mass (*red arrows*). U, urethra; V, vagina.

URETHRAL MALIGNANT MELANOMA

Primary malignant melanoma (MM) of the urethra is rare and accounts for only approximately 4% of urethral neoplasms. Urethral MM is 3 times more common in women than in men. The distal urethra is affected most commonly.[31] The tumors are frequently polypoid, and may be confused with urethral polyps, caruncle, mucosal prolapse, or urethral carcinoma. The clinical signs and symptoms associated with these lesions range from urethral bleeding, dysuria, and difficulty maintaining urinary stream to nonspecific lower urinary tract symptoms.[31]

The imaging features of primary urethral MM depend on melanin content and the presence or absence of hemorrhage. Melanocytic MMs demonstrate both T1 and T2 shortening, whereas amelanotic MMs typically do not exhibit significant T1 or T2 shortening (**Fig. 13**A). The enhancement pattern is commonly homogeneous (**Fig. 13**B). The primary approach to therapy is surgical resection, frequently with bilateral inguinal lymph node dissection. Adjuvant chemotherapy, immunotherapy, radiotherapy, or a combination of these play a role in advanced-stage urethral MMs based on the depth of invasion.[31]

URETHRAL/PERIURETHRAL METASTASIS

Urethral/periurethral metastases are extremely rare. Isolated metastatic urethral lesions noted either at initial presentation of the primary tumor or at follow-up may pose a diagnostic challenge to clinicians.[32] There have been reported cases of metastases to the urethra from the colon, lung, kidney, and prostate cancer. The mode of spread could be lymphatic or hematogenous. Management of urethral metastatic lesions depends on the primary tumor histology. MR imaging findings typically follow those of primary urethral tumor (**Fig. 14**), but the key role of MR is to differentiate urethral metastasis from contiguous urethral/periurethral extension of a lower genital or gastrointestinal tract cancer, as contiguous extension may be amenable to radical surgical excision along with the primary tumor.[33]

MISCELLANEOUS NEOPLASTIC AND NONNEOPLASTIC LESIONS

Urethral fibroepithelial polyps (FEPs) are rare benign growths of mesodermal origin that consist of a fibrovascular core covered by a normal urothelium. FEPs are usually diagnosed during the first decade of life, more often in boys than in girls.[34] Typical clinical manifestations include obstruction, voiding dysfunction, and hematuria. FEPs are most commonly found in the upper third of the urethra.[35] The etiology of FEP is unclear, but may have congenital, infectious, obstructive, and traumatic origins. Surgical resection usually results in cure, and recurrence is rare. Urethral FEPs rarely arise in adults.[36] MR imaging findings of FEPs range from a solitary nonobstructive polypoid lesion confined to the urethra to a polypoid mass with a vascular stalk at the urethral meatus (**Fig. 15**). Differential diagnosis for a mass of urethral meatus is broad, and includes several lesions that may present similarly to FEP, such as caruncle and urethral prolapse. Urethral caruncle is a benign, polypoid mass of the meatus that occurs primarily in postmenopausal women.[37] Urethral prolapse is defined as an eversion of urethral mucosa through the meatal opening. Prolapsed mucosa presents as a polypoid mass at the meatus, often associated with edema and congestion. The most common presentation is with urethral bleeding. The age distribution of urethral prolapse is bimodal: prepubertal girls and postmenopausal women. The exact cause of urethral prolapse remains unknown. Several causes have been proposed, including congenital and acquired conditions leading to hypermobility of the

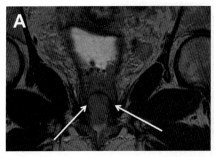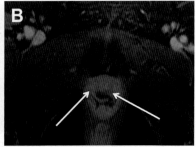

Fig. 13. Urethral melanoma. (*A*) Coronal T2-weighted MR image shows a mildly T2-hyperintense mass (*white arrows*). (*B*) Axial fat-saturated, postcontrast T1-weighted MR image obtained with a pelvic phased-array coil showing homogeneous enhancement of the urethral meatus mass (*white arrows*).

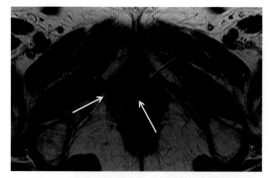

Fig. 14. Urethral metastasis. Axial T2-weighted MR image shows a T2-hyperintense mass lesion (*white arrows*) involving the urethral and periurethral region with associated mass effect on the urethra (*red arrow*) in a patient with carcinoma of cervix.

urethra and weakening of attachment between the inner longitudinal and outer circular–oblique muscle layers of the urethra. Vaginal atrophy and urethral mucosal atrophy caused by decreased levels of estrogens in postmenopausal women are considered to be risk factors for urethral prolapse.[38]

MR IMAGING OF THE URETHRA IN STRESS URINARY INCONTINENCE

Stress urinary incontinence (SUI) is a common problem affecting approximately 4% to 35% of older, parous women. SUI is described as the leakage of urine with any activity associated with an increase in intra-abdominal pressure.[39] There are 3 types of SUI: type I is attributed to loss of posterior urethrovesical angle, type II is due to a combination of loss of posterior urethrovesical angle and urethral hypermobility, and type III is secondary to intrinsic sphincter deficiency.[39] Urethral hypermobility is the downward displacement of the urethra resulting from the weakening of the pelvic-floor muscles and fascia along with horizontal translation of the urethra of 30° or more away from the normal baseline vertical axis at maximal straining.[39] Urethral hypermobility can be diagnosed on dynamic pelvic-floor MR imaging by assessing urethral descent below the pubococcygeal line and measuring the angle of urethral horizontal translation at maximal strain in comparison with baseline urethral axis (**Fig. 16**).[13] Many different surgical options are available for those who fail initial conservative management with

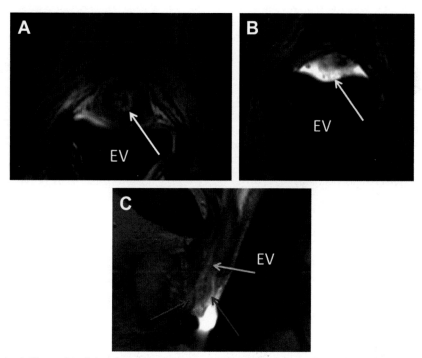

Fig. 15. Urethral fibroepithelial polyp. (*A*) Axial T2-weighted MR image shows hyperintense mucosal layer (*white arrow*) indicating mucosal edema. (*B*) Axial T2-weighted MR image shows a small polypoid mass (*yellow arrow*) at the urethral meatus. (*C*) Sagittal T2-weighted endoluminal MR image showing hyperintense mucosal layer versus stalk (*blue arrow*) associated with a small polypoid mass (*red arrows*) at the urethral meatus. Preoperative differentials included urethral mucosal prolapse versus fibroepithelial polyp. EV, endovaginal coil.

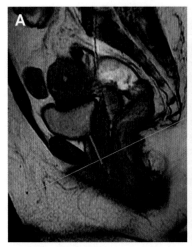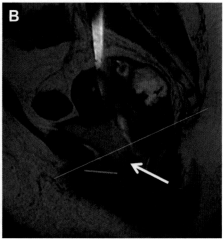

Fig. 16. Urethral hypermobility. Midline sagittal image acquired with fast steady-state free precession imaging (A) at rest, and (B) at maximal strain show urinary bladder neck descent of more than 1 cm below the pubococcygeal line (*green line*) indicating a mild cystocele (*arrow*). Note inferior descent of the urethra (*red line*) along with marked translation of the urethra away from the normal vertical axis, indicating hypermobility of the urethra.

pelvic-floor muscle training and behavioral therapy. Retropubic and transobturator midurethral slings have become the gold standard for treating uncomplicated SUI. These less invasive, novel surgical techniques are less morbid, yet show efficacy comparable with that of traditional surgeries such as Burch colposuspension and pubovaginal slings.[40]

SUMMARY

Patients with urethral disorders manifest a wide spectrum of symptoms. Clinical evaluation and urethrography play a limited role in the evaluation of these patients. High-resolution, multiplanar MR imaging serves as a "one-stop shop" for precise diagnosis of a variety of disorders that involve the urethra and the periurethral region. Accurate detection and characterization of urethral disorders requires understanding of the regional anatomy and meticulous MR imaging technique, and knowledge of a systematic, pattern-based imaging approach.

REFERENCES

1. Macura KJ, Genadry R, Borman TL, et al. Evaluation of the female urethra with intraurethral magnetic resonance imaging. J Magn Reson Imaging 2004; 20(1):153–9.
2. Chou CP, Levenson RB, Elsayes KM, et al. Imaging of female urethral diverticulum: an update. Radiographics 2008;28(7):1917–30.
3. Chaudhari VV, Patel MK, Douek M, et al. MR imaging and US of female urethral and periurethral disease. Radiographics 2010;30(7):1857–74.
4. Rosenblum N, Nitti VW. Female urethral reconstruction. Urol Clin North Am 2011;38(1):55–64, vi.
5. el-Sayed RF, Morsy MM, el-Mashed SM, et al. Anatomy of the urethral supporting ligaments defined by dissection, histology, and MRI of female cadavers and MRI of healthy nulliparous women. AJR Am J Roentgenol 2007;189(5):1145–57.
6. Eilber KS, Raz S. Benign cystic lesions of the vagina: a literature review. J Urol 2003;170(3):717–22.
7. Porten S, Kielb S. Diagnosis of female diverticula using magnetic resonance imaging. Adv Urol 2008;213516.
8. Davis HJ, Telinde RW. Urethral diverticula: an assay of 121 cases. J Urol 1958;80(1):34–9.
9. Dwarkasing RS, Dinkelaar W, Hop WC, et al. MRI evaluation of urethral diverticula and differential diagnosis in symptomatic women. AJR Am J Roentgenol 2011;197(3):676–82.
10. Romanzi LJ, Groutz A, Blaivas JG. Urethral diverticulum in women: diverse presentations resulting in diagnostic delay and mismanagement. J Urol 2000;164(2):428–33.
11. Ganabathi K, Leach GE, Zimmern PE, et al. Experience with the management of urethral diverticulum in 63 women. J Urol 1994;152(5 Pt 1):1445–52.
12. Rawat J, Khan TR, Singh S, et al. Congenital anterior urethral valves and diverticula: diagnosis and management in six cases. Afr J Paediatr Surg 2009; 6(2):102–5.
13. Bennett GL, Hecht EM, Tanpitukpongse TP, et al. MRI of the urethra in women with lower urinary tract

symptoms: spectrum of findings at static and dynamic imaging. AJR Am J Roentgenol 2009;193(6): 1708–15.

14. Leach GE, Bavendam TG. Female urethral diverticula. Urology 1987;30(5):407–15.

15. Siegelman ES, Banner MP, Ramchandani P, et al. Multicoil MR imaging of symptomatic female urethral and periurethral disease. Radiographics 1997;17(2): 349–65.

16. Kim B, Hricak H, Tanagho EA. Diagnosis of urethral diverticula in women: value of MR imaging. AJR Am J Roentgenol 1993;161(4):809–15.

17. Hahn WY, Israel GM, Lee VS. MRI of female urethral and periurethral disorders. AJR Am J Roentgenol 2004;182(3):677–82.

18. Pope TL Jr, Harrison RB, Clark RL, et al. Bladder base impressions in women: "female prostate". AJR Am J Roentgenol 1981;136(6):1105–8.

19. Prasad SR, Menias CO, Narra VR, et al. Cross-sectional imaging of the female urethra: technique and results. Radiographics 2005;25(3):749–61.

20. Agrawal S, Ansari MS, Kapoor R, et al. Congenital posterior urethral diverticula causing bladder outlet obstruction in a young male. Indian J Urol 2008; 24(3):414–5.

21. Nielsen VM, Nielsen KK, Vedel P. Spontaneous rupture of a diverticulum of the female urethra presenting with a fistula to the vagina. Acta Obstet Gynecol Scand 1987;66(1):87–8.

22. Okeke LI, Takure AO, Adebayo SA, et al. Urethral obstruction from dislodged bladder diverticulum stones: a case report. BMC Urol 2012;12:31.

23. Seballos RM, Rich RR. Clear cell adenocarcinoma arising from a urethral diverticulum. J Urol 1995; 153(6):1914–5.

24. Khati NJ, Javitt MC, Schwartz AM, et al. MR imaging diagnosis of a urethral diverticulum. Radiographics 1998;18(2):517–22.

25. Greco A, Giammo A, Tizzani A. Nephrogenic adenoma arising from an urethral diverticulum in a female. Report of a case and review of the literature. Minerva Urol Nefrol 1999;51(1):39–43 [in Italian].

26. Dalbagni G, Zhang ZF, Lacombe L, et al. Female urethral carcinoma: an analysis of treatment outcome and a plea for a standardized management strategy. Br J Urol 1998;82(6):835–41.

27. Miller J, Karnes RJ. Primary clear-cell adenocarcinoma of the proximal female urethra: case report and review of the literature. Clin Genitourin Cancer 2008;6(2):131–3.

28. Gourtsoyianni S, Hudolin T, Sala E, et al. MRI at the completion of chemoradiotherapy can accurately evaluate the extent of disease in women with advanced urethral carcinoma undergoing anterior pelvic exenteration. Clin Radiol 2011; 66(11):1072–8.

29. Hubert KC, Remer EM, Rackley RR, et al. Clinical and magnetic resonance imaging characteristics of vaginal and paraurethral leiomyomas: can they be diagnosed before surgery? BJU Int 2010; 105(12):1686–8.

30. Hwang JH, Lee JK, Oh MJ, et al. A leiomyoma presenting as an exophytic periurethral mass: a case report and review of the literature. J Minim Invasive Gynecol 2009;16(4):507–9.

31. Oliva E, Quinn TR, Amin MB, et al. Primary malignant melanoma of the urethra: a clinicopathologic analysis of 15 cases. Am J Surg Pathol 2000;24(6): 785–96.

32. Noorani S, Rao AR, Callaghan PS. Urethral metastasis: an uncommon presentation of a colonic adenocarcinoma. Int Urol Nephrol 2007;39(3):837–9.

33. Chitale SV, Burgess NA, Sethia KK, et al. Management of urethral metastasis from colorectal carcinomas. ANZ J Surg 2004;74(10):925–7.

34. Demircan M, Ceran C, Karaman A, et al. Urethral polyps in children: a review of the literature and report of two cases. Int J Urol 2006;13(6):841–3.

35. Kumar A, Das SK, Trivedi S, et al. Genito-urinary polyps: summary of the 10-year experiences of a single institute. Int Urol Nephrol 2008;40(4):901–7.

36. Battaglia C, Battaglia B, Ramacieri A, et al. Recurrent postcoital hematuria. A case of fibroepithelial urethral polyp in an adult female. J Sex Med 2011; 8(2):612–6.

37. Conces MR, Williamson SR, Montironi R, et al. Urethral caruncle: clinicopathologic features of 41 cases. Hum Pathol 2012;43(9):1400–4.

38. Holbrook C, Misra D. Surgical management of urethral prolapse in girls: 13 years' experience. BJU Int 2012;110(1):132–4.

39. Shah SM, Gaunay GS. Treatment options for intrinsic sphincter deficiency. Nat Rev Urol 2012; 9(11):638–51.

40. Cox A, Herschorn S, Lee L. Surgical management of female SUI: is there a gold standard? Nat Rev Urol 2013;10(4):188.

Placental Evaluation with Magnetic Resonance

Brian C. Allen, MD*, John R. Leyendecker, MD

KEYWORDS

- Placenta • Accreta • Increta • Percreta • Previa • Magnetic resonance

KEY POINTS

- Ultrasonography is the primary screening modality for the identification of abnormal placentation, but magnetic resonance (MR) imaging is a complementary imaging modality that is useful when ultrasonography is inconclusive.
- As most patients referred for placental evaluation with MR imaging have suspicious findings on ultrasonography, the pretest probability for abnormalities on MR imaging is high.
- Imaging features useful for the diagnosis of abnormal placentation include placental lobulation with uterine contour bulge, interruption of the inner low signal-intensity myometrial layer, and placental heterogeneity resulting from dark intraplacental bands and abnormal vascularity on T2-weighted imaging.
- Reliably differentiating placenta accreta from increta and placenta increta from percreta is difficult, and often not possible.
- Antenatal diagnosis of placental abnormalities is critical in aiding the referring clinician to avoid or mitigate potential complications.

INTRODUCTION

Abnormal placentation is becoming more prevalent, largely attributable to increasing rates of cesarean delivery. Because of the potential maternal morbidity and mortality associated with some undiagnosed placental abnormalities, there is a need for accurate antenatal diagnosis.

Ultrasonography remains the primary method of imaging the placenta, as it is relatively inexpensive and widely available, and evaluation of the placenta is routinely and easily performed during a fetal screening examination at 18 to 20 weeks' gestation. The high negative predictive value of ultrasonography for placental abnormalities relegates magnetic resonance (MR) imaging to a supporting role, reserved for equivocal sonographic findings or incomplete evaluation, as in cases of posterior placenta.

Placenta accreta, increta, and percreta describe a continuum of placental attachment disorders associated with incomplete postpartum detachment of the placenta and postpartum hemorrhage. During the MR imaging evaluation of suspected placenta accreta, other placental and umbilical cord anomalies may be identified, given their reported association with abnormal placentation. These disorders include placenta previa and vascular anomalies, such as velamentous cord insertion and vasa previa.

NORMAL ANATOMY

The normal disc-shaped placenta attaches to the anterior or posterior uterus, with the normal decidua basalis providing a plane of separation between the placenta and the uterine wall. The midportion of the placenta typically measures between

The authors have nothing to disclose.
Abdominal Imaging, Department of Radiology, Wake Forest University School of Medicine, Wake Forest Baptist Medical Center, Medical Center Boulevard, 3rd Floor MRI, Winston-Salem, NC 27157-1088, USA
* Corresponding author.
E-mail address: bcallen2@wakehealth.edu

Radiol Clin N Am 51 (2013) 955–966
http://dx.doi.org/10.1016/j.rcl.2013.07.009

radiologic.theclinics.com

2 and 4 cm in thickness, and the placenta undergoes changes during gestation that are evident on MR imaging.[1] Between 19 and 23 weeks gestational age, the placenta is typically relatively homogeneous on T2-weighted imaging (Fig. 1). Between weeks 24 and 31 the placenta becomes slightly lobulated, and conspicuous septae appear between placental lobules, leading to increased heterogeneity with increasing gestational age (Fig. 2). Following contrast administration, the placenta heterogeneously enhances before the uterus, and becomes more homogeneous over time.[2,3]

The normal myometrium has a trilayered appearance on T2-weighted images (Fig. 3). The middle layer is a heterogeneously hyperintense vascular layer, with thinner low signal-intensity layers on either side.[4] The uteroplacental unit is of uniform, intermediate signal on unenhanced T1-weighted images, affording no opportunity to distinguish the placental-myometrial interface or to examine myometrial architecture.

The myometrium thins at sites of compression, such as adjacent to the spine and aorta, appearing as a single thin layer of uniform signal intensity (Fig. 4). Myometrial contractions are commonly imaged incidentally, visible as rounded or lentiform regions of transient myometrial thickening, demonstrating the low signal intensity typical of smooth muscle on T2-weighted images (Fig. 5). Contractions are easily distinguished from leiomyomas by the intermittent and temporary nature of the former entity. Subplacental contractions can also harmlessly and temporarily deform the overlying placenta.

IMAGING PROTOCOLS

The optimal timing of an MR imaging examination for evaluation of the placenta has not been clearly

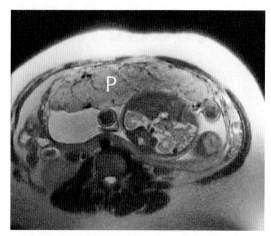

Fig. 2. Normal placenta at 31 weeks' gestation. Axial single-shot fast spin-echo image shows that the placenta (P) appears more heterogeneous and lobulated than at 21 weeks' gestation (see Fig. 1).

established. MR imaging is generally not performed during the first trimester, owing to theoretical concerns for the safety of the fetus and early stage of placental development. During the second trimester, most patients can tolerate supine imaging. However, in the third trimester, lateral decubitus imaging may be required to avoid the risk of impaired systemic venous return caused by uterine compression of the maternal inferior vena cava. Imaging late in the third trimester can be challenging, not only because of difficulties

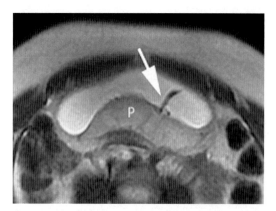

Fig. 1. Normal placenta at 21 weeks' gestation. Axial single-shot fast spin-echo image demonstrates relatively homogeneous signal of the placenta (P) and normal umbilical cord insertion (*arrow*).

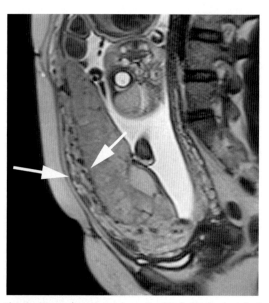

Fig. 3. Normal myometrium. Sagittal single-shot fast spin-echo image demonstrates the heterogeneous, hyperintense middle layer with thin, hypointense layers on either side (*arrows*).

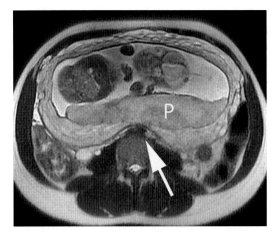

Fig. 4. Normal second-trimester placenta (P) with focal myometrial compression. Axial single-shot fast spin-echo sequence demonstrates compression (*arrow*) of the myometrium over the region of the spine at the level of the aortic bifurcation.

positioning the patient, but also because the placenta becomes more heterogeneous and the myometrium becomes thinner and more stretched late in gestation.

When evaluating the patient for placenta percreta, the bladder should be mildly distended. Anatomic landmarks can be difficult to identify in the setting of a completely collapsed bladder,

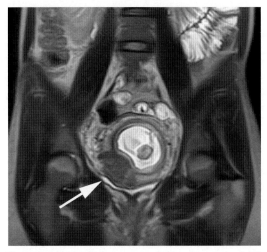

Fig. 5. Myometrial contraction. Coronal half-acquisition single-shot turbo spin-echo (HASTE) image through the uterus of a 25-year-old woman with late first-trimester pregnancy imaged to evaluate suspected appendicitis. A myometrial contraction (*arrow*) appears as a lentiform region of low signal-intensity myometrial thickening, which resolved on subsequent sequences (not shown). A leiomyoma could have a similar appearance, but would persist on all sequences.

and bladder-wall invasion can be difficult to exclude when a full bladder is closely apposed to the uterus. No other patient preparation is typically required.

A multichannel surface coil is used when possible. Initially, single-shot fast spin-echo/turbo spin-echo (ssFSE/ssTSE) or half-acquisition turbo spin-echo (HASTE), or balanced steady-state free-precession (true FISP or FIESTA) sequences are obtained in 3 imaging planes (**Box 1**). These sequences are relatively resistant to both maternal and fetal motion artifacts, and provide sufficient anatomic detail to be diagnostic in many cases. When possible, a radiologist can evaluate these images and decide whether additional imaging planes or sequences are required to further clarify suspicious findings. A fat-suppressed gradient echo T1-weighted sequence can help identify high signal-intensity blood products related to subchorionic hemorrhage or other abnormality (**Fig. 6**).

High-resolution 3-dimensional T2-weighted FSE sequences with isotropic voxel size allow reconstruction of images in any imaging plane, but take several minutes to complete and are more susceptible to image degradation by fetal and maternal motion. Some investigators have used diffusion-weighted imaging to better demonstrate the myometrial-placental interface.[5] Functional imaging of the placenta using intravoxel incoherent motion (IVIM) and blood oxygen level–dependent (BOLD) imaging have been used to evaluate placental perfusion.[6,7] However, these

---

Box 1
MR imaging protocol: sequences for placental imaging

Single-shot fast spin-echo, turbo spin-echo, and half-acquisition turbo spin-echo (ssFSE, ssTSE, HASTE) in the coronal, sagittal, and axial planes with additional imaging planes as needed to evaluate for placental position, attachment, and depth of invasion

Balanced steady-state free precession (true FISP or FIESTA) in the coronal, sagittal, and axial planes with additional imaging planes as needed to evaluate for placental position, attachment, and depth of invasion

High-resolution respiratory-triggered or breath-hold T2-weighted imaging (FSE or TSE) can be performed as needed using a 2-dimensional or 3-dimensional technique for more detailed assessment of the placenta-uterine interface, adjacent structures, and/or cervix

Axial fat-suppressed gradient echo T1-weighted images to assess for blood products

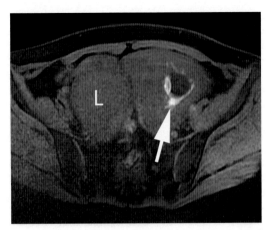

Fig. 6. Subchorionic hemorrhage. Axial T1-weighted, fat-suppressed gradient echo image shows a high signal-intensity rim (*arrow*) surrounding the uterine cavity. A subserosal leiomyoma (L) is also present.

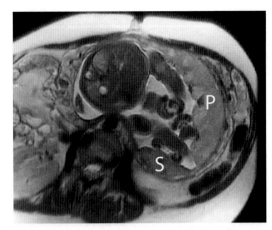

Fig. 7. Succenturiate lobe. Axial single-shot fast spin-echo image in a 40-year-old woman demonstrates the succenturiate lobe (S), clearly separate from the main placenta (P).

methods currently remain research tools, requiring further clinical validation before they assume a role in the routine evaluation of abnormal placentation. Contrast-enhanced MR imaging has been advocated as a means to better delineate the myometrial-placental interface, leading to more accurate assessment of the depth of invasion.[2,8] Although gadolinium-based contrast agents have not been definitively shown to have detrimental effects on the human fetus, these contrast agents do cross the placenta and are generally avoided unless the potential risks to the patient are outweighed by the potential benefits of contrast-enhanced imaging.

IMAGING FINDINGS AND PATHOLOGY
Abnormal Placental Shape

The placenta is usually discoid, but several variant placental shapes have been described.[9] A bilobed placenta has 2 lobes of roughly equal size and has no known associated risks. A succenturiate lobe is an accessory placental lobe that is smaller than the main placenta (**Fig. 7**). This morphology occurs as a result of selective growth in some parts of the placenta and atrophy of other parts, thought to be related to varying uterine blood supply or an underlying local factor such as a leiomyoma or previous uterine surgery.[10] A succenturiate lobe is an important risk factor for postpartum hemorrhage, because the bridging vessels may be subject to trauma and disruption during delivery, and accessory lobes can be retained after delivery.[11,12] In addition, a succenturiate lobe places a patient at risk for vasa previa, which could lead to fetal exsanguination during rupture of membranes.[13,14]

In circumvallate placenta the chorioamniotic membrane insertion is located centrally, away from the edge of the placenta, creating the appearance of a placenta with rolled edges, and such patients are at risk for placental abruption and hemorrhage.[15] Placenta membranacea is an extremely rare anomaly in which all of the fetal membranes are covered by chorionic villi, resulting in a thin, membranous placenta that covers most or all of the uterine wall.[16,17] Placenta membranacea typically presents with vaginal bleeding, and is associated with placenta previa and placenta accreta.

Thinning of the placenta (less than 2 cm thickness) is seen in patients with systemic vascular or hematologic diseases or with major fetal anomalies, such as trisomy 21. Placental thickening (>4 cm) is seen in cases of fetal hydrops, infection, maternal diabetes, and anemia.[9]

Abnormal Location of the Placenta

Typically the placenta implants into the upper uterine segment, but in placenta previa the placenta is located in the lower uterine segment, near or overlying the internal cervical os.[18] There are 4 categories of placenta previa. A low-lying placenta occurs when the placenta extends into the lower uterine segment to within 2 cm of the internal cervical os. A marginal placenta previa occurs when the placenta reaches, but does not cover, the internal os. A partial placenta previa occurs when the placenta partially covers the os, and a complete placenta previa occurs when the placenta completely covers the internal cervical os (**Fig. 8**). The vast majority of low-lying placentas identified during the second trimester are not in

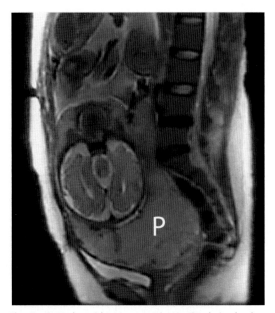

Fig. 8. Complete placenta previa. Sagittal single-shot fast spin-echo image of a 28-year-old woman shows the placenta completely covering the internal cervical os. Placenta percreta was also present. At delivery, the bladder was not invaded but was adherent to the placenta.

the region of the cervix at delivery, as the placenta is thought to grow preferentially toward the well-vascularized fundus, with atrophy of the placental segment near the less vascular cervix.[18,19]

Placenta previa occurs in approximately 0.3% to 0.5% of pregnancies, and the maternal mortality rate related to placenta previa is 0.03% in the United States.[20] Risk factors include prior cesarean delivery or uterine surgery, smoking, advanced maternal age, multiparity and multiple pregnancy.[21–24] Most cases of placenta previa are diagnosed at routine ultrasonography, but when symptomatic, patients typically present with painless bleeding in the late second or early third trimester. Hemorrhagic complications of pregnancy and the need for hysterectomy are associated with placenta previa, and there is an increased risk of preterm birth and perinatal morbidity and mortality.[25,26] Placenta previa is also a risk factor for placenta accreta and more advanced forms of abnormal placentation. In the setting of abnormal placentation, the location of the placenta has implications for surgical management, as methods of vascular control can vary based on whether the lower uterine segment and cervix or the uterine body is involved.[27]

Abnormal Placentation

Normally, the decidua basalis separates placental chorionic villi from the myometrium. During labor,

shearing action between the contracting myometrium and the placenta allows complete separation of the 2 structures during delivery. A defect in the normal decidua basalis, either from prior surgery or instrumentation, allows direct contact of chorionic villi with the myometrium, without intervening decidua basalis. The extent of placental adherence and myometrial penetration varies. In placenta accreta, the chorionic villi directly contact, but do not invade, the uterine wall. In placenta increta, chorionic villi invade the myometrium but do not reach the serosal layer. In placenta percreta, the chorionic villi invade through the myometrium to reach or extend beyond the uterine serosa, with possible invasion of adjacent structures such as the bladder or pelvic side wall. MR imaging has been shown to be accurate in the diagnosis of abnormal placentation, but to consistently and confidently distinguish placenta accreta from increta and increta from percreta remains a challenge, unless there is direct invasion of adjacent organs.[28]

The incidence of abnormal placentation (accreta, increta and percreta) is increasing, largely related to the increasing incidence of cesarean delivery. From 1965 to 2009, the reported cesarean delivery rate in the United States rose from 4.5% to 32.9%.[29,30] Abnormal placentation is currently estimated to occur in from 1 in 2500 to as many as 1 in 500 pregnancies.[31–33]

In addition to prior cesarean delivery, the most common risk factors for abnormal placentation include placenta previa, prior myomectomy or other uterine surgery, and advanced maternal age (**Figs. 9** and **10**).[33–36] As most patients have had an abnormal prenatal ultrasonogram, the pretest probability for abnormal placentation is high.

Abnormal placental attachment to the myometrium may be complicated by postpartum hemorrhage and/or retained products of conception when the placenta fails to cleanly separate from the uterus at the time of delivery (see **Fig. 10**). Up to 95% of patients with abnormal placentation require some form of transfusion support.[37] However, if diagnosed antenatally, steps may be taken to reduce maternal mortality and morbidity.[38] Although definitive management includes planned cesarean section hysterectomy, some institutions request interventional radiology to place embolization or balloon catheters in the internal iliac arteries prophylactically, to be used if necessary.[39] Other approaches to reduce maternal morbidity include segmental myometrial resection or leaving the placenta within the uterus following delivery, and treating with methotrexate or uterine artery embolization.[40–42]

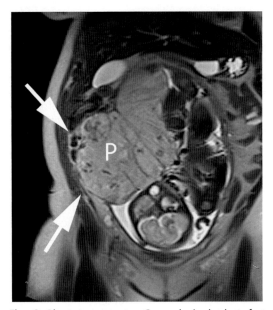

Fig. 9. Placenta percreta. Coronal single-shot fast spin-echo image of a 38-year-old woman at 35 weeks gestational age demonstrates a lateral bulge (*arrows*) in the placenta (P) and lack of identifiable subjacent myometrium at the site of prior resection of a right-sided rudimentary uterine horn. Without the history of prior surgery in this area, this would be an unusual location for abnormal placentation.

Several MR imaging features of abnormal placentation have been described (**Box 2**). Lax and colleagues,[43] in an evaluation of 17 MR imaging features of the placenta and adjacent organs, found 7 features with adequate interobserver variability. Abnormal uterine bulging, the presence of dark intraplacental bands, and placental heterogeneity were considered the most useful features

for the diagnosis of abnormal placentation. In the authors' experience, the combination of dark intraplacental bands and increased vascularity leads to the characteristically heterogeneous placenta, findings that have been confirmed by other investigators.[28,44]

In a similar article, Alamo and colleagues[45] found that the presence of hypointense intraplacental bands was the most useful sign for predicting placental invasion, followed by a focally interrupted myometrial border, invasion of pelvic organs, and tenting of the bladder. Less helpful were uterine contour bulging and heterogeneous intraplacental signal intensity. These investigators also demonstrated higher sensitivity, specificity, and interobserver agreement for more experienced readers in comparison with more junior

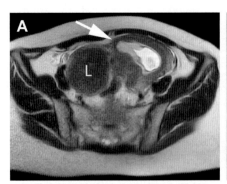
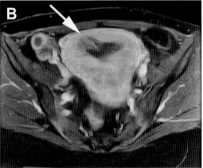

Fig. 10. Abnormal placentation and retained products of conception. (*A*) Axial single-shot fast spin-echo image through the uterus in a 33-year-old woman with a history of prior myomectomy and complicated pregnancy. The 11-week placenta is attached at the myomectomy site (*arrow*). Concern for abnormal placentation and risk of retained products was conveyed to the referring obstetrician. Note a subserosal leiomyoma (L). (*B*) Axial gadolinium-based contrast-enhanced, T1-weighted, fat-suppressed axial image through the uterus after the patient spontaneously aborted, demonstrating retained products of conception (*arrow*) at the prior site of abnormal placentation.

colleagues. Unfortunately, the literature examining the relative value of different MR imaging features for diagnosing abnormal placentation suffers from a relative paucity of cases, and institutions will likely vary in their experience. However, it is reasonable to assume that the likelihood of abnormal placentation increases with the number of described imaging features of placental invasion.

In the authors' experience, disruption of the smooth outer contour of the uterus by outward bulging of a lobulated placenta is a useful sign of abnormal placentation, and is often accompanied by other suspicious findings (Fig. 11).[46] Widening of the lower uterine segment in isolation, resulting in an hourglass-shaped uterus as opposed to an inverted pear-shaped uterus, may be seen occasionally in normal patients but becomes more concerning when additional findings, such as placental lobulation and heterogeneity, are present (Box 3, Fig. 12). Lobulation of the placenta-myometrial interface in the absence of uterine contour deformity can be seen in both normal and abnormal placentation. Although this finding tends to be more exaggerated in the latter setting, other corroborating signs of abnormal placentation should be sought in such cases.

Dark intraplacental bands on T2-weighted imaging contribute to the placental heterogeneity typically seen in abnormal placentation (see Fig. 12; Fig. 13). These dark bands are thicker than the normal placental septae and typically extend

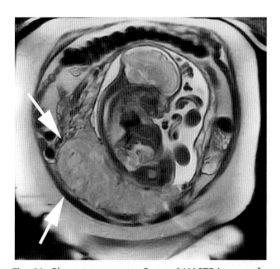

Fig. 11. Placenta percreta. Coronal HASTE image of a 30-year-old woman with history of 2 prior cesarean sections, imaged in the third trimester. No normal myometrium is seen beneath the placenta. Note the deformity (outward bulge) of the uteroplacental complex (*arrows*).

Box 3
Pearls and pitfalls of the MR evaluation of abnormal placentation

Pearls:

There is usually a high pretest probability for abnormal placentation in patients referred for MR imaging

A smooth myometrial-placental interface and trilayered appearance of the myometrium makes a diagnosis of abnormal placentation unlikely

The probability of abnormal placentation increases with the number of risk factors and individual signs on imaging

Suspicious findings should be confirmed in more than 1 imaging plane

Outward placental bulge with distortion/interruption of the external myometrial contour, hypointense intraplacental bands on T2-weighted imaging, and direct invasion of adjacent pelvic organs strongly suggest abnormal placentation

Pitfalls:

Some degree of placenta-myometrial interface lobulation and myometrial thinning may be seen in normal patients

Hourglass-shaped uterus may occasionally be seen in normal patients, particularly when other signs of abnormal placentation are absent

Placental heterogeneity is subjective and difficult to quantify, and normally increases with increasing gestational age during the third trimester

Some imaging planes can lead to a false-positive diagnosis of abnormal placentation or invasion of adjacent structures, owing to the curved shape of the uterus

from the placenta-myometrial interface. The exact reason dark bands form in the setting of abnormal placentation is not well established, and placental heterogeneity is subjective and difficult to quantify. Disorganized, hypertrophied intraplacental blood vessels have also been described as a sign of abnormal placentation.[43] Blood vessels and intraplacental bands can both appear dark on T2-weighted images; the distinction between the two is easily made with steady-state free-precession imaging, as vessels appear bright on this sequence whereas placental bands remain dark (see Fig. 13).

Thinning and/or loss of the normal layered myometrial architecture have been described as a finding of abnormal placentation.[4] However, this

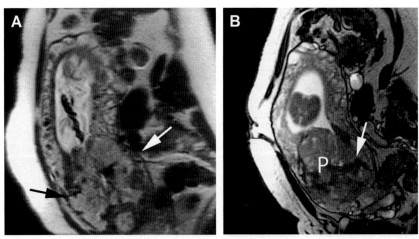

Fig. 12. Placenta previa and placenta percreta in a 25-year-old woman at 21 weeks gestational age. (A) Sagittal single-shot fast spin-echo image shows widening (hourglass appearance) of the lower uterine segment (*black* and *white arrows*). (B) Sagittal steady-state free-precession image at a slightly different location shows a markedly heterogeneous placenta (P) that contains several dark intraplacental bands (*arrow*).

finding is not diagnostic in isolation, as myometrial thinning may be seen beneath a normal placenta and at sites of external compression, such as over the maternal spine (see **Fig. 4**). When present, focal myometrial thinning beneath the placenta in the lower uterine segment in a patient with prior history of cesarean section, in the absence of bulging of the external myometrial contour, often corresponds to superficial myometrial attachment (accreta) without myometrial invasion (**Fig. 14**).

Several studies have compared MR imaging with ultrasonography for the evaluation of abnormal placentation. Warshak and colleagues[8] studied 453 women with placenta previa, previous cesarean delivery, and low-lying anterior placenta, and found 39 patients with confirmed placenta accreta.

Ultrasonography had sensitivity of 77%, specificity of 96%, a positive predictive value of 65%, and a negative predictive value of 98%. In this same study, 42 patients underwent MR imaging for suspicious or inconclusive ultrasonography examinations, revealing sensitivity of 88%, specificity of 100%, a positive predictive value of 100%, and a negative predictive value of 82%. A smaller study of 32 patients clinically at high risk of placenta accreta found that sonography had sensitivity of 93%, specificity of 71%, a positive predictive value of 74%, and a negative predictive value of 92%, whereas MR imaging had sensitivity of 80%, specificity of 65%, a positive predictive value of 67%, and a negative predictive value of 79%.[47] This study found no statistically significant difference

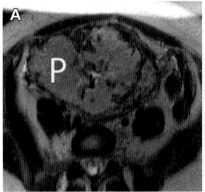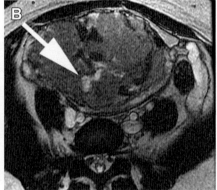

Fig. 13. Heterogeneous placenta with dark placental bands and vessels. (A) Axial single-shot fast spin-echo image through the placenta shows a heterogeneous placenta (P). The distinction between placental bands and vessels is not clear on this sequence. (B) Axial steady-state free-precession sequence shows the vessels to be high signal-intensity structures (*arrow*).

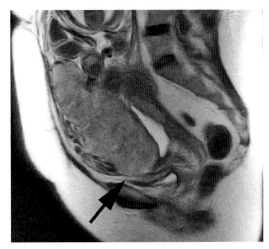

Fig. 14. Placenta accreta in a 36-year-old woman at 31 weeks gestational age. Sagittal single-shot fast spin-echo image through the uterus shows loss of the normal layered myometrium in the lower uterine segment (*arrow*) with focal bulge of the placenta, without distortion of the myometrial contour. Placenta accreta was found at delivery.

between ultrasonography and MR imaging for the diagnosis of abnormal placentation. Based on these results, the investigators concluded that both modalities are complementary and suggested that, if inconclusive findings are found with one modality, the other can be used to clarify the potential abnormality. In another study, Masselli and colleagues[48] found no statistically significant difference in sensitivity or specificity between ultrasonography and MR imaging, but MR imaging performed better at gauging depth of placental invasion.

Vascular Anomalies

The umbilical cord typically inserts centrally on the placenta (see **Fig. 1**). An eccentric, or marginal, insertion occurs when the cord inserts 1 to 2 cm from the placental edge, and this variant has been associated with impairment of fetal growth and preterm delivery.[49–51] A velamentous insertion occurs when the cord inserts on the chorioamniotic membranes, outside the placental margin, resulting in unprotected vessels that are subject to compression or rupture (**Fig. 15**). Velamentous cord insertion is associated with low birth weight, small for gestational age fetuses, and preterm delivery.[52] In addition, intrapartum hemorrhage has been linked to velamentous cord insertion.

Vasa previa, with an incidence of 1 in 2500 deliveries, occurs when fetal vessels course through the membranes between the fetus and the cervix, unprotected by the placenta or the umbilical cord, and often is a result of velamentous or marginal insertion of the cord or vessels running between accessory placental lobes.[53] Vasa previa is a risk factor for hemorrhage, and pressure on the unprotected vessels can lead to decreased fetal blood supply. Risk factors include in vitro fertilization, placenta previa, succenturiate lobed placentas, and multiple pregnancies.[53] Undiagnosed vasa previa is associated with a perinatal mortality as high as 60%.[14,53] Ultrasonography with color Doppler is usually effective at identifying vessels overlying the cervix. Although MR imaging allows global evaluation of the vascular anatomy, it is generally used only when the diagnosis is in question, or if ultrasonographic evaluation is inadequate.[54]

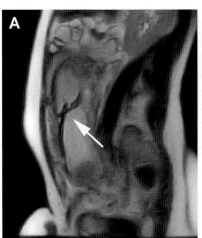
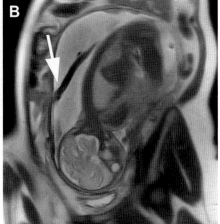

Fig. 15. Velamentous cord insertion in a 32-year-old woman during third trimester of pregnancy. Sagittal (*A*) and coronal (*B*) single-shot fast spin-echo images through the uterus demonstrate insertion of the umbilical cord (*arrows*) into the fetal membranes remote from the placenta (not visible on these images).

> **Box 4**
> **What the referring physician needs to know: abnormal placentation**
>
> Placental location with respect to the uterus and cervix
>
> Placental anomalies
>
> Anomalous umbilical cord insertion site or evidence of vasa previa
>
> If the placenta is confined to uterus (accreta, increta) or if it invades adjacent organs or structures (percreta)

SUMMARY

As abnormal placentation becomes more prevalent, primarily because of increasing rates of cesarean delivery, there is a need for accurate antenatal diagnosis to prevent the high morbidity and mortality of undiagnosed placental abnormalities. Ultrasonography remains the primary screening modality for the identification of abnormal placentation, but MR imaging is a complementary imaging modality that is useful when ultrasonography is inconclusive. When abnormal placentation is confirmed with MR, a detailed description of the findings should be provided to the referring physician (**Box 4**).

Because MR imaging is often used as an adjunctive imaging modality when ultrasonography has already identified a potential abnormality, the pretest probability for MR imaging is generally high. Risk factors for abnormal placentation that may be identified with MR imaging include abnormal placental morphology and placental location. A variety of MR imaging features has been associated with abnormal placentation, and identification of multiple features improves confidence. Determining the depth of placental invasion with any imaging modality remains a challenge unless gross extension beyond the uterine serosa is present.

REFERENCES

1. Blaicher W, Brugger PC, Mittermayer C, et al. Magnetic resonance imaging of the normal placenta. Eur J Radiol 2006;57(2):256–60.
2. Tanaka YO, Sohda S, Shigemitsu S, et al. High temporal resolution dynamic contrast MRI in a high risk group for placenta accreta. Magn Reson Imaging 2001;19(5):635–42.
3. Marcos HB, Semelka RC, Worawattanakul S. Normal placenta: gadolinium-enhanced dynamic MR imaging. Radiology 1997;205(2):493–6.
4. Kim JA, Narra VR. Magnetic resonance imaging with true fast imaging with steady-state precession and half-Fourier acquisition single-shot turbo spin-echo sequences in cases of suspected placenta accreta. Acta Radiol 2004;45(6):692–8.
5. Morita S, Ueno E, Fujimura M, et al. Feasibility of diffusion-weighted MRI for defining placental invasion. J Magn Reson Imaging 2009;30(3):666–71.
6. Chalouhi GE, Deloison B, Siauve N, et al. Dynamic contrast-enhanced magnetic resonance imaging: definitive imaging of placental function? Semin Fetal Neonatal Med 2011;16(1):22–8.
7. Moore RJ, Issa B, Tokarczuk P, et al. In vivo intravoxel incoherent motion measurements in the human placenta using echo-planar imaging at 0.5 T. Magn Reson Med 2000;43(2):295–302.
8. Warshak CR, Eskander R, Hull AD, et al. Accuracy of ultrasonography and magnetic resonance imaging in the diagnosis of placenta accreta. Obstet Gynecol 2006;108(3 Pt 1):573–81.
9. Elsayes KM, Trout AT, Friedkin AM, et al. Imaging of the placenta: a multimodality pictorial review. Radiographics 2009;29(5):1371–91.
10. Baergen RN, Benirschke K. Manual of pathology of the human placenta. 2nd edition. New York: Springer; 2011.
11. Chihara H, Otsubo Y, Ohta Y, et al. Prenatal diagnosis of succenturiate lobe by ultrasonography and color Doppler imaging. Arch Gynecol Obstet 2000;263(3):137–8.
12. Hata K, Hata T, Aoki S, et al. Succenturiate placenta diagnosed by ultrasound. Gynecol Obstet Invest 1988;25(4):273–6.
13. Lee W, Lee VL, Kirk JS, et al. Vasa previa: prenatal diagnosis, natural evolution, and clinical outcome. Obstet Gynecol 2000;95(4):572–6.
14. Oyelese KO, Schwarzler P, Coates S, et al. A strategy for reducing the mortality rate from vasa previa using transvaginal sonography with color Doppler. Ultrasound Obstet Gynecol 1998;12(6):434–8.
15. Harris RD, Wells WA, Black WC, et al. Accuracy of prenatal sonography for detecting circumvallate placenta. AJR Am J Roentgenol 1997;168(6):1603–8.
16. Ahmed A, Gilbert-Barness E. Placenta membranacea: a developmental anomaly with diverse clinical presentation. Pediatr Dev Pathol 2003;6(2):201–2.
17. Greenberg JA, Sorem KA, Shifren JL, et al. Placenta membranacea with placenta increta: a case report and literature review. Obstet Gynecol 1991;78(3 Pt 2):512–4.
18. Oyelese Y, Smulian JC. Placenta previa, placenta accreta, and vasa previa. Obstet Gynecol 2006;107(4):927–41.

19. Benirschke K, Baergen RN, Burton G. Pathology of the human placenta. 6th edition. Heidelberg (Germany): Springer; 2012.

20. Iyasu S, Saftlas AK, Rowley DL, et al. The epidemiology of placenta previa in the United States, 1979 through 1987. Am J Obstet Gynecol 1993;168(5): 1424–9.

21. Ananth CV, Smulian JC, Vintzileos AM. The association of placenta previa with history of cesarean delivery and abortion: a metaanalysis. Am J Obstet Gynecol 1997;177(5):1071–8.

22. Ananth CV, Savitz DA, Luther ER. Maternal cigarette smoking as a risk factor for placental abruption, placenta previa, and uterine bleeding in pregnancy. Am J Epidemiol 1996;144(9): 881–9.

23. Ananth CV, Wilcox AJ, Savitz DA, et al. Effect of maternal age and parity on the risk of uteroplacental bleeding disorders in pregnancy. Obstet Gynecol 1996;88(4 Pt 1):511–6.

24. Ananth CV, Demissie K, Smulian JC, et al. Placenta previa in singleton and twin births in the United States, 1989 through 1998: a comparison of risk factor profiles and associated conditions. Am J Obstet Gynecol 2003;188(1):275–81.

25. Crane JM, van den Hof MC, Dodds L, et al. Neonatal outcomes with placenta previa. Obstet Gynecol 1999;93(4):541–4.

26. Crane JM, Van den Hof MC, Dodds L, et al. Maternal complications with placenta previa. Am J Perinatol 2000;17(2):101–5.

27. Palacios-Jaraquemada JM, Bruno CH, Martin E. MRI in the diagnosis and surgical management of abnormal placentation. Acta Obstet Gynecol Scand 2013;92(4):392–7.

28. Teo TH, Law YM, Tay KH, et al. Use of magnetic resonance imaging in evaluation of placental invasion. Clin Radiol 2009;64(5):511–6.

29. Taffel SM, Placek PJ, Liss T. Trends in the United States cesarean section rate and reasons for the 1980-85 rise. Am J Public Health 1987;77(8): 955–9.

30. Martin JA, Hamilton BE, Ventura SJ, et al. Births: final data for 2009. Natl Vital Stat Rep 2011;60(1): 1–70.

31. Khong TY. The pathology of placenta accreta, a worldwide epidemic. J Clin Pathol 2008;61(12): 1243–6.

32. Wu S, Kocherginsky M, Hibbard JU. Abnormal placentation: twenty-year analysis. Am J Obstet Gynecol 2005;192(5):1458–61.

33. Miller DA, Chollet JA, Goodwin TM. Clinical risk factors for placenta previa-placenta accreta. Am J Obstet Gynecol 1997;177(1):210–4.

34. Clark SL, Koonings PP, Phelan JP. Placenta previa/accreta and prior cesarean section. Obstet Gynecol 1985;66(1):89–92.

35. Gielchinsky Y, Rojansky N, Fasouliotis SJ, et al. Placenta accrete—summary of 10 years: a survey of 310 cases. Placenta 2002;23(2–3):210–4.

36. Silver RM, Landon MB, Rouse DJ, et al. Maternal morbidity associated with multiple repeat cesarean deliveries. Obstet Gynecol 2006;107(6): 1226–32.

37. Stotler B, Padmanabhan A, Devine P, et al. Transfusion requirements in obstetric patients with placenta accreta. Transfusion 2011;51(12):2627–33.

38. Warshak CR, Ramos GA, Eskander R, et al. Effect of predelivery diagnosis in 99 consecutive cases of placenta accreta. Obstet Gynecol 2010;115(1): 65–9.

39. Carnevale FC, Kondo MM, de Oliveira Sousa W Jr, et al. Perioperative temporary occlusion of the internal iliac arteries as prophylaxis in cesarean section at risk of hemorrhage in placenta accreta. Cardiovasc Intervent Radiol 2011;34(4):758–64.

40. Allahdin S, Voigt S, Htwe TT. Management of placenta praevia and accreta. J Obstet Gynaecol 2011;31(1):1–6.

41. Timmermans S, van Hof AC, Duvekot JJ. Conservative management of abnormally invasive placentation. Obstet Gynecol Surv 2007;62(8): 529–39.

42. Doumouchtsis SK, Arulkumaran S. The morbidly adherent placenta: an overview of management options. Acta Obstet Gynecol Scand 2010;89(9): 1126–33.

43. Lax A, Prince MR, Mennitt KW, et al. The value of specific MRI features in the evaluation of suspected placental invasion. Magn Reson Imaging 2007;25(1):87–93.

44. Derman AY, Nikac V, Haberman S, et al. MRI of placenta accreta: a new imaging perspective. AJR Am J Roentgenol 2011;197(6):1514–21.

45. Alamo L, Anaye A, Rey J, et al. Detection of suspected placental invasion by MRI: do the results depend on observer' experience? Eur J Radiol 2013;82(2):e51–7.

46. Leyendecker JR, DuBose M, Hosseinzadeh K, et al. MRI of pregnancy-related issues: abnormal placentation. AJR Am J Roentgenol 2012;198(2): 311–20.

47. Dwyer BK, Belogolovkin V, Tran L, et al. Prenatal diagnosis of placenta accreta: sonography or magnetic resonance imaging? J Ultrasound Med 2008; 27(9):1275–81.

48. Masselli G, Brunelli R, Casciani E, et al. Magnetic resonance imaging in the evaluation of placental adhesive disorders: correlation with color Doppler ultrasound. Eur Radiol 2008;18(6):1292–9.

49. Rolschau J. The relationship between some disorders of the umbilical cord and intrauterine growth retardation. Acta Obstet Gynecol Scand Suppl 1978;72:15–21.

50. Davies BR, Casanueva E, Arroyo P. Placentas of small-for-dates infants: a small controlled series from Mexico City, Mexico. Am J Obstet Gynecol 1984;149(7):731–6.

51. Brody S, Frenkel DA. Marginal insertion of the cord and premature labor. Am J Obstet Gynecol 1953; 65(6):1305–12.

52. Heinonen S, Ryynanen M, Kirkinen P, et al. Perinatal diagnostic evaluation of velamentous umbilical cord insertion: clinical, Doppler, and ultrasonic findings. Obstet Gynecol 1996;87(1): 112–7.

53. Oyelese KO, Turner M, Lees C, et al. Vasa previa: an avoidable obstetric tragedy. Obstet Gynecol Surv 1999;54(2):138–45.

54. Oyelese Y, Jha RC, Moxley MD, et al. Magnetic resonance imaging of vasa praevia. BJOG 2003; 110(12):1127–8.

Imaging of Female Infertility
A Pictorial Guide to the Hysterosalpingography, Ultrasonography, and Magnetic Resonance Imaging Findings of the Congenital and Acquired Causes of Female Infertility

Katherine Kaproth-Joslin, MD, PhD*, Vikram Dogra, MD

KEYWORDS

- Female infertility • Fallopian tube • Ovary • Uterus • Imaging • Müllerian duct anomalies

KEY POINTS

- Hysterosalpingography is the gold standard in assessing the patency of the fallopian tubes, which is among the most common causes of female factor infertility, making this technique the most frequent first-choice imaging modality in the assessment of female infertility.
- Ultrasonography and magnetic resonance imaging are typically used for evaluation of indeterminate or complicated cases of female infertility and for presurgical planning.
- Müllerian duct anomalies are most commonly classified by the American Fertility Society classification scheme, divided into 7 classes: Class I, uterine hypoplasia and/or agenesis; Class II, unicornuate uterus; Class III, uterus didelphys; Class IV, bicornuate; Class V, septate uterus; Class VI, arcuate uterus; and Class VII, diethylstilbestrol-related anomalies.
- Acquired abnormalities of the uterus include submucosal fibroids, endometrial polyps, adenomyosis, uterine synechiae, and cervical stenosis.
- Acquired abnormalities of the fallopian tube include tubal occlusion, hydrosalpinx, and salpingitis isthmica nodosa.
- Imaging plays a role in the detection of secondary causes of ovarian factor infertility, including endometriosis and polycystic ovarian syndrome.

INTRODUCTION

Infertility affects approximately 15% of couples, and is defined as the inability to conceive after a 12-month period of regular unprotected intercourse. Causes include ovulation dysfunction occurring in 20% of cases, male factor infertility occurring in 30% of cases, and tubal and pelvic abnormalities occurring in approximately 30% of cases, with a combination of factors occurring in 20% of cases.[1,2] Based on the guidelines established by the European Society of Human Reproduction and Embryology in 2008, couples who have not achieved pregnancy after 1 year of unprotected intercourse should be offered additional clinical workup for infertility. First-line

The authors have nothing to disclose.
Department of Imaging Sciences, University of Rochester Medical Center, 601 Elmwood Avenue, Box 648, Rochester, NY 14642, USA
* Corresponding author.
E-mail address: Katherine_kaproth-joslin@urmc.rochester.edu

radiologic.theclinics.com

studies should include semen analysis and ovulation assessment. If normal or if there is a suspicion of tubal damage based on clinical history, tubal patency can then be performed with hysterosalpingography (HSG).[3] For cases in which ovarian abnormality is assumed, transvaginal ultrasonography (US) is the recommended imaging modality for ovarian evaluation. Magnetic resonance (MR) imaging is reserved for indeterminate or complicated cases.

This article reviews the normal anatomy of the uterus, fallopian tubes, and ovaries. The imaging techniques best used to study these structures are discussed, as well as the normal imaging characteristics of each organ. The imaging findings for the congenital causes of female infertility are reviewed, including the müllerian duct anomalies and gonadal dysgenesis. Finally, the authors examine the acquired causes of female infertility, addressing the common uterine, fallopian tube, and ovarian abnormalities that lead to this condition.

ANATOMY

The uterus is a thick-walled fibromuscular structure that serves as an incubation chamber, allowing for implantation of a fertilized ovum and housing for the fetus during gestation. Its size and shape depend on patient age and parity. The uterus is divided into 2 major sections, the body and the cervix. The uterine body can further be divided into 3 parts: the fundus, which is the superiormost portion above the level of the fallopian tube ostia; the main body, which is the largest part of the uterus; and the isthmus, which is the inferior portion directly above the internal cervical os.[4] The cervix serves as the connection between the uterine body and the vagina.

Fallopian tubes provide the conduit for the ovum to journey from the ovary to the uterus, measuring 10 to 12 cm in length and positioned along the superior aspect of the broad ligaments bilaterally. Each fallopian tube is divided into 3 parts on imaging. The interstitial/corneal portion is a short proximal segment, which courses through the muscular portion of the uterine wall. The isthmic portion is the long narrow segment that connects the interstitial and ampullary regions of the fallopian tube. The ampullary portion is where the distal fallopian tube widens at the level of the ovary.[4]

The ovaries are the ovum-producing paired organs typically located in the lateral pelvic wall adjacent to the bifurcation of the common iliac vessels, posterior to the broad ligament and anterior to the ureter. Ovarian size and location are dependent on age, menstrual status, and parity. The ovarian parenchyma is divided into 2 parts: the medulla, where the blood supply enters and exits the ovary, and the cortex, which contains multiple follicles in varying stages of development.

IMAGING TECHNIQUES

HSG is the gold standard in assessing the patency of the fallopian tubes, which is among the most common causes of female factor infertility, making this technique the most frequent imaging choice in the assessment of female infertility.[5] This study can also be used for evaluation of the endometrial cavity contour and to detect the presence of müllerian anomalies. In this procedure, radiopaque contrast is injected into the uterine cavity and fallopian tubes, and fluoroscopic images are obtained of the endometrial canal and fallopian tube lumens, with limited to no evaluation of the external uterine contour. Using this imaging modality, the uterus should appear as a smooth-walled inverted triangle, with the bilateral fallopian tubes appearing as thin smooth lines that widen at the ampullary region; free spillage of contrast should be observed bilaterally (**Fig. 1**A).[2,4]

US also plays an important role in the initial evaluation of female infertility, allowing for morphologic characterization of the uterus and ovaries, with limited evaluation of the fallopian tubes. Transvaginal US evaluation of the uterine contour and morphology, including endometrial and myometrial defects, can be performed. US is also optimal for the evaluation of the ovarian stroma, follicles, and overall ovarian volume, especially in the setting of polycystic ovarian syndrome. In addition, sonohysterography allows for the instillation of saline into the endometrial canal, permitting a detailed examination of the endometrial lumen and assessment any lesions if present. On US imaging, the myometrium demonstrates a homogeneous hypoechoic echotexture. The endometrium is hyperechoic, with a variable appearance and thickness that is dependent on the phase of the menstrual cycle, measuring up to 1.6 cm in thickness. Depending on the phase of the cycle, cystic regions may be present within the endometrium, representing regions of blood and/or endometrial breakdown (see **Fig. 1**B). The ovaries are typically hypoechoic to the adjacent myometrium, with the medulla slightly hyperechoic to the cortex (see **Fig. 1**C). Developing follicles are anechoic; however, corpus luteal cysts can have a thick, echogenic vascular ring.

MR imaging is typically reserved for intricate or indeterminate cases, providing detailed assessment of the pelvic soft tissues and assisting in differentiating between causes detected during HSG and US examination. In addition, MR often

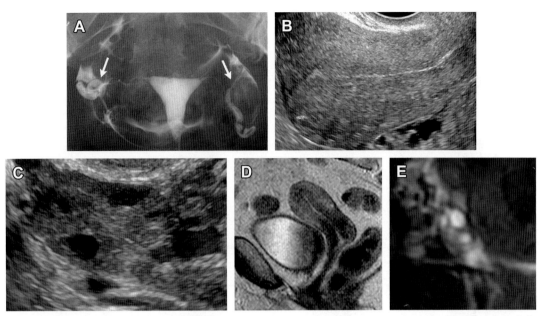

Fig. 1. Normal anatomy of uterus, fallopian tube, and ovary. (*A*) Hysterosalpingography (HSG) image of the normal uterus and fallopian tubes. Note free spillage of contrast bilaterally (*arrows*). (*B*) Ultrasonography (US) image of a normal uterus. (*C*) US image of a normal ovary. (*D*) Magnetic resonance (MR) imaging of a normal uterus. (*E*) MR imaging of a normal ovary.

plays a key role in presurgical planning.[6] On MR imaging, the uterus and cervix demonstrate intermediate signal on T1-weighted imaging. On T2-weighted imaging the endometrium is high signal, with a lower-signal junctional zone, and an intermediate myometrium (see **Fig. 1**D). On T1-weighted images, the ovaries are homogeneous intermediate signal with low-signal follicles. These follicles are high signal on T2-weighted imaging, with intermediate-signal cortex (see **Fig. 1**E).

CONGENITAL UTERINE AND FALLOPIAN TUBE ANOMALIES

Müllerian duct anomalies occur secondary to failure of organogenesis, failure of fusion, or failure of reabsorption, causing incomplete development of one or both of the uterine horns. These anomalies are most commonly classified by the American Fertility Society (AFS) classification scheme.[7] The scheme is based on the embryologic development of the müllerian ducts and is divided into 7 classes: Class I, uterine hypoplasia and/or agenesis; Class II, unicornuate uterus; Class III, uterus didelphys; Class IV, bicornuate; Class V, septate uterus; Class VI, arcuate uterus; and Class VII, diethylstilbestrol (DES)-related anomalies (**Fig. 2**).

Class I: Uterine Hypoplasia and Agenesis

Uterine hypoplasia and/or agenesis occur when both müllerian ducts fail to or incompletely develop, causing absence or rudimentary development of the uterus and proximal vagina. Mayer-Rokitansky-Küster-Hauser syndrome is the most common form of the condition, in which a genetic female (46,XX) with normal external genitalia presents with primary amenorrhea and dyspareunia, vaginal agenesis, and a partial or absent uterus.[8] Additional renal anomalies may also be present. US and MR imaging demonstrates a fibrous remnant/connective tissue and vessels in the expected region of the uterus in the setting of agenesis, and small hypoplastic uterine soft-tissue remnant in the setting of hypoplasia. The upper two-thirds of the vagina are absent or atretic in both conditions. Ovaries appear normal, but may be more superiorly located. HSG evaluation is not indicated for this condition.

Class II: Unicornuate Uterus

Incomplete or failed development of one of the müllerian ducts results in a functional uterine cavity with a single uterine horn, representing approximately 4% of the uterine anomalies.[9] There may be an associated rudimentary horn on the contralateral side, with or without a communication with the dominant uterine horn. This condition is often asymptomatic and is found during the workup for infertility; however, it may also be associated with cyclic pelvic pain when the rudimentary horn is noncommunicating and contains functional

Congenital Müllerian Anommalies

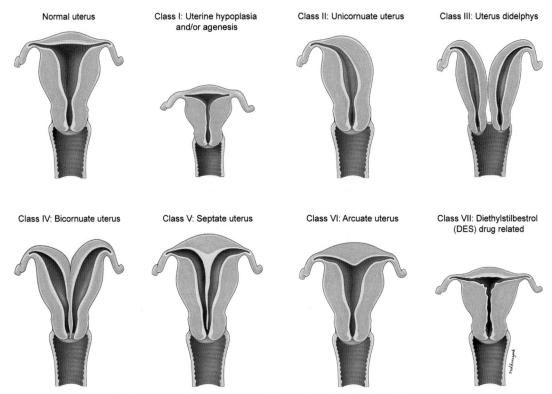

Fig. 2. Uterine anomalies based on the American Fertility Society Classification Scheme.

endometrium. Imaging with HSG, US, and MR demonstrates a fusiform "banana-shaped" endometrial canal, which is laterally deviated with a single fallopian tube (**Fig. 3**). When detected, MR imaging should be performed to evaluate for a rudimentary horn, as this structure is often resected secondary to an increased risk of endometriosis and/or ectopic pregnancy (see **Fig. 3**B).[10] In addition, urinary tract anomalies are often associated with this condition, with renal agenesis contralateral to the dominant uterine horn most commonly seen.

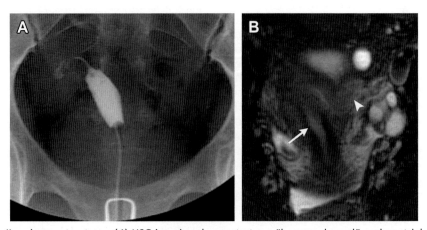

Fig. 3. Class II: unicornuate uterus. (*A*) HSG imaging demonstrates a "banana-shaped" endometrial canal, laterally deviated to the right with a single fallopian tube. (*B*) MR T2-weighted image of the same patient demonstrates a unicornuate uterus (*arrow*) on the right with rudimentary horn on the left, not detected by HSG (*arrowhead*).

Class III: Didelphys Uterus

Didelphys uterus occurs when there is complete failure of fusion of the müllerian ducts, resulting in a duplicated pair of uteri and cervices, and represents approximately 11% of uterine anomalies.[9] Imaging with HSG, US, and MR demonstrates 2 symmetric, widely spaced uterine horns each with its own cervix (**Fig. 4**). A longitudinal vaginal septum is present in approximately 75% of cases, and a unilateral horizontal septum may also be present, which can lead to ipsilateral hematometrocolpos. Failure to identify and cannulate both cervices during HSG may lead to the false diagnosis of unicornuate uterus. This condition is also associated with urinary tract anomalies, which

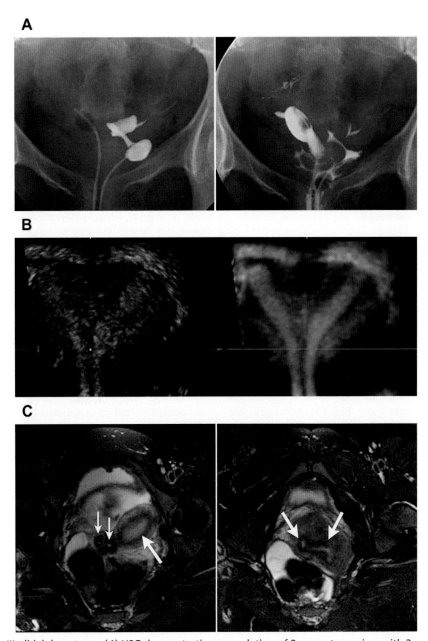

Fig. 4. Class III: didelphys uterus. (*A*) HSG demonstrating cannulation of 2 separate cervices with 2 separate endometrial canals. (*B*) 3-dimensional US, gray-scale on the left and B-mode on the right, demonstrating 2 separate endometrial cavities and 2 separate cervical canals. (*C*) MR axial T2-weighted fat-suppressed images. Left image shows 2 cervices (*thin arrows*) with the left uterine cavity (*thick arrow*) partially visualized. Right image is slightly more superior and shows 2 separate uterine cavities (*thick arrows*).

are present in 23% of women with didelphys uterus.[9]

Class IV: Bicornuate Uterus

Bicornuate uterus occurs when the superior portions of the müllerian ducts fail to fuse with normal fusion of the inferior uterine segment, and represents approximately 46% of the uterine anomalies.[9] The central myometrium can extend to the level of the internal cervical os (bicornuate unicollis) or external uterine os (bicornuate bicollis). US and MR imaging demonstrate a fundal uterine cleft larger than 1 cm separating divergent uterine horns (**Fig. 5**A). HSG, US, and MR imaging demonstrate fusiform symmetric size and appearance of the endometrial canals, with possible visualization of a communication between the inferior segments of the uterine horns (see **Fig. 5**). A widened angle (>105°) between the uterine horns with a widened intercornual distance of greater than 4 cm is suggestive of bicornuate uterus on HSG; however, the imaging technique is limited in its differentiation from a septate uterus, as the external uterine contour is not evaluated.

Class V: Septate Uterus

Failure of the fibromuscular septum between the two müllerian ducts to resorb after ductal fusion leads to the development of a septate uterus, one of the most common müllerian duct anomalies (55%).[5] The resulting partition may be fibrous or contain myometrium, and a vaginal septum can also be present. Imaging demonstrates symmetric endometrial cavities, which are narrower and smaller than normal. US and MR demonstrate a normal, flat, or contour depression of the uterine fundus of less than 1 cm (**Fig. 6**A). Although HSG is limited in its ability to differentiate this from bicornuate uterus, a narrow angle of less than 75° between the uterine horns and/or an intercornual

distance of less than 4 cm is suggestive of septate uterus (see **Fig. 6**B).[11] Transvaginal US and MR imaging have improved the diagnostic accuracy for septate uterus, with hysteroscopy and laparoscopy serving as gold standards for diagnosis.[9] Composition and extent of the septum can be evaluated with MR imaging, with the thin fibrous septum demonstrating a low T2 signal and the thicker myometrial septum demonstrating an intermediate T2 signal (see **Fig. 6**A).[5] Of the müllerian duct anomalies, this condition is associated with the highest rate of reproductive failures, is associated with infertility and miscarriage, and is thought to be secondary to the poor blood supply of the septum providing unsuitable support for the implanted embryo.[12]

Class VI: Arcuate Uterus

The arcuate uterus is considered a normal variant of uterine morphology, where near but incomplete resorption of the septum results in a focal bulge at the level of the uterine fundus. HSG, US, and MR imaging demonstrate a single endometrial canal, with a smooth, broad indentation of the myometrium (<1 cm) at the uterine fundus (**Fig. 7**). The external uterine contour is normal on US and MR imaging (see **Fig. 7**B). HSG may be limited in distinguishing arcuate from septate uterus; therefore in a patient with recurrent pregnancy loss, additional imaging with MR or US may be needed for further evaluation.

Class VII: Infantile Uterus (T-Shaped, DES-Related Uterine Anomalies)

DES, a nonsteroidal estrogen, was widely used in the United States in the 1950s to treat a variety of obstetric conditions, including miscarriage and preeclampsia. It was later discovered that compared with the general population, the daughters of these patients had both a higher rate of

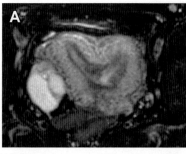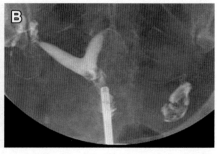

Fig. 5. Class IV: bicornuate uterus. Symmetric size and appearance of 2 divergent endometrial canals with a communication between the inferior segments of the uterine horns. (*A*) MR image demonstrates a fundal uterine cleft, which is greater than 1 cm, separating divergent uterine horns. (*B*) HSG examination of the same patient is suggestive of bicornuate uterus, as there is a widened angle (>105°) between the uterine horns with a widened intercornual distance of more than 4 cm.

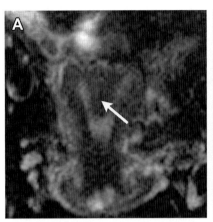
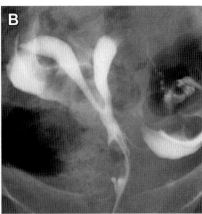

Fig. 6. Class V: septate uterus. (*A*) MR image demonstrating a normal external uterine contour with 2 symmetric endometrial cavities, which are narrower and smaller than normal. Note the thickened septum with intermediate T2-weighted signal isointense with the adjacent myometrium (*arrow*). (*B*) HSG demonstrating a double endometrial canal with an acute uterine horn angle of less 75°.

vaginal clear-cell carcinoma and a higher incidence of having a hypoplastic, infantile-shaped (T-shaped) uterus.[13] HSG is the imaging modality of choice for this condition. Cannulation of the uterus may be difficult secondary to stenosis/hypoplasia of the cervical canal. Once cannulated, the uterus demonstrates a single, narrowed irregular endometrial canal with a shortened upper uterine segment and a characteristic T-shape. Myometrial constriction bands may be present and are typically midfundal in location. The fallopian tubes are shortened with an irregular contour (**Fig. 8**).

CONGENITAL OVARIAN ANOMALIES
Gonadal Dysgenesis

Gonadal dysgenesis is a congenital condition characterized by abnormal gonadal organization and function, whereby the gonadal tissue is replaced by fibrous stroma with no germ cells present, referred to as streak gonads.[14] The most common form of this condition is secondary to Turner syndrome (45 XO karyotype), although variable karyotypes may be present. Imaging is not typically performed to identify this condition, with diagnosis typically based on clinical, biochemical, and karyotype identification. When performed, imaging demonstrates small oval to linear fibrous tissue within the broad ligament with absence of normal-appearing ovaries. This condition is best seen with MR imaging, although detection is limited, with the gonads found in only approximately 40% to 65% of cases. On MR, the streak gonads are seen as a small linear to oval structure in the broad ligament, which is isointense or slightly hypointense to muscle on T1-weighted imaging. US has limited utility in detecting streak gonads, but may be useful for assessment of associated müllerian duct abnormalities.

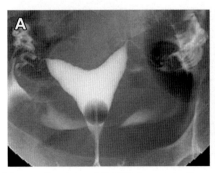
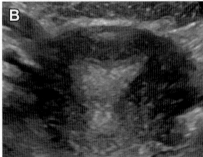

Fig. 7. Class VI: arcuate uterus. (*A*) HSG demonstrating a single endometrial canal with a smooth broad indentation of the myometrium (<1 cm) at uterine fundus. (*B*) US image demonstrating a single endometrial canal with a smooth broad indentation of the myometrium (<1 cm) at the uterine fundus. Note the smooth external uterine contour.

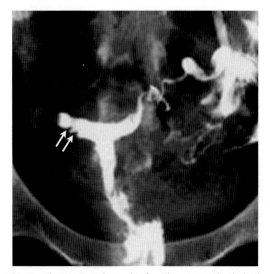

Fig. 8. Class VII: T-shaped/infantile uterus/diethylstilbestrol exposure. HSG demonstrates a single narrowed irregular endometrial canal with a shortened upper uterine segment with a classic T-shape. Note the appearance of the myometrial constriction bands indenting on the right (*arrows*).

ACQUIRED ABNORMALITIES
Uterine Abnormalities

Submucosal fibroids

Fibroids, also known as leiomyomas or myomas, are benign estrogen-dependent smooth-muscle lesions that originate from the uterine myometrium, occurring in 20% to 40% of women in their reproductive years.[15,16] These lesions can be either solitary or multifocal, and can arise from any part of the uterus. When the mass protrudes into the endometrial canal, it is considered submucosal in location and is thought to cause infertility by interfering with embryo implantation.[9,16] Though often asymptomatic, individuals may experience abnormal uterine bleeding, dysmenorrhea, and pelvic pressure.[16] Imaging of a submucosal fibroid shows a mass projecting into the endometrial cavity. Transvaginal US is the recommended initial imaging modality, demonstrating a focal heterogeneous mass that is hypoechoic to the myometrium and may have acoustic shadowing (**Fig. 9**A). When imaged during HSG, the lesion is best visualized early in uterine filling, and is

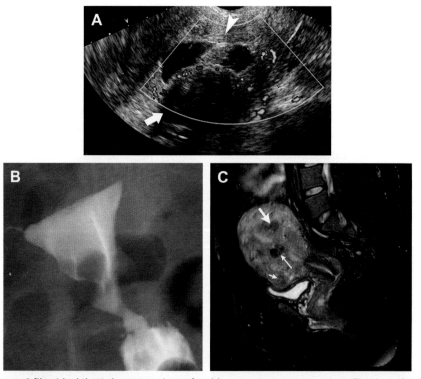

Fig. 9. Submucosal fibroids. (*A*) US demonstrating a focal heterogeneous mass protruding into the endometrial canal, which is hypoechoic to the myometrium with acoustic shadowing (*thick arrow*). Also present is a hyperechoic focal protrusion of the endometrium consistent with a polyp (*arrowhead*). (*B*) HSG showing an intraluminal mass projecting into the endometrial cavity. (*C*) MR T2-weighted images demonstrating multiple uterine fibroids, with low signal intensity compared with myometrium. (Locations: submucosal, *thin arrow*; mural, *thick arrow*; subserosal, *short arrow*.)

depicted as an intraluminal mass projecting into the endometrial cavity. However, this finding is nonspecific and differentiation from other causes, such as endometrial polyps, may be needed (see **Fig. 9**B). If further imaging is required, MR imaging and/or sonohysterography are the recommended modalities to further evaluate these lesions, and can be performed before surgical resection to determine the number, location, and extent of lesions. MR imaging findings of myoma depend on its level of degeneration, normally demonstrating low signal intensity in comparison with myometrium on T2-weighted images; however, it may show a high T2 signal with cystic degeneration (see **Fig. 9**C).[16]

Endometrial polyps

Endometrial polyps are a focal overgrowth of the endometrial glands and stroma, surrounded by normal endometrium. Classically these lesions are divided into 3 subtypes: hyperplastic polyps, which have glands similar to those seen in endometrial hyperplasia; atrophic polyps, which occur in postmenopausal woman and have atrophic cystically dilated glands; and functional polyps, which follow the menstrual cycle.[16] Imaging demonstrates an intraluminal pedunculated endometrial mass, measuring between 1 mm and 2 cm in size, which may distort the uterine cavity. Transvaginal US and/or sonohysterography are considered the imaging modalities of choice, demonstrating a focal echogenic mass protruding into the endometrial lumen from the endometrium, with an intact endometrial stripe and a feeding vessel identified on Doppler imaging (see **Fig. 9**A; **Fig. 10**A). MR imaging is used for indeterminate lesions with variable appearance based on subtype. Polyps are best seen during early filling on HSG; however, differentiation from other origins, such as submucosal fibroids, is limited (see **Fig. 10**B).

Adenomyosis

Adenomyosis is a benign process whereby the endometrial glands and stroma invade the myometrium, causing hyperplastic and hypertrophic changes of the myometrium. The process may be diffuse, whereby the uterus takes on an enlarged globular shape or focal area, referred to as an adenomyoma, which presents in 1 of 3 ways: as a localized version of the diffuse form; as a well-circumscribed nodule of smooth-muscle cells, endometrial glands, and stroma; or as a cyst secondary to repetitive bleeding, leading to cavitation.[17] US is the initial imaging modality of choice, demonstrating an enlarged globular uterus with loss of the junctional zone. Striated regions of or overall increase in echogenicity of the myometrium is seen secondary to endometrial extension, with additional small hypodense myometrial cysts noted (**Fig. 11**A). MR imaging demonstrates diffuse enlargement (>12 mm) of the junctional zone with poorly defined margins and small T2 bright foci, consistent with dilated endometrial glands or foci of hemorrhage projecting into the myometrium (see **Fig. 11**B).[17] In addition, MR aids in the differentiation of fibroma from focal adenoma, with adenomas demonstrating a more oval shape with an ill-defined margin, whereas fibromas are more rounded with a well-circumscribed margin (see **Fig. 11**C).[17]

Uterine synechiae

Uterine synechiae, also known as intrauterine adhesions, intrauterine webs, or intrauterine scarring, are permanent adhesions of the endometrial canal leading to partial or complete loss of the uterine cavity and/or intrauterine cervical os. The condition is thought to arise from any cause that is destructive of the endometrial lining, including previous pregnancy, infection, missed abortion, and previous curettage.[4,18] When the finding is associated with clinical symptoms of infertility,

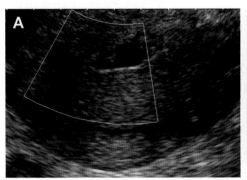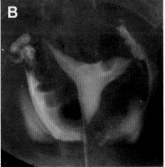

Fig. 10. Endometrial polyps. (*A*) Sonohysterographic image demonstrating a focal echogenic mass protruding into the endometrial lumen, with an intact endometrial stripe and a feeding vessel identified on Doppler imaging. (*B*) HSG shows a small filling defect within the left uterine horn.

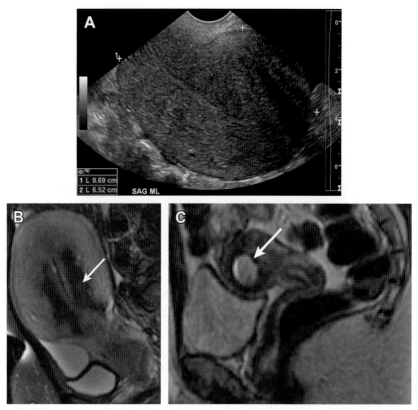

Fig. 11. Adenomyosis. (*A*) US image demonstrates diffuse uterine enlargement with heterogeneous myometrium and loss of the junctional zone without focal mass. (*B*) Sagittal T2-weighted fat-saturated MR image demonstrates an enlarged uterus with diffuse thickening of the junctional zone greater than 12 mm (*arrow*). (*C*) Sagittal T2-weighted fat-saturated MR image demonstrates a focal mass with an ill-defined hypointense rim and hyperintensity centrally (*arrow*).

menstrual abnormalities, and/or recurrent pregnancy loss, the term Asherman syndrome may be applied.[18] HSG is the imaging technique of choice for the diagnosis of this condition, demonstrating irregular, well-defined, angular, and/or straight linear filling defects within the endometrial canal (**Fig. 12**A). Depending of the extent of adhesions, the canal may not be distensible, and contrast injection may be painful. In addition, there may be partial or complete obliteration of the endometrial canal.[18] US is limited in the detection of adhesions, which if detected can show irregular

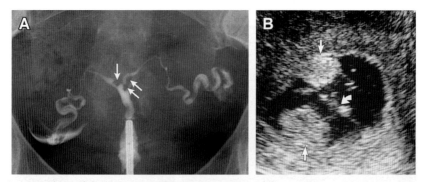

Fig. 12. Uterine synechiae. (*A*) HSG demonstrating permanent filling defects within the endometrial canal (*arrows*). (*B*) Sonohysterogram demonstrating linear filling defect within the endometrial canal, consistent with intrauterine adhesions (*curved arrow*). Additional focal echogenic masses protrude into the endometrial lumen, consistent with polyps (*thick arrows*).

thickness of the endometrium with regions of hypoechogenicity consistent with areas of fibrosis. Sonohysterography is as effective as HSG in the detection of synechiae, with the added benefit of approximating the size of the endometrial cavity (see **Fig. 12B**).

Cervical stenosis

Cervical stenosis is defined by the inability to insert a 2.5-mm or thinner dilator into the cervical canal.[19] This finding can be congenital in nature or can occur secondary to infection, DES exposure in utero, or iatrogenic trauma such as previous cone biopsy, cryotherapy, or laser vaporization of the cervix, causing scarring and fibrosis.[5,19] The consequences of cervical stenosis are directly proportional to the severity of the narrowing, with higher-grade stenoses leading to obstructive symptoms by preventing outflow of menstrual blood and restricting sperm entry into the uterus. Best seen on HSG, the cervical canal may be narrowed in length (normally measuring 0.5–3 cm with size depending on age and parity); or in the cases of near complete to complete obstruction, insertion of the HSG catheter is blocked, preventing imaging of the canal or uterus.[5,19] Additional imaging with MR or US can be performed to look for secondary signs of obstruction, including hematometra and hydrometra.[19]

Fallopian Tube Abnormalities

Tubal occlusion

Tubal occlusion is defined as the blockage of the fallopian tube, and most commonly occurs secondary to infection, with causes such as pelvic inflammatory disease, septic abortion, and/or abdominal infection. Additional causes include sequelae of trauma to the abdomen and pelvis, endometriosis, and/or inflammatory conditions such as inflammatory bowel disease.[4] HSG is the gold-standard imaging modality in the diagnosis of tubal occlusion, demonstrating an abrupt cutoff in contrast within the fallopian tube; nonopacification of the distal tube, which can occur at any point

along the length of the tube; and lack of intraperitoneal free spillage of contrast (**Fig. 13**).[20] If the obstruction is identified within the proximal/corneal portion of the fallopian tube, differentiation from spasm must be considered, with delayed imaging or administration of a spasmolytic agent such as scopolamine or glucagon to determine whether the obstruction is permanent or temporary.[2,4,20]

Hydrosalpinx

Hydrosalpinx occurs when the ampullary portion of the fallopian tube becomes blocked, causing dilatation of the proximal tube, taking on a classic sausage-shaped appearance. The condition is often bilateral and is caused by scarring and/or adhesions of the distal tube, with the major source secondary to pelvic inflammatory disease, and with additional abnormalities including adhesions from prior pelvic surgery or trauma, endometriosis, and tubal neoplasm.[21] HSG demonstrates a dilated proximal tube with absence of free intraperitoneal spillage of contrast (**Fig. 14A**). If detected on HSG, postprocedural antibiotic prophylaxis is recommended to prevent infection from stasis of contrast material within the obstructed tube. US and MR imaging show a fluid-filled tubular structure measuring greater the 3 mm arising from the lateral uterine fundus, separate from the adjacent ovary, which may fold over on itself, making a C- or S-shaped cystic mass with the appearance of incomplete septae (see **Fig. 14B, C**).[21,22] The imaging characteristics of the fluid vary depending on whether the fluid is simple, hemorrhagic, protein, or pus filled.[21,22]

Salpingitis isthmica nodosa

Salpingitis isthmica nodosa is an inflammatory process of the fallopian tube of unknown etiology, whereby small outpouchings develop on the isthmic portion, caused by nodular thickening of the hypertrophic myosalpinx enclosing cystically dilated glandular spaces lined by tubular epithelium.[23] The condition is often associated with pelvic inflammatory disease, infertility, and

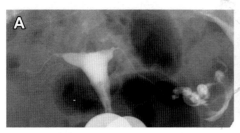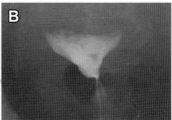

Fig. 13. Tubal occlusion. (*A*) HSG demonstrating tubal occlusion on the right and free spill of contrast on the left. (*B*) HSG demonstrating bilateral tubal occlusion, which persisted after administration of spasmolytic agent.

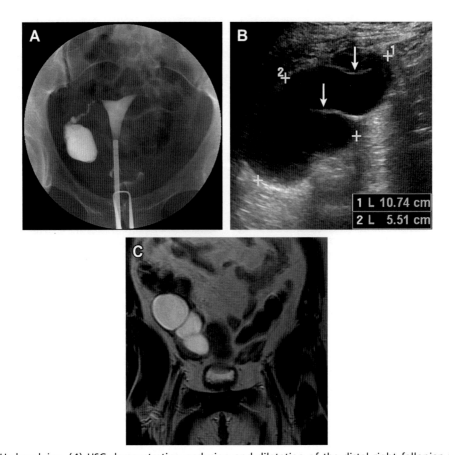

Fig. 14. Hydrosalpinx. (*A*) HSG demonstrating occlusion and dilatation of the distal right fallopian tube with absence of free intraperitoneal spillage of contrast. (*B*) US image demonstrates an enlarged hypoechoic tubular structure in the region of the right adnexa with the appearance of incomplete septa (*arrow*). (*C*) T2-weighted MR image shows an enlarged fluid signal mass in the region of the right adnexa.

occasionally ectopic pregnancy.[4,5] HSG demonstrates subcentimeter diverticula of the isthmus extending from the lumen into the wall of the fallopian tube (**Fig. 15**).[4] The condition is often bilateral, and there may be decreased free spillage of contrast depending on increasing severity of the condition. Proximal tubal occlusion may be present; if suspected, selective fallopian tube catheterization beyond the tubal occlusion may be performed to further evaluate the fallopian tube lumen.

Ovarian Abnormalities

The primary causes of ovarian factor infertility are typically diagnosed based on clinical and

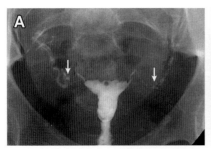
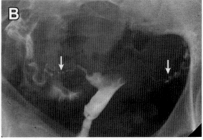

Fig. 15. Salpingitis isthmica nodosa. (*A, B*) Two HSG images demonstrating bilateral subcentimeter diverticula of the fallopian tube isthmus extending from the lumen into the wall of the fallopian tube (*arrows*).

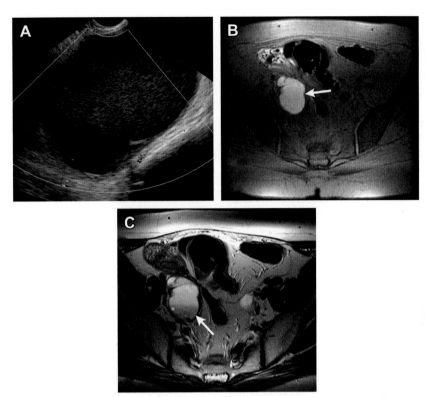

Fig. 16. Endometriosis. US image demonstrates a diffusely homogeneous cystic structure of the left adnexa with low-level internal echo and no internal flow (*A*). MR imaging demonstrates an endometrioma (*arrows*) with high signal intensity on T1-weighted image (*B*) and intermediate signal on T2-weighted image (*C*), with shading consistent with layering blood products (*asterisk*).

biochemical findings, with imaging typically not playing a significant role in diagnosis. Causes include nonfunctional ovaries, premature ovarian failure, and gonadal dysgenesis. Imaging, however, can play a significant role in detecting the secondary causes of ovarian factor infertility, including endometriosis and polycystic ovarian syndrome.

Endometriosis

Endometriosis is defined as the presence of endometrial glands and stroma outside of the uterus, primarily affecting the ovaries and peritoneal surfaces of the pelvis. The condition often presents as chronic pelvic pain and infertility, and affects approximately 10% of women of reproductive age.[24] Ovarian lesions often present as cysts with hemorrhage, called an endometrioma, and deep invasion of endometriosis on the peritoneum greater than 5 mm can cause fibrosis and muscular hyperplasia. US of an endometrioma demonstrates a thick-walled complex cyst with homogeneous low-level echoes, often referred to as a chocolate cyst, and may have small calcifications along the wall of the cyst (**Fig. 16**). Peritoneal implants are difficult to visualize with US, but can be suspected if tethering of the bowel is seen

or if the ovaries are in close approximation to the uterus.[5] MR imaging has improved detection of peritoneal implants, but sensitivity is still low (13%). If seen these lesions demonstrate an intermediate signal with high signal foci on T1-weighted images, and hypointense signal on T2-weighted images also with high signal foci. MR imaging of endometrioma demonstrate high signal intensity on T1-weighted images, and intermediate signal with shading consistent with layering blood products on T2-weighted images (see **Fig. 16**B, C).

Polycystic ovary syndrome

Polycystic ovary syndrome is a condition in which 2 of 3 conditions must be present: oligo-ovulation and/or anovulation, hyperandrogenism without other cause, and polycystic ovaries without other cause. Imaging therefore plays an important role in this diagnosis, assisting in the quantification of ovarian volume and assessment of follicle size and number. Transvaginal US is the imaging modality of choice, demonstrating ovarian volumes greater than 10 mL, more than 12 cysts measuring 2 to 9 mm in diameter per ovary, and increased echogenicity of the ovarian stroma;

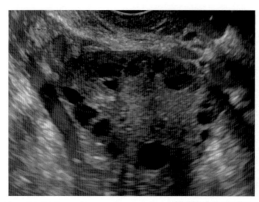

Fig. 17. Polycystic ovarian syndrome. US image demonstrates an enlarged left ovary with numerous follicles (>12), with an overall volume of 20 cm³.

however, there is great overlap of these findings with normal ovarian ranges (**Fig. 17**).[5] MR imaging demonstrates low signal in the stroma on T2-weighted images with small peripheral high-signal cysts.

SUMMARY

Female causes of infertility are both congenital and acquired, affecting the uterus, fallopian tubes, and ovaries. Imaging plays an important role in the evaluation of female infertility, with HSG, US, sonohysterography, and MR imaging each playing a complementary role in the screening, diagnosis, and/or management of the various disorders. The workup of female factor infertility often begins with HSG, evaluating the uterus and fallopian tubes for congenital and acquired abnormalities, transitioning to US or MR imaging when further characterization is needed. Normal findings on HSG can indicate ovarian or hormonally related causes of infertility, whereas failure to cannulate the cervix can indicate stenosis or obstruction of the cervical canal.

ACKNOWLEDGMENTS

Illustrations were created by Nadezhda D. Kiriyak, Medical Imager, Department of Imaging Sciences, University of Rochester, Rochester, NY. Figures were created by Margaret Kowaluk, Graphic Designer, Department of Imaging Sciences, University of Rochester, Rochester, NY.

REFERENCES

1. Fritz MA. The modern infertility evaluation. Clin Obstet Gynecol 2012;55(3):692–705.
2. Schankath AC, Fasching N, Urech-Ruh C, et al. Hysterosalpingography in the workup of female infertility: indications, technique, and diagnostic findings. Insights Imaging 2012;3:475–83.
3. Good clinical treatment in assisted reproduction-An ESHRE position paper. Eur Soc Hum Reprod Embryol 2008. Available at: http://www.eshre.eu/~/media/emagic%20files/Guidelines/GCT%20English.pdf. Accessed August 14, 2013.
4. Simpson WL, Beitia LG, Mester J. Hysterosalpingography: a reemerging study. Radiographics 2006;26: 419–31.
5. Steinkeler JA, Woodfield CA, Lazarus E, et al. Female infertility: a systematic approach to radiologic imaging and diagnosis. Radiographics 2009; 29:1353–70.
6. Behr SC, Courtier JL, Qayyum A. Imaging of müllerian duct anomalies. Radiographics 2012;32: E233–50.
7. The American Fertility Society classification of adnexal adhesions, distal tubal occlusion, tubal occlusion secondary to tubal ligation, tubal pregnancies, müllerian anomalies and intrauterine adhesions. Fertil Steril 1988;49(6):944–55.
8. Morcel K, Camborieux L, Guerrier D. Mayer-Rokitansky-Küster-Hauser (MRKH) syndrome. Orphanet J Rare Dis 2007;2:13.
9. Taylor E, Gomel V. The uterus and fertility. Fertil Steril 2008;89(1):1–16.
10. Khati NJ, Fraizer AA, Brindle KA. The unicornuate uterus and its variants. J Ultrasound Med 2012;31: 319–31.
11. Reuter KL, Daly DC, Cohen SM. Septate versus bicornuate uteri: errors in imaging diagnosis. Radiology 1989;172(3):749–52.
12. Homer HA, Ij TC, Cooke ID. The septate uterus: a review of management and reproductive outcomes. Fertil Steril 2000;73:1–14.
13. Riberio SC, Tormena RA, Peterson TV, et al. Müllerian duct anomalies: review of current management. Sao Paulo Med J 2009;127(2):92–6.
14. Choi HK, Cho KS, Lee HW, et al. MR imaging of intersexuality. Radiographics 1998;18:83–96.
15. Ciarmela P, Islam S, Reis FM, et al. Growth factors and myometrium: biologic effects in uterine fibroid and possible clinical implications. Hum Reprod Update 2011;17(6):772–90.
16. Griffin Y, Sudigali V, Jacques A. Radiology of benign disorders of menstruation. Semin Ultrasound CT MR 2010;116(3):747–58.
17. Valentini AL, Gul SS, Sogali BG, et al. Adenomyosis: from the sign to the diagnosis, Imaging, diagnostic pitfall and differential diagnosis: a pictorial review. Radiol Med 2011;116:1267–87.
18. Deans R, Abborr J. Review of Intrauterine adhesions. J Minim Invasive Gynecol 2010;17(5):555–69.
19. Valle RF, Sankpal R, Marlow JL, et al. Cervical stenosis: a challenging clinical entity. J Gynecol Surg 2002;18:129–43.

20. Eng CW, Tang PH, Ong CL. Hysterosalpingography: current applications. Singapore Med J 2007;48(4): 368–74.

21. Kim MY, Rha SE, Oh SN. MR imaging findings of hydrosalpinx: a comprehensive review. Radiographics 2009;29:495–507.

22. Patel MD, Acord DL, Young SW. Likelihood ratio of sonographic findings in discriminating hydrosalpinx from other adnexal masses. AJR Am J Roentgenol 2006;186:1033–8.

23. Chawla N, Kudesia S, Azad S, et al. Salpingitis isthmica nodosa. Indian J Pathol Microbiol 2009;52: 434–5.

24. Chamié LP, Blasbalg R, Pereira RM, et al. Findings of pelvic endometriosis at transvaginal US, MR imaging, and laparoscopy. Radiographics 2011;31:E77–100.

Obstetric (Nonfetal) Complications

Alampady K.P. Shanbhogue, MD[a],*,
Christine O. Menias, MD[b], Neeraj Lalwani, MD[c],
Chandana Lall, MD[d], Ashish Khandelwal, MD[e],
Arpit Nagar, MD[f]

KEYWORDS

- Obstetric emergency • Placental abruption • Uterine rupture • Postpartum complications • MDCT
- MR imaging

KEY POINTS

- Ultrasonography is the investigation of choice for evaluation of obstetric complications. Both the American Congress of Obstetricians and Gynecologists and American College of Radiology guidelines indicate that computed tomography should be performed only if clinical workup indicates that it is beneficial, and the radiation dose should be as low as reasonably achievable.
- Magnetic resonance imaging, especially with a combination of T1-weighted and diffusion-weighted imaging, is 100% sensitive for establishing the diagnosis of placental abruption.
- Ultrasonography has high negative predictive value but low positive predictive value for the diagnosis of retained products of conception (RPOC). A normal appearance of the endometrium excludes the diagnosis, and false-positive diagnosis of RPOC has been reported to occur in 17% to 51% cases.
- A recent meta-analysis of 14 prospective studies (12,101 patients) in pregnant women with abdominal pain or vaginal bleeding evaluated with history, physical examination, laboratory analyses, and transvaginal ultrasonography showed that transvaginal ultrasonography is the single best modality for evaluation of suspected ectopic pregnancy.
- Most adnexal torsion in pregnancy occurs before 20 weeks of gestation, and mostly in the first trimester. Mature cystic teratoma is the most common underlying disease, followed by corpus luteal cyst and other lead points such as paraovarian cysts.

INTRODUCTION

Each year more than half a million women die worldwide as a result of complications related to pregnancy or childbirth. The burden of pregnancy-related complications is increasingly being recognized both in terms of escalating health care costs and effect of hospitalization on the women and their families. In the United States alone, pregnancy-related complications in the antepartum period alone account for an average of more than 2 million hospital days of care per year, with an annual estimated cost of more than 1 billion dollars. Pathophysiology of several of these complications is directly

Conflicts of Interest: The authors have no conflicts of interest to declare.
[a] Department of Radiology, Beth Israel Medical Center, 16th Street and 1st Avenue, New York, NY 10003, USA;
[b] Mayo Clinic LL Radiology, 13400 East Shea Blvd, Scottsdale, AZ 85259, USA; [c] Department of Radiology, University of Washington, Seattle, WA 98104, USA; [d] Department of Radiology, University of California, Irvine, Orange, CA 92697, USA; [e] Department of Radiology, Brigham and Women's Hospital, Harvard Medical School, Boston, MA 02115, USA; [f] Department of Radiology, Ohio State University Medical Center, Columbus, OH, USA
* Corresponding author.
E-mail address: kshanbhogue@chpnet.org

Radiol Clin N Am 51 (2013) 983–1004
http://dx.doi.org/10.1016/j.rcl.2013.07.012

related to anatomic and physiologic changes of pregnancy. Being the primary site of these changes, the female reproductive tract is thus the system that is most frequently affected by these complications. Although select complications such as placental abruption, HELLP syndrome, molar pregnancy, and ectopic pregnancy are unique to pregnancy, others such as uterine infections, uterine rupture, hyperreactio luteinalis, ovarian torsion, and fibroid growth/degeneration are more common during pregnancy. In addition, unique pregnancy subtypes such as molar pregnancy predispose to choriocarcinoma; and ectopic pregnancy can rupture, which can be life threatening. Postpartum period complications are distinct, including hemorrhage, infection, uterine rupture, and gonadal vein thrombosis. Imaging plays a crucial role in diagnosis and management of these pregnancy-related obstetric and gynecologic complications. With the advent of interventional radiology, an armamentarium of new therapeutic options is available to treat these complications. In this article, a comprehensive update is provided on epidemiology, natural history, clinical manifestations, and imaging features of a wide spectrum of pregnancy-related obstetric and gynecologic complications, with discussion on implications on management.

IMAGING MODALITIES AND IMAGING PROTOCOL

Perhaps no issue has undergone as much recurring debate in the radiology community in the last decade as the appropriateness of imaging in pregnant patients. Increasing awareness of the risk of radiation exposure to the fetus demands an optimum imaging protocol that aims to attain maximum diagnostic benefit with minimal justifiable radiation risk. This protocol is necessary given that computed tomography (CT) is the largest source of medical radiation exposure in the United States, accounting for up to 24% of radiation exposure to the US population from all sources.[1]

Universally, it is accepted that ultrasonography should be the initial modality for evaluation of the pregnant patient, with other modalities used only in cases in which ultrasonography is nondiagnostic. Ultrasonography is fast, can be performed at the bedside, and confers no known risk to the mother or the fetus. Ultrasonography can be performed transabdominally or transvaginally, and both these approaches have advantages and disadvantages. Transvaginal ultrasonography scanning is typically performed with a tight-radius, small-footprint curvilinear probe with a frequency

range of 7.0 to 10 MHz and is performed with an empty bladder. Transvaginal scanning provides superior imaging of the uterus and adnexa and is likely better tolerated by the pregnant patient than transabdominal scanning. However, transvaginal ultrasonography is not always necessary and may not provide a panoramic view of the uterus and adnexa in advanced pregnancy. The transabdominal approach is particularly useful in this setting because it is easier to perform and provides a broader view of the uterus, adnexa, and other abdominal/pelvic viscera in the immediate vicinity.[2] Transabdominal ultrasonography is performed using a curvilinear probe in the frequency range of 2.5 to 5.0 MHz and requires a full bladder as an acoustic window to better visualize the pelvic organs. Ultrasonography is the modality of choice to confirm the presence of a living intrauterine pregnancy in the first trimester, and to evaluate for placental, uterine, and cervical diseases in the second and third trimesters. Ultrasonography is fairly accurate in depicting first-trimester complications such as ectopic pregnancy and molar pregnancy as well as select second-trimester and third-trimester complications such as placenta previa and abruptio placenta. Ultrasonography is also the best initial investigation for evaluation of postpartum complications such as postpartum hemorrhage (PPH), endometritis, and retained products of conception (RPOC).

Multidetector CT (MDCT) and magnetic resonance (MR) imaging serve as problem-solving tools in difficult cases. Both the American Congress of Obstetricians and Gynecologists and American College of Radiology (ACR) guidelines indicate that CT should be performed only if clinical workup indicates that it is beneficial, and the radiation dose should be as low as reasonably achievable.[3] The mother should be counseled on the risks of radiation exposure. Adverse events related to administration of iodinated contrast agent have not been reported, and hence it is safe to use them when necessary. Some of the recommended protocol modifications to be used in pregnant women include decreasing kVp in small patients, decreasing mAs, using automated tube current modulation, limiting the field of view, avoiding multiphasic examinations, and using lead shielding or internal barium shielding with 30% of orally administered barium.[3] CT is mostly reserved for pregnant patients presenting with abdominal trauma. Routine contrast-enhanced CT can be safely used in accurate assessment of select suspected postpartum gynecologic complications such as endometritis, pelvic abscess, septic thrombophlebitis, bladder flap hematoma, uterine rupture, and hepatic or perihepatic complications of eclampsia. MR imaging has several advantages, including multiplanar capability, superior tissue contrast resolution, and, most importantly, lack of ionizing radiation. MR imaging is therefore the next best investigation for evaluation of pregnancy-related obstetric complications with indeterminate ultrasonography findings. According to the ACR guidelines, use of intravenous gadolinium is not recommended in pregnant patients. MR imaging accurately depicts the presence and extent of more complex placental abnormalities such as placenta accreta, increta, and percreta and provides excellent anatomic delineation in cases such as uterine rupture. MR imaging can usually be performed in the supine position in the second trimester of pregnancy. However, a left lateral decubitus position might be preferred in the third trimester for improved patient comfort and reduced risk of impaired venous return. Multichannel phased array surface coils are usually used to ensure maximum signal. However, with advanced pregnancy, a body coil may be necessary. The scans are usually performed with a moderately distended bladder. This strategy allows accurate detection of conditions such as placenta percreta. Typical protocol includes multiplanar steady-state free-precession sequences (true fast imaging with steady-state precession or balanced fast field echo), multiplanar T2-weighted single-shot echo train spin-echo sequences (half-Fourier rapid acquisition with relaxation enhancement, or half-Fourier acquisition single-shot turbo spin-echo) and fat-suppressed T1-weighted gradient-echo sequence (volumetric interpolated breath-hold examination).[4] Diffusion-weighted imaging has been shown to be beneficial in identifying placental hemorrhages and improves the sensitivity and specificity of diagnosis of placental abruption.

PLACENTAL COMPLICATIONS
Abruptio Placenta

Abruptio placenta, which refers to premature separation of a normally implanted placenta, occurs in an estimated 1% of childbirths.[5] Several maternal conditions such as chronic hypertension, preeclampsia, cocaine use, smoking, and multiple gestations predispose for placental abruption.[6] History of previous abruption increases the risk, with the estimated risk of abruption increasing from 1% to 5% in patients with history of 1 previous episode of abruption to 20% to 25% with history of more than 2 previous episodes of abruption.[7] Placental abruption can also occur as a result of shearing forces in the setting of trauma,

affecting 5% to 6% of patients sustaining minor abdominal trauma and up to 40% to 50% of patients sustaining major abdominal trauma.[8,9] Placental abruption can be of 3 subtypes based on the location of the blood: retroplacental, marginal or subchorionic, and preplacental or subamniotic. Clinically, most placental abruptions present with second-trimester or third-trimester vaginal bleeding, pain, and uterine tenderness. In placental abruptions after abdominal trauma, clinical symptoms and signs usually manifest within 6 to 48 hours, with rare instances of initial clinical presentation extending for up to 5 days after trauma.[8–10]

Ultrasonography is the initial investigation of choice for patients presenting with third-trimester vaginal bleeding with clinical suspicion of placental abruption. Ultrasonographic appearance of abruption largely depends on the location and duration of hemorrhage. Presence of a hyperechoic or hypoechoic layer of tissue in the retroplacental plane, subchorionic region, or preplacental region or an abnormally thick and heterogeneous placenta (>5 cm thick) suggests the diagnosis of placental abruption in the appropriate clinical settings (**Fig. 1**). Care should be taken to distinguish retroplacental abruption from normal retroplacental complex comprising normal vascular complex of uterine vessels, myometrium, and decidua, which appear hypoechoic and usually measure less than 20 mm thick.[11] In addition, lack of mass effect and presence of vascular channels within help differentiate the normal retroplacental complex from a true hematoma.[11–14] Other entities that can mimic retroplacental hematoma are normal myometrial contractions and myometrial mass lesions, such as leiomyomas.[11–14] Myometrial contractions are transient and leiomyomas are homogenous, without evolution of echo patterns on serial imaging. Subchorionic hematoma is more readily seen on ultrasonography and appears as an intraplacental region of variable echogenicity that is marginal in location and elevates the amniochorionic membrane. The elevated amniochorionic membrane may appear as a free-floating intrauterine membrane, a finding classically described in subchorionic abruption. Associated intra-amniotic hemorrhage or hematoma can also be seen. However, acute hemorrhage can have similar echotexture to that of the placenta, and subacute hemorrhage can seep retroplacentally in to the cervix without forming a sonographically detectable retroplacental clot, resulting in an overall poor accuracy of ultrasonography in detecting placental abruption.[11,15] A recent study[16] showed that ultrasonography can miss the diagnosis of placental abruption in up to 50% cases. Several

A   **B**

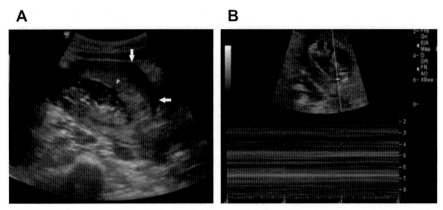

Fig. 1. Placental abruption with fetal demise. Grayscale sonographic image (*A*) shows a hypoechoic layer (*arrows*) behind the placenta (P) consistent with retroplacental hematoma. M-mode ultrasonography shows (*B*) no fetal cardiac activity consistent with fetal demise.

other studies have shown that the sensitivity of ultrasonography can be as low as 24% for detection of placental abruption.[17,18] However, ultrasonography is highly specific for this diagnosis, with specificity and positive predictive value of up to 96% and 88%, respectively.[17] Ultrasonography can also assess for fetal viability and detect other causes of third-trimester vaginal bleeding, such as placenta previa. In patients with a high index of suspicion for abruption and a negative ultrasonographic evaluation, MR imaging is the imaging modality of choice for further evaluation if necessary. MR imaging, especially with a combination of T1-weighted and diffusion-weighted imaging, is shown to be 100% sensitive for establishing the diagnosis.[16] Blood breakdown products create susceptibility artifacts on diffusion-weighted imaging and cause signal alterations that can be detected on T1-weighted images. Presence of intra-amniotic hemorrhage can also be readily detected on T1-weighted imaging (**Fig. 2**). Diagnosis of placental abruption on CT is often

challenging, given the normal heterogeneous enhancement of the placenta on CT. It is thus important to carefully analyze placenta in every pregnant patient who has sustained abdominal trauma for evidence of abruption. Typically, placental abruptions manifest as retroplacental or full-thickness areas of hypoenhancement, which form acute angles with myometrium (**Fig. 3**).[19]

Management of placental abruption depends on the clinical presentation, the gestational age, and the presence or absence of maternal and fetal compromise. Prompt diagnosis and treatment of severe placental abruption are essential given the significant increased adverse maternal and fetal outcomes, with perinatal mortality of up to 25%.[5,20] Fetal mortality has been reported to be even higher at 75% with placental abruption after maternal abdominal trauma.[21] Conservative management with serial ultrasonographic imaging/surveillance can be adopted in partial placental abruption without maternal or fetal compromise or distress.[20]

A   **B**

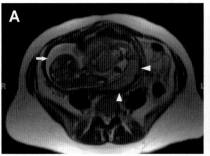 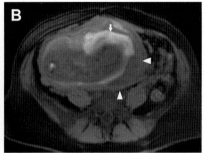

Fig. 2. Placental abruption. Axial T2-weighted (*A*) and T1-weighted (*B*) MR images show linear low T2-weighted signal intensity signal in the retroplacental region, with corresponding mild increased T1 signal (*arrowheads*) consistent with retroplacental hemorrhage. Also seen is the high T1-weighted signal intensity within the uterine cavity consistent with intra-amniotic hemorrhage (*arrows*).

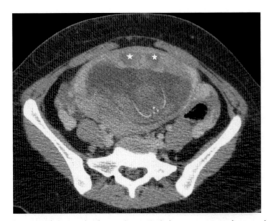

Fig. 3. Placental abruption. Axial contrast-enhanced CT image shows focal hypodense areas in the retroplacental region (*asterisk*) in a pregnant patient presenting with blunt abdominal trauma consistent with placental abruption.

Placental Implantation Abnormalities

Placenta previa

Placenta previa refers to placental implantation in the lower uterine segment and can be of complete/central, partial, or marginal subtypes.[22] The reported incidence of placenta previa in the United States is variable, and it is estimated to occur in 0.3% to 1% of deliveries.[23] Placenta previa is more frequently seen with multiparity, multiple gestations, advanced maternal age (>40 years), large placenta, previous cesarean delivery (1.5-fold–5-fold risk), previous abortions, and previous placenta previa.[24] Incidence of placenta previa increases from 1% after 1 cesarean delivery to 3.7% after 5 cesarean deliveries.[25] It is thought to occur because of implantation of fertilized ovum in to the lower uterine segment. Appropriate monitoring and management of patients with placenta previa are necessary, given the increased incidence of complications such as placental abruption, hemorrhage, fetal malpresentation, fetal malformations, fetal growth restriction, preterm births, cervical outlet obstruction, and need for cesarean delivery or hysterectomy.[26,27] Abnormal cord insertion, circumvallate placenta, and placenta accreta (occurs in 3%–5% of patients with placenta previa) also frequently coexist with placenta previa. Overall, placenta previa can increase perinatal mortality by up to 3 to 4 times compared with that of normal pregnancy.[27]

Clinically, painless bright red vaginal bleeding in the second or third trimester is the hallmark clinical presentation of placenta previa (seen in 70% cases). Patients can also present with heavy PPH. On imaging, the diagnosis is established by showing placenta partially or completely covering the internal os on transvaginal ultrasonography (**Fig. 4**). Transvaginal ultrasonography is safe for evaluation of placenta previa without increased risk of bleeding, because the angle between the probe and the cervix prevents the probe from entering the cervix and injuring the placenta itself.[28] The sensitivity of transvaginal ultrasonography is up to 100% and the specificity is up to 98.8% for the diagnosis of placenta previa. Accurate assessment of posterior placenta previa on transabdominal ultrasonography may require manual elevation of the fetal head (to eliminate acoustic shadowing from the fetal calvarium) or assessment of the relationship between the posterior fetal calvarium and the maternal sacrum. Postvoid scans with an empty urinary bladder are necessary to accurately diagnose placenta previa, because an overly distended bladder can push an anterior low-lying placenta posteriorly, giving it a false impression of complete placenta previa. Also, it is important to consider the gestational age at the time of diagnosis because most (>90%) placenta previas diagnosed at 20 weeks of gestation resolve by term. MR imaging can serve as a problem-solving tool, because it

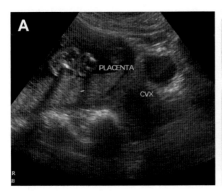
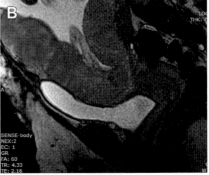

Fig. 4. Placenta previa in 2 different patients. Grayscale sonographic image (*A*) and sagittal T2-weighted MR images (*B*) show placenta completely covering the internal os, consistent with placenta previa.

accurately depicts the abnormality, including a posterior placenta previa, and depicts coexistent abnormalities, including placenta accreta, percreta, or placental abruption. Management of placenta previa involves careful maternal and fetal monitoring until term or fetal maturity, and an elective cesarean delivery. Vaginal delivery is advocated in placenta previa only if the os-placental distance is more than 2 cm at 35 weeks of gestation.

Placenta accreta, increta, and percreta

Placenta accreta, increta, and percreta belong to a spectrum of placental implantation abnormalities that result from failure of normal process of decidual formation and placental implantation, affecting a portion of, or the entire, placenta. The placental villi may adhere directly to (accreta, 78%), invade into (increta, 17%), or through (percreta, 5%) the myometrium.[29] Estimated incidence of placental implantation abnormalities ranges widely from 1 in 1667 pregnancies to 1 in 70,000 pregnancies, with a recent reported incidence of 1 in 2500 deliveries.[30,31] Risk factors for placenta increta, accreta, and percreta include abnormal sites of placental implantation (such as placenta previa) and previous cesarean delivery, which together account for approximately 50% of incidence of placenta accreta.[32] The incidence increases from 5% in patients without previous uterine surgery to 15% to 70% in patients with history of previous uterine surgery.[31,33,34] Other risk factors include number of pregnancies (risk increases from 1 in 500,000 for <3 previous pregnancies to 1 in 2500 for >6 pregnancies) and advanced maternal age.

Placenta accreta is suspected sonographically when the placental parenchyma shows placental lacunae, which are vascular structures of varying size and shape, creating a Swiss-cheese appearance.[35] Presence of turbulent Doppler flow within the lacunae and disruption of the normal continuous retroplacental color flow also indicate placenta accreta. Other sonographic findings such as loss of retroplacental clear space, myometrial thinning, and lack of visualization of myometrium are of questionable importance in the diagnosis of placenta accreta. Ultrasonographic findings of numerous vascular channels surrounding the uterine myometrium, irregular bladder, or rectal wall, with extensive vascularity, favor placenta percreta.[35] Reported sensitivity and specificity of ultrasonography for the diagnosis of placental implantation abnormalities (placenta accreta and percreta) range widely from sensitivities of 50% to 100% and specificities of 50% to 98%.[31,36] MR imaging serves as a problem-solving tool and is fairly sensitive (80%–85%) and specific (65%–100%) for establishing the diagnosis.[31,36] MR imaging findings of placenta accreta include abnormal uterine bulge, heterogeneous T2-weighted signal, and randomly oriented T2 dark intraplacental bands (**Fig. 5**).[35] Placenta percreta can be more readily detected because the placenta bulges out of the normal myometrial contour with focal myometrial interruption and with or without invasion of the urinary bladder, rectum, or small intestine (**Fig. 6**). Presence of placenta previa is more readily detectable on ultrasonography and MR imaging and should raise the suspicion for an underlying placenta accreta or percreta.

Complications of placenta accreta and percreta include massive hemorrhage, which may necessitate cesarean hysterectomy, and damage to pelvic organs such as bladder, ureter, or rectum because of direct placental invasion. Timely prenatal diagnosis is hence necessary for planning the delivery, including ensuring the surgical expertise, availability of blood products, prepartum and postpartum uterine artery embolization (UAE), and intensive postpartum care.[36]

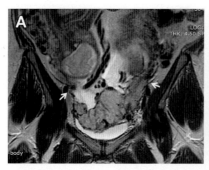 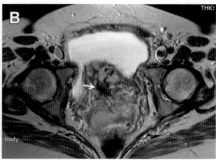

Fig. 5. Placenta previa with placenta increta. Coronal (*A*) and axial (*B*) T2-weighted MR images show loss of normal pear shape of the uterus (*arrows*) with randomly distributed dark intraplacental bands anteroinferiorly, raising the suspicion for placenta increta. Surgical pathology confirmed the diagnosis.

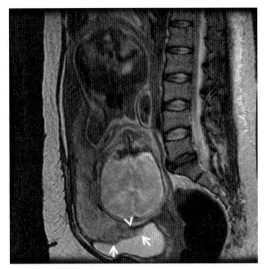

Fig. 6. Placenta previa with placenta percreta. Coronal T2-weighted MR images show invasion of placenta beyond the contour of the myometrium into the urinary bladder (*arrows*) consistent with placenta percreta. There is loss of normal T2 hypointense signal of the dome of the urinary bladder at the site of placental invasion (*arrowhead*).

Placental Neoplasms

Gestational trophoblastic disease

Placental neoplasms can be classified as gestational trophoblastic disease or nontrophoblastic neoplasms. Gestational trophoblastic disease (GTD) is a spectrum of tumors with varied biological behavior, natural history, prognosis, and imaging appearances. Please refer to the article on GTD elsewhere in this issue by Shanbhogue and colleagues for further details.

Nontrophoblastic neoplasms

Nontrophoblastic neoplasms are rare and include placental chorioangioma, teratoma, yolk sac tumor, hepatocellular adenoma, leiomyoma, lymphoma, and metastases. Placental chorioangiomas have been assigned a plethora of names, including placental hemangioma and placental hamartoma, and are rare, with an estimated incidence of 0.6% to 1% in retrospective analysis of placental specimens.[37] These chorioangiomas are usually solitary and can occur on the maternal or fetal surface. Large externally visible hemangiomas appear as well-encapsulated tumors with glistening surface and show histologic features similar to hemangiomas elsewhere in the body, with numerous blood vessels in a moderately abundant perivascular stroma.[38] Histogenesis of placental hemangiomas is unclear and these are variably classified as true neoplasms, hamartomas, or hyperplasias. Although most pathologists believe

this hemangioma to be a true neoplasm or hamartoma, increased incidence of placental hemangioma in high-altitude pregnancies points toward underlying vascular proliferation as a possible cause. Malignant histologic types (placental chorangiocarcinoma) have also been rarely described.[39] Clinically, placental hemangiomas are usually asymptomatic. Association with preeclampsia, fetal growth restriction (likely because of increased fetal circulation), polyhydramnios, and premature delivery have been described, which are likely to occur in large tumors (>5 cm).[40] A few patients have associated placentomegaly resulting from vascular stasis. On ultrasonography, chorioangioma manifests as a well-defined complex echogenic mass that protrudes into the amniotic cavity, with increased flow on color Doppler interrogation (**Fig. 7**).[41] On MR imaging, placental chorioangiomas manifest as T2 hyperintense, hypervascular lesions that protrude from the fetal surface of the placenta.[42] However, signal intensity on T1-weighted and T2-weighted imaging may vary depending on the degree of hemorrhage.[43] Differential diagnosis of placental chorioangioma includes blood clot, uterine leiomyoma, and other tumors of the placenta such as teratomas. Blood clots do not show flow on Doppler imaging, and leiomyomas are seen along the maternal surface of the placenta. Placental teratomas are rare, almost always incidentally discovered, mature teratomas with nonspecific imaging appearance (**Fig. 8**).

UTERINE COMPLICATIONS
Rupture

Uterine rupture accounts for up to 20% of maternal deaths from hemorrhage in the

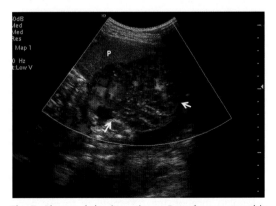

Fig. 7. Placental chorioangioma. Doppler sonographic images show a heterogeneously hypoechoic mass protruding from the surface of the placenta into the amniotic cavity with increased vascular flow (*arrows*). Surgical pathology confirmed the diagnosis of placental chorioangioma. P, placenta.

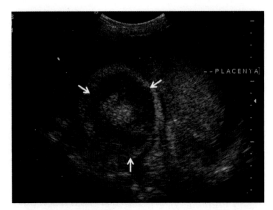

Fig. 8. Placental teratoma. Grayscale sonographic images show a heterogeneously hypoechoic mass protruding from the surface of the placenta with an echogenic rim (*arrows*). Surgical pathology confirmed the diagnosis of placental teratoma.

antepartum and postpartum period.[44] Most uterine ruptures (≥90%) are associated with a previous cesarean delivery; incidence of uterine rupture with low transverse incision is approximately 0.2% to 1.5% and with the classic incision is 4% to 9%.[45–47] Other risk factors for uterine rupture include previous uterine surgeries such as myomectomy and septoplasty, multiple gestation, grand multiparity, polyhydramnios, manual removal of placenta, and other invasive procedures such as dilatation and curettage performed for premature termination of pregnancy or retained placenta in the postpartum period.

Clinically, patients with uterine rupture present with abrupt fetal distress, bleeding, pelvic pain, and circulatory collapse. Manual examination may reveal evidence of rupture in some but not all patients. Imaging plays a major role in establishing the diagnosis. On ultrasonography, uterine rupture frequently manifests as intraperitoneal or extraperitoneal hematoma in relation to the uterus with evidence of uterine dehiscence in some cases.[48] Other sonographic features include fetal parts in an extrauterine location, intra-amniotic hemorrhage, and focal bulging of membranes through the site of dehiscence.[49] Presence of an empty uterus with free intraperitoneal fluid, and free-floating fetus and placenta within the maternal abdomen, is an uncommon but most specific finding of uterine rupture. MDCT findings may vary from a focal hypoenhancing area extending through the myometrium to complete myometrial disruption with massive hemoperitoneum (Fig. 9A–C). MR imaging acts as a problem-solving tool, showing the presence and extent of rupture in indolent cases with atypical presentation (see Fig. 9D). In contrast to uterine

rupture, scar dehiscence refers to separation of an old myometrial scar without penetrating the uterine serosa or resulting in complications. MR imaging can also delineate the presence and extent of scar dehiscence (see Fig. 9E).[50,51] Management of uterine rupture involves immediate operative delivery, repair of the rupture, or removal of the uterus. Up to 50% of uterine ruptures from dehiscent scars may be missed during the pregnancy, resulting in increased fetal mortality (of up to 22%) and increased postpartum complications, such as bladder flap hematoma.[49,52] Fetal demise can occur in 50% to 70% of fundal incision ruptures and 10% to 15% of lower uterine segment incision ruptures. Once repaired, there is up to 20% recurrence risk in subsequent pregnancy.

Bladder flap hematoma refers to postpartum hematomas that occur beneath the surgically incised and reapproximated peritoneal fold adjacent to the lower uterine segment cesarean delivery incision. On ultrasonography and CT, bladder flap hematomas manifest as heterogeneous lesions of varying echogenicity/density and size extending between the urinary bladder and the lower segment of the uterus (vesicouterine space) (Fig. 10). Surgical transvaginal evacuation, laparotomy, and evacuation and laparoscopic drainage are some of the treatment options, depending on the size of the hematoma and preference and expertise of the surgeon.[53] Percutaneous ultrasonography and CT-guided drainage can be attempted in large infected hematomas.[53]

Acute Fibroid Degeneration

Uterine fibroids are common, affecting 20% to 30% of women in the reproductive age group. Reported prevalence of fibroids in pregnancy ranges from 0.3% to 2.6%.[49] Uterine fibroids can be symptomatic in pregnancy because of rapid growth, torsion, or acute red degeneration. Red degeneration is a hemorrhagic infarction caused by either venous thrombosis or rupture of intratumoral arteries and commonly occurs in the second half of pregnancy or in the puerperium. Growth of fibroids during the pregnancy is believed to be a major contributing factor that predisposes to red degeneration. Overall, less than one-third of the fibroids show significant growth (>10% volume change) during pregnancy.[54] An estimated 10% of pregnant women with fibroids need hospitalization for fibroid-related complications. Clinically, most patients present with acute-onset pain, tenderness on palpation, low-grade fever, and leukocytosis.

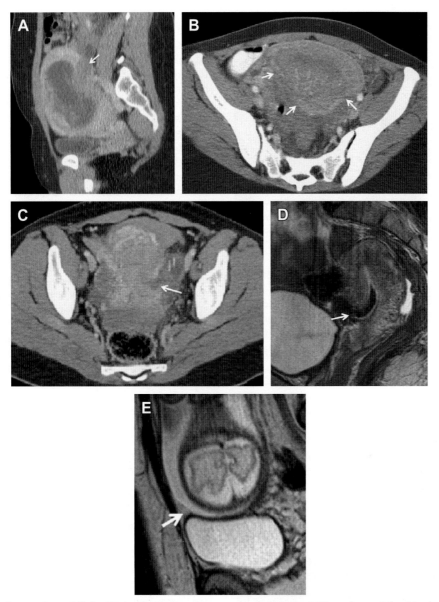

Fig. 9. Uterine rupture. (*A*) Sagittal reformation from contrast-enhanced CT performed for blunt abdominal trauma shows focal hypodensity along the posterior myometrial wall consistent with rupture (*arrow*). (*B*) Axial contrast-enhanced CT shows hemoperitoneum with a defect in the posterior myometrium (*arrows*). (*C*) Axial contrast-enhanced CT image post abortion demonstrates a focal defect along the left posterolateral wall of lower uterine segment (*arrow*) with hemoperitoneum. (*D*) Sagittal T2-weighted MR image in a patient with history of previous cesarean delivery, presenting with acute pelvic pain and vaginal bleeding, shows a large defect in the lower anterior uterine segment consistent with uterine rupture (*arrow*). (*E*) Sagittal T2-weighted MR image shows marked myometrial thinning in the lower uterine segment in a patient with previous cesarean delivery suggestive of scar dehiscence (*arrow*).

On imaging, point tenderness with the ultrasonographic probe in the region of the fibroid can be helpful in supporting the diagnosis. This entity needs to be differentiated from other potential causes of acute abdomen in the second half of pregnancy, including abruptio placenta, acute hydramnios, and ovarian torsion. In difficult cases MR imaging serves as a problem-solving tool because it shows diffuse or peripheral high signal intensity at T1-weighted images with variable signal intensity at T2-weighted images depending on the degree of intralesional hemorrhage (**Figs. 11** and **12**). Diffuse high T2 signal caused by edema may precede acute degeneration.

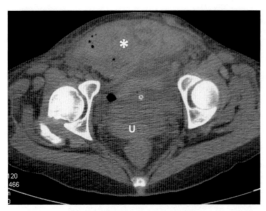

Fig. 10. Bladder flap hematoma and large hematoma in the prevesical space (*asterisk*) in the patient with history of recent cesarean delivery. U, uterus.

Management of red degeneration is conservative and involves bed rest, sedation, analgesia, and in some cases, antibiotics to prevent secondary infection. The pain usually resolves over 7 to 10 days. Severe cases of red degeneration of fibroid can result in second-trimester abortion.

RPOC

RPOC represent failure of the uterus to evacuate part of the placenta or the entire placenta after delivery. It may complicate a terminated pregnancy or a normal vaginal or cesarean delivery. Factors that predispose for RPOC include adhesions, uterine atony, uterine scarring, succenturate lobe, and placenta accreta. Clinically, the presentation is variable, most common being prolonged PPH or endometritis. Imaging appearance of RPOC depends on the type and extent of retained tissue

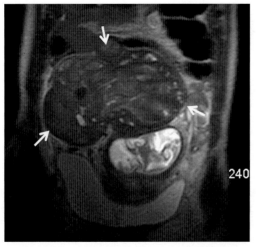

Fig. 11. Degenerating uterine fibroid. Coronal T2-weighted MR image shows a large uterine fibroid with multiple foci of high T2 signal intensity (*arrows*).

and degree of necrosis. Ultrasonographic appearances of RPOC include heterogeneous echotexture soft tissue mass within the uterine cavity, complex endometrial fluid, or thickened endometrium (**Fig. 13**).[55,56] Color Doppler interrogation may aid in the diagnosis by showing perfusion, 75% of patients with RPOC had color Doppler flow in the endometrium compared with 40% of normal patients.[54] Normal postpartum endometrial thickness varies from 0.4 to 1.3 cm.[57] It may be indistinguishable from GTD on imaging alone. However, correlation with serum β-human chorionic gonadotropin (β-HCG) level is useful for differentiation. Sensitivity of ultrasonography for diagnosis of RPOC varies from 44% to 93.8%, with the specificity ranging from 73.9% to 92%.[55,58,59] Durfee and colleagues[55] in their study on the role of pelvic ultrasonography in 163 cases of RPOC conclude that presence of an endometrial mass was the most sensitive (79%) and specific (89%) sonographic feature of RPOC. These investigators reported that isolated findings of either complex fluid in the endometrial canal or a thick endometrium measuring greater than 10 mm had low sensitivity, specificity, and negative and positive predictive value for this diagnosis. The investigators also concluded that absence of Doppler flow does not exclude the diagnosis of RPOC. Ultrasonography has high negative predictive value, and a normal appearance of the endometrium (either a thin endometrial lining <10 mm or simple endometrial fluid) excludes the diagnosis of RPOC.[55] Reported false-positive diagnosis of RPOC on ultrasonography varies from 17% to 51%,[59–61] with blood clots being most commonly mistaken for RPOC. Saline infusion sonography can be used to differentiate RPOC from blood clots because the former remain adherent to the endometrial lining, whereas the latter float once the saline is infused. MR imaging may help in indeterminate cases by showing heterogeneously enhancing endometrial mass or soft tissue lesion (see **Fig. 13**). MR imaging can also depict coexistent or predisposing underlying disease such as placenta percreta. Management of RPOC involves curettage of the uterine cavity.

Endometritis/Wound Infection

Postpartum endometritis refers to the infection of endometrium or decidua (RPOC) with or without extension in to the myometrium and parametrial tissues. It is polymicrobial in nearly three-quarters of cases and arises from ascending infection from vaginal flora. Incidence of postpartum infection has significantly decreased with the routine use of antibiotic prophylaxis in the

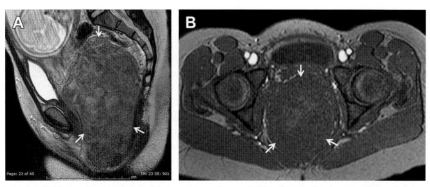

Fig. 12. Red degeneration of a primary pelvic retroperitoneal fibroid. Sagittal T2-weighted (*A*) and axial T1-weighted (*B*) MR images shows a large fibroid with few foci of high T1 signal intensity within a rapidly growing pelvic retroperitoneal fibroid (*arrows*).

peripartum period. An estimated 10% to 20% of patients on antibiotic prophylaxis and 50% to 90% of patients without antibiotic prophylaxis develop postpartum infection.[62] Estimated incidence of endometritis after vaginal delivery is as low as 1% to 3% and the incidence after cesarean delivery is approximately 20%.[63] Common risk factors for development of pelvic infections in the postpartum phase include cesarean delivery (10-fold–20-fold increase), invasive procedure

during labor, premature rupture of membranes, prolonged labor, retained placenta, extremes of age, and low socioeconomic status. Postpartum endometritis is classified as early (occurring within 48 hours) or late (3 days–6 weeks after delivery). If untreated, endometritis may progress to myometritis, pelvic abscess, or septic thrombophlebitis.

Clinically, presence of fever, lower abdominal pain, foul-smelling vaginal discharge, vaginal bleeding, tachycardia, and leukocytosis are some of

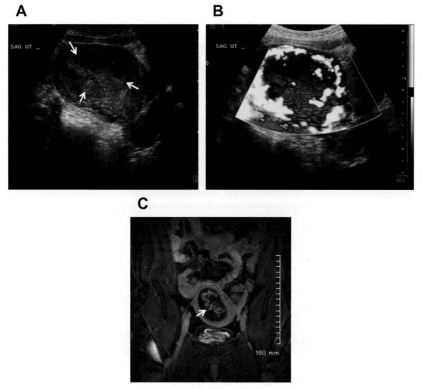

Fig. 13. RPOC. Grayscale (*A*) and color Doppler (*B*) ultrasonography images of the uterus shows a heterogeneously echogenic endometrial mass with increased vascular flow (*arrow* in *A*). (*C*) Coronal gadolinium-enhanced MR image shows heterogeneously enhancing endometrial contents (*arrow*) consistent with RPOC.

the symptoms/signs that indicate presence of endometritis. Most cases present within the first week after delivery. Ultrasonography is the initial investigation of choice when endometritis is suspected. A diffusely heterogeneous appearance of endometrium with or without evidence of gas on ultrasonography in a postpartum patient presenting with fever and other signs of infection indicates endometritis (Fig. 14). MDCT and MR imaging show fluid and air within the endometrial cavity, thick abnormally enhancing and heterogeneous endometrium, parametrial stranding, myometrial, parametrial, or broad ligament abscesses, and coexistent septic pelvic or ovarian thrombophlebitis (see Fig. 14).[64] Evidence of infection at the incision site within the uterus or anterior abdominal wall is also readily shown on MDCT and MR imaging. Management of endometritis involves use of broad-spectrum antibiotics, dilatation and curettage for RPOC, and an aggressive surgical approach for large myometrial or parametrial abscess.

PPH

PPH is defined as excessive vaginal bleeding within 24 hours (primary PPH) or 24 hours to 6 weeks (secondary PPH) after delivery.[65] Defined as blood loss exceeding 500 mL after vaginal delivery and 1000 mL after cesarean delivery, this is an uncommon but potentially lethal obstetric emergency, which accounts for up to 35% of maternal deaths in the puerperium.[65,66] Causes of PPH include uterine atony (most common cause of primary PPH), RPOC (most common cause of secondary PPH), uterocervical injury, subinvolution of the placenta, placenta accreta, endometritis, pseudoaneurysms or arteriovenous malformations (AVMs) of the uterine artery, and rarely, choriocarcinoma.[65,67,68] Ultrasonography is the imaging investigation of choice for initial evaluation of PPH. Presence of RPOC or evidence of endometritis can be detected on ultrasonography with reasonable accuracy (see earlier discussion). Uterine vascular malformations can also be instantly recognized on ultrasonography by evidence of myometrial vascular lakes, which show low resistance, high diastolic flow, and color aliasing (Fig. 15). A normal postpartum imaging appearance without evidence of RPOC favors the diagnosis of uterine atony or uterine subinvolution. The normal postpartum uterus measures about 7 to 10 cm anteroposteriorly, 14.5 to 25 cm long, and 7 to 14 cm wide.[69] MDCT and MR imaging can be performed in doubtful cases to evaluate for occult disease such as uterine injury or infection as well as to evaluate for vascular causes such as pseudoaneurysms and AVMs (Fig. 16). Pelvic

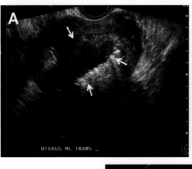
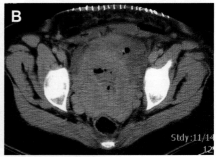
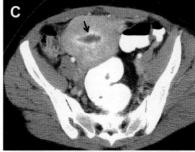

Fig. 14. Postpartum endometritis in 3 different patients. (A) Grayscale ultrasonographic image shows diffusely heterogeneous endometrium with foci of gas (arrows) in a patient with postpartum fever and vaginal bleeding. (B) Axial contrast-enhanced CT image of the uterus shows a heterogeneous enhancement of the endometrial canal with foci of gas. (C) Axial contrast-enhanced CT image shows abnormal enhancement of the endometrium (black arrow) in a patient with postpartum fever.

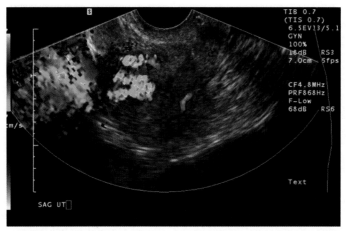

Fig. 15. PPH caused by postcesarean delivery uterine AVM. Color Doppler image shows serpiginous vascular structures, which show increased Doppler flow in the right lateral myometrium.

angiography is reserved for cases with indeterminate cause on noninvasive imaging techniques and is able to simultaneously diagnose and treat vascular complications such as AVM and pseudoaneurysm (**Fig. 17**). Accurate antenatal imaging diagnosis of predisposing factors such as placenta previa and placenta accreta is necessary to avoid potentially life-threatening PPH.

Interventional radiology plays a significant role in treatment of PPH. UAE can be used as a definite treatment option for entities such as vascular malformations (uterine, cervical, or vaginal aneurysms and AVMs), uterine atony, and placenta accreta. It is the preferred first-line treatment strategy in hemodynamically stable patients with refractory PPH and can be used as a second-line treatment in hemodynamically unstable patients with failed surgical management or contraindication for surgery.[70] UAE has been found to be effective in stopping hemorrhage in up to 95% of cases.[65]

OVARIAN COMPLICATIONS
Ovarian/Adnexal Torsion

Pregnancy increases the risk of adnexal torsion caused by laxity of ligamentous structures and enlargement of ovary related to luteal cyst. Reported incidence of adnexal masses in pregnancy varies widely, from 1 in 81 to 1 in 8000 pregnancies.[71] Reported incidence of torsion also varies widely, from 5.4% to 13.8% of all adnexal masses in pregnancy.[71–75] Most adnexal torsion in pregnancy occurs before 20 weeks of gestation, and mostly in the first trimester.[76] A recent study[76] reported that up to 60% of adnexal torsion occurred between the 10th and 17th weeks of gestation, with the highest risk at 15 to 16 weeks. Mature cystic teratoma is the most common underlying cause of torsion, followed by corpus luteum cysts; paraovarian cysts account for only a small percentage of adnexal torsions in pregnancy. Adnexal torsion in pregnancy commonly occurs in tumors

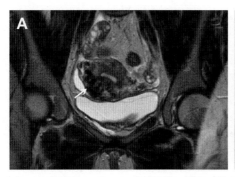
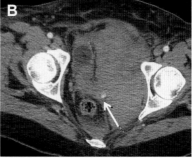

Fig. 16. Usefulness of MR imaging and MDCT in PPH. (*A*) Uterine AVM. Coronal T2-weighted MR image shows serpiginous vascular structures as low signal intensity regions/signal void on T2-weighted images (*arrow*). (*B*) Vaginal artery pseudoaneurysm. Axial contrast-enhanced CT image shows a large left hemipelvic extraperitoneal hematoma with a focus of arterial enhancement (*arrow*) consistent with pseudoaneurysm.

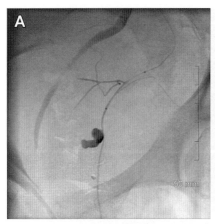
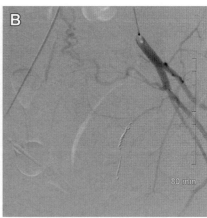

Fig. 17. Digital subtraction angiographic image before (*A*) and after (*B*) embolization shows a vaginal artery pseudoaneurysm, which was successfully embolized.

between 5 and 10 cm in diameter, with most torsion occurring in tumors measuring 6 to 8 cm in diameter (odds ratio 2.8).[76] Clinically, patients present with acute-onset abdominal or pelvic pain. On imaging, ultrasonography may show an enlarged morphologically abnormal ovary with lack of flow, abnormal position of the ovary, twisted pedicle sign, and presence of free fluid. Adnexal torsion can be intermittent. Hence, evidence of normal flow on Doppler sonography has low negative predictive value to rule out torsion. However, the diagnosis of torsion is favored if the flow is absent or markedly reduced on the symptomatic side. Findings that favor adnexal torsion on MR imaging include enlargement of the ovary, hemorrhage, twisted vascular pedicle, periovarian fat stranding, and free fluid (**Fig. 18**). Management of ovarian torsion includes emergent detorsion, preferably with a laparoscopic approach, which often involves surgical removal of the tumor itself.

Hyperreactio Luteinalis

Hyperreactio luteinalis (synonym: theca lutein cysts) refers to multilocular cystic ovarian mass commonly seen in patients with high HCG stimulation, such as in molar pregnancy, choriocarcinoma, or multiple gestations.[77] Occasionally, this entity can also be seen with patients without high HCG levels.[78] Clinically, most are asymptomatic; when symptomatic, these manifest in the third trimester of pregnancy with abdominal distension or acute pain resulting from bleeding, rupture, or torsion. Up to 30% patients with hyperreactio luteinalis may present with maternal virilization. Patients with polycystic ovarian syndrome are at higher risk for this complication, which is believed to be caused by increased sensitivity of the ovarian

stroma to the circulating β-HCG levels.[79] On imaging, this complication typically manifests as bilateral moderate to massive enlargement of the ovaries (≤35 cm) with multiple simple or hemorrhagic follicular cysts (**Fig. 19**). Occasionally, cysts are unilateral and may mimic ovarian malignancy.[79] MR imaging can be used in doubtful cases to assess for presence of peritoneal metastases, which, if present, favor a diagnosis of ovarian malignancy.[78] Most of the lesions are managed conservatively.[80] Surgery is reserved for patients presenting with ovarian torsion, rupture, or hemorrhage. Spontaneous regression of cysts usually occurs after delivery; however, persistence of the

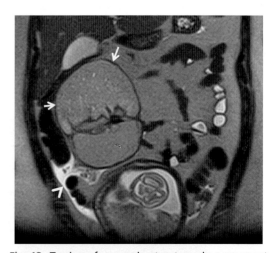

Fig. 18. Torsion of an ovarian teratoma in a pregnant patient presenting with acute right lower quadrant pain. A predominantly solid fat-containing mass is seen in the right midabdomen (*arrows*) with surrounding fluid (*arrowhead*). Surgical pathology confirmed the diagnosis of torsion of an ovarian teratoma.

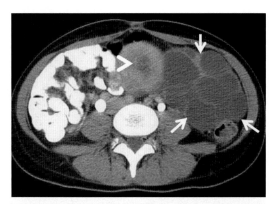

Fig. 19. Multicystic left ovarian mass (*arrows*) consistent with hyperreactio luteinalis in a patient with choriocarcinoma (*arrowhead*).

cyst after a long period of β-HCG regression has been reported.[80]

Ovarian Vein Thrombophlebitis

Ovarian vein thrombosis is most commonly seen as a postpartum complication. Ovarian vein thrombophlebitis may complicate a bland thrombus, especially in patients with endometritis. Ovarian vein thrombosis is estimated to occur in 1 in 600 term pregnancies and predominantly is right sided (≤90% of cases).[64] Compression and stasis of flow in ovarian veins caused by enlarging uterus, uterine infection, and peripartum hypercoagulability are believed to account for an increased incidence of ovarian vein thrombosis/thrombophlebitis in the postpartum period. Clinically, presence of fever, increased white blood cell count, and acute flank pain in the immediate postpartum period with absence of an obvious source of

infection should alert the radiologist to vigilantly evaluate ovarian veins for the presence of thrombosis/thrombophlebitis. A timely diagnosis is essential to institute anticoagulant therapy and prevent extension of the clot into the inferior vena cava (IVC) and subsequent pulmonary thromboembolism. Ultrasonography may show thrombus within the abdominal portion of the ovarian vein.[49] On contrast-enhanced CT or MR imaging, filling defects can be readily identified within the ovarian veins, with or without extension in to the IVC (**Fig. 20**). Presence of enhancement of the wall of the ovarian vein with central low attenuating thrombus and perivenous stranding favors thrombophlebitis.[64] Treatment primarily involves antibiotic and anticoagulant therapy.

Ectopic Pregnancy

Ectopic pregnancy refers to pregnancy outside the endometrial cavity. Ectopic pregnancy has been estimated to account for 1.3% to 2% of all reported pregnancies in the United States, affecting more than 100,000 women each year.[81,82] There has been a nearly 6-fold increase in the incidence of ectopic pregnancy since the 1970s, primarily because of delayed childbearing, increasing incidence of sexually transmitted infections, and increasing use of contraceptive procedures.[83] Women with tubal damage related to pelvic inflammatory disease or surgery, intrauterine contraceptive devices, endometriosis, or history of previous ectopic pregnancies are at the highest increased risk for development of ectopic pregnancy.[81] Early and accurate diagnosis of ectopic pregnancy is essential to reduce maternal morbidity and mortality. Clinically, the classic triad of amenorrhea,

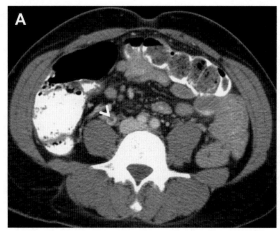
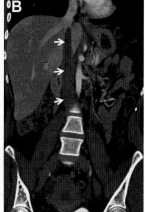

Fig. 20. Gonadal vein thrombosis in 2 different postpartum women presenting with fever and leukocytosis. (*A*) Axial contrast-enhanced CT image shows a filling defect within the right gonadal vein (*arrowhead*). (*B*) Coronal reformatted image from contrast-enhanced CT shows thrombosis of the inferior vena cava (*arrows*).

abdominal pain, and vaginal bleeding are seen in less than half of all patients with ectopic pregnancy.[84] A high index of clinical suspicion is hence necessary in early diagnosis of ectopic pregnancy. Overall, vaginal bleeding is seen in most (50%–80%) patients with ectopic pregnancy, and when it coexists with abdominal pain, it is highly sensitive for this diagnosis.[85,86] Specific signs on physical examination that can be helpful in the diagnosis of ectopic pregnancy include cervical motion tenderness, peritoneal signs, and in less than 10% cases, a palpable adnexal mass.[87] Most ectopic pregnancies occur in the fallopian tube (98%), with the ampullary region being the most common location (80%).[88] Other uncommon locations include the ovarian (<1%), abdominal (1%–2%), and cervical (0.15%) region. Implantation within a cesarean delivery scar/fibrous tissue is the rarest form, and the most life threatening, given the high risk of uterine rupture. Cesarean scar pregnancy can be of 2 types: the first type is one in which the gestational sac implants on the scar with progression toward either the cervicoisthmic space or the uterine cavity; the second type is the deep implantation of the sac into the cesarean delivery defect, with resultant high risk of rupture or bleeding.[89]

A recent meta-analysis[90] of 14 prospective studies (12,101 patients) in pregnant women with abdominal pain or vaginal bleeding evaluated with history, physical examination, laboratory analyses, and transvaginal ultrasonography showed that transvaginal ultrasonography is the single best modality for evaluation of suspected ectopic pregnancy. The investigators of this study concluded that presence of an adnexal mass in the absence of an intrauterine pregnancy on transvaginal sonography has the highest likelihood ratio (likelihood ratio of 111) for the diagnosis of ectopic pregnancy (**Fig. 21**). Lack of adnexal abnormalities on transvaginal sonography favors against ectopic pregnancy, with a negative likelihood ratio of 0.12. In general, ectopic pregnancy is suspected if no intrauterine gestational sac is seen with serum β-HCG levels of more than 1000 to 1500 mIU/mL. Sensitivity and specificity for this finding is 40% to 99% and 84% to 100%, respectively.[91–93] Presence of a complex adnexal mass with serum β-HCG levels of more than 1500 mIU/mL is considered to be highly specific (≤96%) for ectopic pregnancy.[81] Presence of a yolk sac or fetal pole within a gestational sac outside the uterine endometrial cavity is the characteristic sonographic finding. MDCT findings of ectopic pregnancy include a complex high-density adnexal mass with or without surrounding stranding and

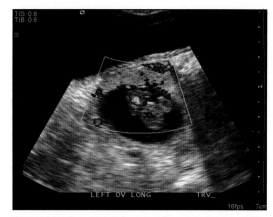

Fig. 21. Left adnexal ectopic pregnancy. Color Doppler image shows a fetal pole within a gestational sac in the left adnexa.

hemoperitoneum (**Fig. 22**). MR imaging with its high tissue contrast resolution is able to detect both ruptured and unruptured ectopic pregnancies with high accuracy (**Fig. 23**). A complex hemorrhagic adnexal mass with hemoperitoneum should raise the suspicion for ectopic pregnancy in the appropriate clinical settings (acute pain and increased β-HCG level). MR imaging is able to accurately delineate the precise location of the ectopic pregnancy, especially in cases with indeterminate on ultrasonographic findings. Gestational sac and fetal pole of early ectopic pregnancy are well depicted on T2-weighted MR images. MR imaging is also highly accurate in showing the anatomic details of the gestational sac in unusual locations such as the cesarean scar (**Fig. 24**).

Treatment of ectopic pregnancy is predominantly surgical, which is the mainstay therapy

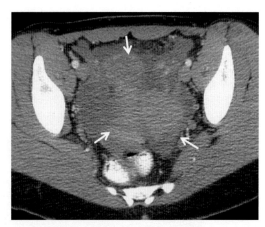

Fig. 22. Ruptured left adnexal ectopic pregnancy. Axial contrast-enhanced CT image shows a heterogeneously hyperdense mass in the left adnexa (*arrows*), with surrounding fluid/hemoperitoneum.

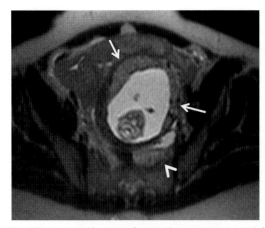

Fig. 23. Ruptured cornual ectopic pregnancy. Axial T2-weighted MR images show a fetus within the left cornual region (*arrows*) with hemoperitoneum with fluid-fluid level in the pelvis (*arrowhead* showing dependent low signal intensity) consistent with rupture cornual ectopic pregnancy.

in patients with hemodynamic instability and hemoperitoneum. Medical therapy with systemic methotrexate has been successfully used for uncomplicated cases without rupture. Methotrexate therapy is generally not indicated in patients with a β-HCG level greater than 5000, adnexal mass measuring greater than 3.5 cm, live fetus, and evidence of rupture with free peritoneal fluid seen on ultrasonography.[94–96] Ultrasound-guided chemical ablation of the ectopic implant by injecting methotrexate, potassium chloride, and hyperosmolar glucose has been found to be successful in treatment of tubal pregnancy without evidence rupture, hemodynamic instability, or hemoperitoneum.[97,98] UAE has been successfully used in treatment of cornual and cervical ectopic pregnancies. Expectant management has been used in

nonviable tubal pregnancies with downtrending β-HCG.[99] Cesarean scar pregnancy can also be managed by medical (systemic or local methotrexate therapy) or surgical approaches (laparotomy and excision of gestational sac).[89] Ultrasound-guided chemical ablation with or without UAE has also been used to treat cesarean scar pregnancy in the first trimester, with a success rate of up to 80%.[100]

Abdominal Pregnancy

Abdominal pregnancy is the least common location of ectopic pregnancy, where the implantation occurs outside the uterus and fallopian tubes within the maternal peritoneal cavity. Abdominal pregnancy accounts for 1 in 6000 to 10,000 births and approximately 1% to 1.6% of all ectopic pregnancies.[101–103] Abdominal pregnancies can be of primary (primary implantation in peritoneal cavity) or secondary (primary implantation in tube/ovary with subsequent erosion in to peritoneal cavity) types. Abdominal pregnancies can occur on or within the omentum, posterior cul-de-sac, uterine serosa, pelvic side wall, and solid or hollow visceral organs, such as the bowel, liver, or spleen.[104] Studdiford[105] established criteria for diagnosis of primary peritoneal pregnancy, which include: (1) pregnancy exclusively related to peritoneal surface, (2) normal fallopian tubes and ovaries, (3) no evidence of uteroperitoneal fistula. Abdominal pregnancy carries high mortality (≤90 times normal pregnancy and 7 times higher than other ectopic pregnancies), primarily related to hemorrhage from abnormal placental implantation and separation.[102] The fetus in abdominal pregnancy can survive in up to 10% cases; however, up to 50% of surviving fetuses show significant morphologic deformity. Given the potential catastrophic consequences and dismal maternal-fetal outcome, abdominal pregnancies are terminated at the time of diagnosis. Diagnosis can be established on ultrasonography by showing the fetus posterior or superior to the uterus, absence of myometrium surrounding the fetus, or no myometrial tissue between the fetus and the urinary bladder and a separate normal uterus (**Fig. 25**). Ancillary findings of abnormal lie of the fetus and oligohydramnios are also useful in establishing the diagnosis. Increase of maternal serum α-fetoprotein levels has been reported in select cases of abdominal pregnancy, believed to be secondary to extensive visceral implantation of the placenta.[106] Abdominal pregnancy detected before the twentieth week of gestation is managed with termination immediately after the diagnosis to reduce maternal mortality. Traditionally, surgical

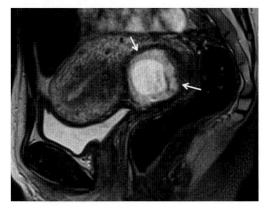

Fig. 24. Cesarean scar pregnancy. Sagittal T2-weighted MR image shows a gestational sac with fetal pole within a cesarean delivery scar (*arrows*).

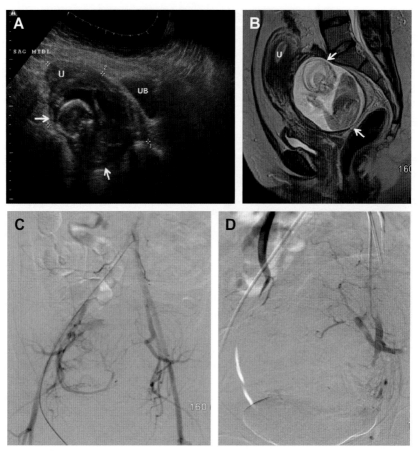

Fig. 25. Primary abdominal pregnancy treated with embolization to reduce intraoperative blood loss. Grayscale sonographic (*A*) and sagittal T2-weighted MR images (*B*) show a gestational sac with fetus within the cul-de-sac (*arrows*). (*C*) Preembolization and (*D*) postembolization digital subtraction angiographic images show successful bilateral internal iliac artery embolization. U, uterus; UB, urinary bladder.

ligation of the placental blood supply has been performed to reduce blood loss during the surgery. Endovascular embolization of the blood supply before the laparoscopic removal of the gestational mass or laparotomy has also been shown to reduce blood loss during the surgery. Varma and colleagues[107] reported a case of viable abdominal pregnancy with placental implantation to the omentum successfully managed at the 35th week of gestation. These investigators indicate that more than 100 cases of live births have been reported in advanced abdominal pregnancy and suggest that expectant management with close surveillance can possibly be used in advanced abdominal pregnancies detected in the late second or the third trimester.

SUMMARY

Imaging plays a vital role in the diagnosis of a wide array of nonfetal obstetric and gynecologic complications. Ultrasonography and MR imaging are the mainstay imaging modalities in the antepartum phase. Knowledge of epidemiologic and clinical features and usefulness of an appropriate imaging and interventional technique are necessary for timely diagnosis and management.

REFERENCES

1. Schauer DA, Linton OW. National Council on Radiation Protection and Measurements report shows substantial medical exposure increase. Radiology 2009;253:293–6.
2. Moore C, Promes SB. Ultrasound in pregnancy. Emerg Med Clin North Am 2004;22:697–722.
3. Wieseler KM, Bhargava P, Kanal KM, et al. Imaging in pregnant patients: examination appropriateness. Radiographics 2010;30:1215–29 [discussion:1230–3].

4. Masselli G, Gualdi G. MR imaging of the placenta: what a radiologist should know. Abdom Imaging 2013;38(3):573–87.

5. Ananth CV, Berkowitz GS, Savitz DA, et al. Placental abruption and adverse perinatal outcomes. JAMA 1999;282:1646–51.

6. Tikkanen M. Placental abruption: epidemiology, risk factors and consequences. Acta Obstet Gynecol Scand 2011;90:140–9.

7. Toivonen S, Heinonen S, Anttila M, et al. Obstetric prognosis after placental abruption. Fetal Diagn Ther 2004;19:336–41.

8. Pearlman MD, Tintinallli JE, Lorenz RP. A prospective controlled study of outcome after trauma during pregnancy. Am J Obstet Gynecol 1990;162: 1502–7 [discussion: 1507–10].

9. Vaizey CJ, Jacobson MJ, Cross FW. Trauma in pregnancy. Br J Surg 1994;81:1406–15.

10. Curet MJ, Schermer CR, Demarest GB, et al. Predictors of outcome in trauma during pregnancy: identification of patients who can be monitored for less than 6 hours. J Trauma 2000;49:18–24 [discussion: 24–5].

11. Nyberg DA, Cyr DR, Mack LA, et al. Sonographic spectrum of placental abruption. AJR Am J Roentgenol 1987;148:161–4.

12. Fleming AD. Abruptio placentae. Crit Care Clin 1991;7:865–75.

13. Gottesfeld KR. The clinical role of placental imaging. Clin Obstet Gynecol 1984;27:327–41.

14. McGahan JP, Phillips HE, Reid MH, et al. Sonographic spectrum of retroplacental hemorrhage. Radiology 1982;142:481–5.

15. Nyberg DA, Mack LA, Benedetti TJ, et al. Placental abruption and placental hemorrhage: correlation of sonographic findings with fetal outcome. Radiology 1987;164:357–61.

16. Masselli G, Brunelli R, Di Tola M, et al. MR imaging in the evaluation of placental abruption: correlation with sonographic findings. Radiology 2011;259: 222–30.

17. Glantz C, Purnell L. Clinical utility of sonography in the diagnosis and treatment of placental abruption. J Ultrasound Med 2002; 21:837–40.

18. Sholl JS. Abruptio placentae: clinical management in nonacute cases. Am J Obstet Gynecol 1987; 156:40–51.

19. Wei SH, Helmy M, Cohen AJ. CT evaluation of placental abruption in pregnant trauma patients. Emerg Radiol 2009;16:365–73.

20. Oyelese Y, Ananth CV. Placental abruption. Obstet Gynecol 2006;108:1005–16.

21. Shah KH, Simons RK, Holbrook T, et al. Trauma in pregnancy: maternal and fetal outcomes. J Trauma 1998;45:83–6.

22. Elsayes KM, Trout AT, Friedkin AM, et al. Imaging of the placenta: a multimodality pictorial review. Radiographics 2009;29:1371–91.

23. Harper LM, Odibo AO, Macones GA, et al. Effect of placenta previa on fetal growth. Am J Obstet Gynecol 2010;203:330.e1–5.

24. Oyelese Y, Smulian JC. Placenta previa, placenta accreta, and vasa previa. Obstet Gynecol 2006; 107:927–41.

25. Marshall NE, Fu R, Guise JM. Impact of multiple cesarean deliveries on maternal morbidity: a systematic review. Am J Obstet Gynecol 2011;205:262. e1–8.

26. Iyasu S, Saftlas AK, Rowley DL, et al. The epidemiology of placenta previa in the United States, 1979 through 1987. Am J Obstet Gynecol 1993;168: 1424–9.

27. Salihu HM, Li Q, Rouse DJ, et al. Placenta previa: neonatal death after live births in the United States. Am J Obstet Gynecol 2003;188: 1305–9.

28. Timor-Tritsch IE, Yunis RA. Confirming the safety of transvaginal sonography in patients suspected of placenta previa. Obstet Gynecol 1993;81:742–4.

29. Mazouni C, Gorincour G, Juhan V, et al. Placenta accreta: a review of current advances in prenatal diagnosis. Placenta 2007;28:599–603.

30. ACOG Committee on Obstetric Practice. ACOG committee opinion. Number 266, January 2002: placenta accreta. Obstet Gynecol 2002;99: 169–70.

31. Warshak CR, Eskander R, Hull AD, et al. Accuracy of ultrasonography and magnetic resonance imaging in the diagnosis of placenta accreta. Obstet Gynecol 2006;108:573–81.

32. Miller DA, Chollet JA, Goodwin TM. Clinical risk factors for placenta previa–placenta accreta. Am J Obstet Gynecol 1997;177:210–4.

33. Clark SL, Koonings PP, Phelan JP. Placenta previa/accreta and prior cesarean section. Obstet Gynecol 1985;66:89–92.

34. To WW, Leung WC. Placenta previa and previous cesarean section. Int J Gynaecol Obstet 1995;51: 25–31.

35. Baughman WC, Corteville JE, Shah RR. Placenta accreta: spectrum of US and MR imaging findings. Radiographics 2008;28:1905–16.

36. Dwyer BK, Belogolovkin V, Tran L, et al. Prenatal diagnosis of placenta accreta: sonography or magnetic resonance imaging? J Ultrasound Med 2008; 27:1275–81.

37. Wou K, Chen MF, Mallozzi A, et al. Pregnancy outcomes and ultrasonographic diagnosis in patients with histologically-proven placental chorioangioma. Placenta 2011;32:671–4.

38. Amer HZ, Heller DS. Chorangioma and related vascular lesions of the placenta–a review. Fetal Pediatr Pathol 2010;29:199–206.

39. Faes T, Pecceu A, Van Calenbergh S, et al. Choriogiocarcinoma of the placenta: a case report and clinical review. Placenta 2012;33:658–61.

40. Zanardini C, Papageorghiou A, Bhide A, et al. Giant placental chorioangioma: natural history and pregnancy outcome. Ultrasound Obstet Gynecol 2010;35:332–6.

41. Prapas N, Liang RI, Hunter D, et al. Color Doppler imaging of placental masses: differential diagnosis and fetal outcome. Ultrasound Obstet Gynecol 2000;16:559–63.

42. Mochizuki T, Nishiguchi T, Ito I, et al. Case report. Antenatal diagnosis of chorioangioma of the placenta: MR features. J Comput Assist Tomogr 1996;20:413–6.

43. Kawamotoa S, Ogawa F, Tanaka J, et al. Chorioangioma: antenatal diagnosis with fast MR imaging. Magn Reson Imaging 2000;18:911–4.

44. Nagaya K, Fetters MD, Ishikawa M, et al. Causes of maternal mortality in Japan. JAMA 2000;283: 2661–7.

45. Brill Y, Kingdom J, Thomas J, et al. The management of VBAC at term: a survey of Canadian obstetricians. J Obstet Gynaecol Can 2003;25:300–10.

46. Miller DA, Goodwin TM, Gherman RB, et al. Intrapartum rupture of the unscarred uterus. Obstet Gynecol 1997;89:671–3.

47. Neuhaus W, Bauerschmitz G, Gohring U, et al. Risk of uterine rupture after cesarean section–analysis of 1,086 births. Zentralbl Gynakol 2001; 123:148–52 [in German].

48. Sherer DM, Abulafia O, Anyaegbunam AM. Intra- and early postpartum ultrasonography: a review. Part II. Obstet Gynecol Surv 1998;53:181–90.

49. Di Salvo DN. Sonographic imaging of maternal complications of pregnancy. J Ultrasound Med 2003;22:69–89.

50. Leyendecker JR, Gorengaut V, Brown JJ. MR imaging of maternal diseases of the abdomen and pelvis during pregnancy and the immediate postpartum period. Radiographics 2004;24:1301–16.

51. Nishino M, Hayakawa K, Iwasaku K, et al. Magnetic resonance imaging findings in gynecologic emergencies. J Comput Assist Tomogr 2003;27: 564–70.

52. Shrout AB, Kopelman JN. Ultrasonographic diagnosis of uterine dehiscence during pregnancy. J Ultrasound Med 1995;14:399–402.

53. Malvasi A, Tinelli A, Tinelli R, et al. The post-cesarean section symptomatic bladder flap hematoma: a modern reappraisal. J Matern Fetal Neonatal Med 2007;20:709–14.

54. Rosati P, Exacoustos C, Mancuso S. Longitudinal evaluation of uterine myoma growth during pregnancy. A sonographic study. J Ultrasound Med 1992;11:511–5.

55. Durfee SM, Frates MC, Luong A, et al. The sonographic and color Doppler features of retained products of conception. J Ultrasound Med 2005; 24:1181–6 [quiz: 1188–9].

56. Hertzberg BS, Bowie JD. Ultrasound of the postpartum uterus. Prediction of retained placental tissue. J Ultrasound Med 1991;10:451–6.

57. Wachsberg RH, Kurtz AB, Levine CD, et al. Real-time ultrasonographic analysis of the normal postpartum uterus: technique, variability, and measurements. J Ultrasound Med 1994;13:215–21.

58. Carlan SJ, Scott WT, Pollack R, et al. Appearance of the uterus by ultrasound immediately after placental delivery with pathologic correlation. J Clin Ultrasound 1997;25:301–8.

59. Shen O, Rabinowitz R, Eisenberg VH, et al. Trans-abdominal sonography before uterine exploration as a predictor of retained placental fragments. J Ultrasound Med 2003;22:561–4.

60. Malvern J, Campbell S, May P. Ultrasonic scanning of the puerperal uterus following secondary postpartum haemorrhage. J Obstet Gynaecol Br Commonw 1973;80:320–4.

61. Sadan O, Golan A, Girtler O, et al. Role of sonography in the diagnosis of retained products of conception. J Ultrasound Med 2004;23:371–4.

62. Swartz WH, Grolle K. The use of prophylactic antibiotics in cesarean section. A review of the literature. J Reprod Med 1981;26:595–609.

63. Dinsmoor MJ, Newton ER, Gibbs RS. A randomized, double-blind, placebo-controlled trial of oral antibiotic therapy following intravenous antibiotic therapy for postpartum endometritis. Obstet Gynecol 1991;77:60–2.

64. Menias CO, Elsayes KM, Peterson CM, et al. CT of pregnancy-related complications. Emerg Radiol 2007;13:299–306.

65. Pelage JP, Soyer P, Repiquet D, et al. Secondary postpartum hemorrhage: treatment with selective arterial embolization. Radiology 1999;212:385–9.

66. Kirby JM, Kachura JR, Rajan DK, et al. Arterial embolization for primary postpartum hemorrhage. J Vasc Interv Radiol 2009;20:1036–45.

67. Dildy GA 3rd. Postpartum hemorrhage: new management options. Clin Obstet Gynecol 2002;45: 330–44.

68. Varner M. Postpartum hemorrhage. Crit Care Clin 1991;7:883–97.

69. Kawamura DM. Sonography of postpartum uterus. 2nd edition. Philadelphia: Lippincott Williams & Wilkins; 1997.

70. Thabet A, Kalva SP, Liu B, et al. Interventional radiology in pregnancy complications: indications, technique, and methods for minimizing radiation exposure. Radiographics 2012;32:255–74.

71. Whitecar MP, Turner S, Higby MK. Adnexal masses in pregnancy: a review of 130 cases undergoing surgical management. Am J Obstet Gynecol 1999;181:19–24.

72. Bromley B, Benacerraf B. Adnexal masses during pregnancy: accuracy of sonographic diagnosis and outcome. J Ultrasound Med 1997;16:447–52 [quiz: 453–4].

73. Chiang G, Levine D. Imaging of adnexal masses in pregnancy. J Ultrasound Med 2004;23:805–19.

74. Descargues G, Tinlot-Mauger F, Gravier A, et al. Adnexal torsion: a report on forty-five cases. Eur J Obstet Gynecol Reprod Biol 2001;98:91–6.

75. Mashiach S, Bider D, Moran O, et al. Adnexal torsion of hyperstimulated ovaries in pregnancies after gonadotropin therapy. Fertil Steril 1990;53:76–80.

76. Yen CF, Lin SL, Murk W, et al. Risk analysis of torsion and malignancy for adnexal masses during pregnancy. Fertil Steril 2009;91:1895–902.

77. Lawrence PH, Lyons EA, Levi CS. Hyperreactio luteinalis. J Ultrasound Med 1983;2:375–6.

78. Ghossain MA, Buy JN, Ruiz A, et al. Hyperreactio luteinalis in a normal pregnancy: sonographic and MRI findings. J Magn Reson Imaging 1998;8:1203–6.

79. Yapar EG, Vural T, Ekici E, et al. Hyperreactio luteinalis masquerading as an ovarian neoplasm in a triplet pregnancy. Eur J Obstet Gynecol Reprod Biol 1996;65:177–80.

80. Montz FJ, Schlaerth JB, Morrow CP. The natural history of theca lutein cysts. Obstet Gynecol 1988;72:247–51.

81. Ramakrishnan K, Scheid DC. Ectopic pregnancy: forget the "classic presentation" if you want to catch it sooner. J Fam Pract 2006;55:388–95.

82. Saraiya M, Berg CJ, Shulman H, et al. Estimates of the annual number of clinically recognized pregnancies in the United States, 1981-1991. Am J Epidemiol 1999;149:1025–9.

83. Carr RJ, Evans P. Ectopic pregnancy. Prim Care 2000;27:169–83.

84. Stovall TG, Kellerman AL, Ling FW, et al. Emergency department diagnosis of ectopic pregnancy. Ann Emerg Med 1990;19:1098–103.

85. Buckley RG, King KJ, Disney JD, et al. Derivation of a clinical prediction model for the emergency department diagnosis of ectopic pregnancy. Acad Emerg Med 1998;5:951–60.

86. Fylstra DL. Tubal pregnancy: a review of current diagnosis and treatment. Obstet Gynecol Surv 1998;53:320–8.

87. Dart RG, Kaplan B, Varaklis K. Predictive value of history and physical examination in patients with suspected ectopic pregnancy. Ann Emerg Med 1999;33:283–90.

88. Bouyer J, Coste J, Fernandez H, et al. Sites of ectopic pregnancy: a 10 year population-based study of 1800 cases. Hum Reprod 2002;17:3224–30.

89. Maymon R, Halperin R, Mendlovic S, et al. Ectopic pregnancies in caesarean section scars: the 8 year experience of one medical centre. Hum Reprod 2004;19:278–84.

90. Crochet JR, Bastian LA, Chireau MV. Does this woman have an ectopic pregnancy?: the rational clinical examination systematic review. JAMA 2013;309:1722–9.

91. Braffman BH, Coleman BG, Ramchandani P, et al. Emergency department screening for ectopic pregnancy: a prospective US study. Radiology 1994;190:797–802.

92. Kaplan BC, Dart RG, Moskos M, et al. Ectopic pregnancy: prospective study with improved diagnostic accuracy. Ann Emerg Med 1996;28:10–7.

93. Mol BW, Hajenius PJ, Engelsbel S, et al. Serum human chorionic gonadotropin measurement in the diagnosis of ectopic pregnancy when transvaginal sonography is inconclusive. Fertil Steril 1998;70:972–81.

94. Lipscomb GH, Bran D, McCord ML, et al. Analysis of three hundred fifteen ectopic pregnancies treated with single-dose methotrexate. Am J Obstet Gynecol 1998;178:1354–8.

95. Menon S, Colins J, Barnhart KT. Establishing a human chorionic gonadotropin cutoff to guide methotrexate treatment of ectopic pregnancy: a systematic review. Fertil Steril 2007;87:481–4.

96. Barnhart KT, Gosman G, Ashby R, et al. The medical management of ectopic pregnancy: a meta-analysis comparing "single dose" and "multidose" regimens. Obstet Gynecol 2003;101:778–84.

97. Levine D. Ectopic pregnancy. Radiology 2007;245:385–97.

98. Nama V, Manyonda I. Tubal ectopic pregnancy: diagnosis and management. Arch Gynecol Obstet 2009;279:443–53.

99. Kirk E, Bourne T. The nonsurgical management of ectopic pregnancy. Curr Opin Obstet Gynecol 2006;18:587–93.

100. Jurkovic D, Hillaby K, Woelfer B, et al. First-trimester diagnosis and management of pregnancies implanted into the lower uterine segment cesarean section scar. Ultrasound Obstet Gynecol 2003;21:220–7.

101. Alto WA. Abdominal pregnancy. Am Fam Physician 1990;41:209–14.

102. Atrash HK, Friede A, Hogue CJ. Abdominal pregnancy in the United States: frequency and maternal mortality. Obstet Gynecol 1987;69:333–7.

103. Bajo JM, Garcia-Frutos A, Huertas MA. Sonographic follow-up of a placenta left in situ after delivery of the fetus in an abdominal pregnancy. Ultrasound Obstet Gynecol 1996;7:285–8.

104. Costa SD, Presley J, Bastert G. Advanced abdominal pregnancy. Obstet Gynecol Surv 1991;46:515–25.

105. Studdiford WE. Primary peritoneal pregnancy. Am J Obstet Gynecol 1942;44:487–91.

106. Shumway JB, Greenspoon JS, Khouzami AN, et al. Amniotic fluid alpha fetoprotein (AFAFP) and maternal serum alpha fetoprotein (MSAFP) in abdominal pregnancies: correlation with extent and site of placental implantation and clinical implications. J Matern Fetal Med 1996;5:120–3.

107. Varma R, Mascarenhas L, James D. Successful outcome of advanced abdominal pregnancy with exclusive omental insertion. Ultrasound Obstet Gynecol 2003;21:192–4.

Imaging of Acute Abdomen in Pregnancy

Ashish Khandelwal, MD[a],*, Najla Fasih, MD[b],
Ania Kielar, MD[b]

KEYWORDS

- Pregnancy • Acute abdomen • Radiation exposure • Appendicitis • Cholecystitis • Pancreatitis
- Bowel obstruction • Abdominal trauma

KEY POINTS

- Physiologic changes during pregnancy can alter presentations of common pathology.
- Women should be counseled that x-ray exposure from a single diagnostic procedure, typically less than 5 rad, has not been associated with an increase in fetal anomalies or pregnancy loss.
- Concern about possible effects of high-dose ionizing radiation exposure should not prevent medically indicated imaging modalities from being performed on a pregnant woman.
- The principle of as low as reasonably achievable (ALARA) should be followed while using imaging modalities that use ionizing radiation.
- During pregnancy, imaging procedures not associated with ionizing radiation such as ultrasonography and magnetic resonance imaging should be used in preference to modalities using ionizing radiation when appropriate.

INTRODUCTION

Acute abdomen develops during 1 in 500 to 635 pregnancies.[1] Assessment of the pregnant woman with abdominal pain should be undertaken in a practical and scrupulous manner. Causes of acute abdomen in pregnant women can be classified into obstetric or nonobstetric entities, and may require surgical exploration. The delay in diagnosis and intervention only worsens the outcome for the mother and the fetus. Appropriate deployment of imaging in pregnant females is challenging and requires careful analysis of risk/benefit ratio, with the need for a diagnostic test which will be precise and of lowest risk to both mother and fetus.

This article reviews the role of imaging in non-obstetric conditions causing acute abdominal pain in pregnant patients. Also appraised are the areas of general concern with regard to the use of appropriate modalities in common diagnostic scenarios, current recommendations for use of contrast agents in pregnancy, imaging appearance of acute abdominal processes, and the general consensus on the management approach to these conditions.

ANATOMIC AND PHYSIOLOGIC CHANGES IN PREGNANCY

The physiologic and anatomic changes of various organs, secondary to hormonal fluctuations during the course of pregnancy, result in major diagnostic challenges for the clinician. The enlarged gravid uterus causes compression or displacement of surrounding viscera and laxity of the anterior abdominal wall. As a result, there is often a delay

Funding Sources: None.
Conflict of Interest: None.
[a] Department of Radiology, Brigham and Women's Hospital, Harvard Medical School, 75 Francis Street, Boston, MA 02115, USA; [b] Department of Medical Imaging, The Ottawa Hospital, University of Ottawa, 501 Smyth Road, Ottawa, Ontario K1H 8L6, Canada
* Corresponding author.
E-mail address: akhandelwal1@partners.org

radiologic.theclinics.com

in the clinical diagnosis of intra-abdominal abnormalities secondary to their atypical location and often-delayed peritoneal signs.

Because of biliary stasis and increased concentration of bile during pregnancy under the enhanced hormonal milieu, there is an increased risk of cholelithiasis and biliary colic.[2] Higher levels of progesterone cause a decrease in pressure in the lower esophageal sphincter and reduce both small-bowel and large-bowel motility. This process may lead to gastroesophageal reflux and constipation.[3] There is ureteric dilatation secondary to compression of the lower ureter from the gravid uterus, and decreased peristalsis of the ureter as a result of the smooth-muscle relaxation effects of progesterone. These factors increase the risk of stone formation and infection.[4] Pregnancy is also associated with an increased propensity for thrombosis arising from hyperestrogenemia. Later in gestation, the compressive effects of the uterus on the inferior vena cava can lead to a reduction in venous return. This phenomenon is associated with increased occurrence of venous thrombosis in the extremities and, rarely, development of Budd-Chiari syndrome.[5]

CURRENT CONSENSUS ON THE USE OF IMAGING DURING PREGNANCY

"Don't penalize her for being pregnant!" is the appropriate approach of radiologists and clinicians to the management of pregnant patients with acute abdominal pain. Delay in diagnosis may lead to poor outcomes. The lack of awareness about choice of imaging modality for a particular clinical scenario is not uncommon. Ultrasonography (US) and magnetic resonance (MR) imaging, which do not expose the patient and her fetus to ionizing radiation, should be used when feasible. However, when deemed necessary the use of computed tomography (CT) should not be delayed, because of concern for exposure of the fetus to ionizing radiation. Single CT use for triaging the pregnant patient in acute distress has been shown to lead to favorable maternal and fetal outcomes.[6]

EFFECTS OF IONIZING RADIATION

Exposure to ionizing radiation can lead to 2 types of effects, namely deterministic and stochastic effects.[7] Estimated fetal exposure from common radiologic procedures is shown in **Table 1**. Deterministic effects, also known as threshold phenomena, have a "no-adverse-effect level" for a particular outcome on the fetus, meaning that if

Table 1 Estimated fetal exposure from common radiologic procedures	
Procedure	**Exposure**
Chest radiograph (2 views)	0.02–0.07 mrad
Abdominal film (single view)	100 mrad
Hip film (single view)	200 mrad
Mammography	7–20 mrad
Barium enema or small-bowel series	2–4 rad
CT scan of head or chest	<1 rad
CT scan of abdomen and lumbar spine	3.5 rad
CT pelvimetry	250 mrad

Data from American College of Obstetricians and Gynecologists. Guidelines for diagnostic imaging during pregnancy. ACOG Committee opinion No. 299. Obstet Gynecol 2004;104:649.

there is less than a predetermined exposure to radiation, no adverse outcome is expected. Pregnancy loss, congenital malformations, neurobehavioral abnormalities, and fetal growth retardation are deterministic effects. A summary of suspected in utero induced deterministic radiation effects is given in **Table 2**. By contrast, stochastic effects do not have a threshold and can occur at any radiation dose. Risks of cancer and genetic defects are stochastic effects.[7] Overall, the total fetal dose from background radiation sources is less than 0.1 rad (1 mSv) during the entire pregnancy.[6,8] According to the American College of Radiology, no single diagnostic imaging study results in radiation exposure to a degree that would threaten the well-being of the developing fetus.[9] Exposure to less than 5 rad (50 mSv) has not been associated with an increase in fetal anomalies or pregnancy loss.[6]

Irradiation during early pregnancy may result in spontaneous abortion; however, if the gestation continues, there are no known long-term deleterious effects. The most vulnerable period is 8 to 15 weeks' gestation, with effects of ionizing radiation on the developing fetus that can lead to intrauterine growth retardation and central nervous system defects (microcephaly, mental retardation). After 15 weeks the developing fetus is much less sensitive to radiation effects.

The carcinogenic hazard of ionizing radiation is less well understood. According to the International Commission on Radiological Protection, the best quantitative estimate of risk is about 1 cancer per 500 fetuses exposed to 30 mGy of radiation.[6] It is estimated that 1 to 2 rad of fetal

Table 2
Summary of suspected in utero induced deterministic radiation effects

Gestational Age (wk)	Radiation Dose 50–100 mGy (5–10 rad)	Radiation Dose >100 mGy (>10 rad)
0–2	None	None
3–4	Probably none	Possible spontaneous abortion
5–10	Potential effects too subtle to be clinically detectable	Possible malformations increasing in likelihood as dose increases
11–17	Potential effects too subtle to be clinically detectable	Increased risk of deficits in IQ or mental retardation that increase in frequency and severity with increasing dose
18–27	None	IQ deficits not detectable at diagnostic doses
>27	None	None applicable to diagnostic medicine

Exposure to less than 5 rad has not been associated with an increase in fetal anomalies or pregnancy loss.
Data from International Commission on Radiological Protection. Pregnancy and medical radiation. Ann ICRP 2000;30(1):iii–viii, 1–43; and Streffer C, Shore R, Konermann G, et al. Biological effects after prenatal irradiation (embryo and fetus). A report of the International Commission on Radiological Protection. Ann ICRP 2003;33(1–2):5–206.

exposure may increase the risk of leukemia by a factor of 1.5 to 2.0 over the natural incidence, and that an estimated 1 in 2000 children exposed to ionizing radiation in utero will develop childhood leukemia.[10,11] The fetal dose from a CT scan depends on maternal abdominal girth and the depth of the fetus from the anterior maternal skin surface.[12] The larger the maternal diameter and greater the depth of the fetus from the anterior maternal skin surface, the smaller the resulting fetal dose. The fetal dose will also vary depending on scanning parameters. A fetal radiation exposure of at least 100 mGy is necessary before counseling about possible pregnancy termination.[13]

significantly, as the majority of the fetal dose is related to scatter of photons within the exposed maternal tissues.[14] Radiation exposure in imaging must be applied at levels as low as reasonably achievable (ALARA), with medical benefit exceeding the well-managed levels of risk. Different measures such as limiting the scanned volume, widening the beam collimation, increasing pitch, decreasing kilovoltage, and decreasing milliamperage are encouraged to reduce the radiation dose.[15] The fetal radiation dose in pregnant patients should be estimated by placing a thermoluminescent dosimeter on the abdomen during imaging, particularly when repeated imaging may be required.

STRATEGIES TO DECREASE THE RADIATION DOSE

The first step in decreasing radiation exposure during pregnancy is to consult with the referring clinician about the indications and the need for any radiologic examination for evaluation of abdominal pain in pregnancy. Utility of any available nonionizing alternative imaging should also be assessed. If examination with radiation is deemed necessary, the imaging technologist and the imaging physician should work together to optimize the study and minimize the radiation dose. Establishment of a sound strategy for imaging the acute abdomen in pregnancy can expedite patient evaluation. Providing lead shielding to wrap the pelvis of the pregnant patient during nonpelvic CT may psychologically benefit the patient but has not been shown to reduce radiation dose

COUNSELING THE PREGNANT PATIENT FOR IMAGING PROCEDURES

Exposure to diagnostic radiation during pregnancy is associated with high levels of anxiety among pregnant women and their health care providers. Physicians should use evidence-based counseling to allay misperceptions of risk. When counseling women and families of reproductive age, it is important to notify them about the background risks of developmental effects for which all healthy women are at risk.[7,16,17] Women should be counseled that x-ray exposure from a single diagnostic procedure does not result in harmful fetal effects. Specifically, exposure to less than 5 rad has not been associated with an increase in fetal anomalies or pregnancy loss.[18,19] It is simpler to counsel families concerning the deterministic risks because if the exposure is below the level of adverse effect, it is appropriate to inform the family that their risks are not increased. For the oncogenic or mutagenic risks, the radiologist can inform the family that the risk is negligibly small. Obtaining consent from the pregnant patient is of pivotal importance in providing comprehensive medical care.

ULTRASONOGRAPHY AND MR IMAGING SAFETY

US and MR imaging have been traditionally considered safe in pregnancy because of their lack of ionizing radiation. However, energy exposure from US has been arbitrarily restricted to 94 mW/cm^2 by the United States Food and Drug Administration (FDA).[10] MR imaging, with its varying magnetic fields and pulsed radiofrequency gradients, may theoretically increase the risk of hazardous biological effects, miscarriage, and heating effects in the fetus.[20,21] Present data have not conclusively documented any deleterious effects of MR imaging exposure on the developing fetus.[22] The American College of Radiology (ACR) approves imaging of pregnant patients in any trimester, although discourages unnecessary MR use.[6,23] Typically, single-shot fast spin-echo sequences cause increased specific absorption rate, in comparison with gradient-recalled echo sequences. In MR exposures up to 1 hour, the total body exposure should be limited to a total energy deposition of 120 Wmin/kg in order not to overload the thermoregulatory system in the normal individual.[24] For exposures to pregnant women, a reduction of these values by a factor of 2 is recommended.[24]

USE OF CONTRAST AGENTS DURING PREGNANCY

Iodinated contrast material crosses the placenta and enters the fetal circulation. However, no teratogenic effects have been reported with these contrast agents. Although paramagnetic contrast agents are unlikely to cause harm, these agents should be used during pregnancy only if the potential benefit justifies the potential risk to the fetus. Gadolinium has been shown to have teratogenic effects in animal studies.[6] Gadolinium-based contrast agents are classified as pregnancy category C drugs by the FDA, and their routine use is not approved.[25] The current ACR guideline for safe MR imaging practices suggests that MR imaging contrast agents should not be routinely administered to pregnant patients, and that a decision should be made by the attending radiologist

only on a case-by-case basis with a risk/benefit analysis.[22]

APPROACH TO COMMON NONOBSTETRIC CONDITIONS CAUSING ACUTE ABDOMEN IN PREGNANCY

Various conditions other than appendicitis can cause abdominal pain during pregnancy, including abnormalities of gastrointestinal, hepatobiliary, genitourinary, vascular, and gynecologic origin.

Appendicitis

Appendicitis affects 1 in 1500 pregnancies, and is the most common reason for nonobstetric surgical intervention in pregnancy.[26,27] The incidence is thought to be similar in the pregnant and the nonpregnant population. It occurs most often in the second trimester. There is often delay in diagnosis because the presentation is variable, owing to lack of typical pain features of appendicitis, pregnancy-associated nausea/vomiting confusing the clinical presentation, and nonspecific leukocytosis of pregnancy making laboratory values more unreliable. An unruptured appendicitis is associated with a fetal loss of 3% to 5%, with little effect on maternal mortality. By contrast, in the case of ruptured appendicitis there is an associated rate of fetal loss of 20% to 25%.[28,29] These data emphasize the need for accurate early diagnosis and timely surgical intervention.

US with graded compression is often the preferred initial imaging modality for suspected appendicitis in pregnant women. It is safe, inexpensive, and easily accessible. The appendix is often superiorly displaced from its normal position within the right lower quadrant, especially later in gestation. Scanning patients in the left posterior oblique or left lateral decubitus position, rather than in the supine position, has been advocated to increase the success of visualizing the appendix.[30] As in nonpregnant patients, appendicitis is diagnosed when a tubular, noncompressible, nonperistaltic, blind-ending, tender structure with a diameter of greater than 6 mm is localized arising from cecal base. The major limitation of US is suboptimal assessment of alternative diagnoses, limitations of body habitus, and operator dependency.[31] US also has limited utility for diagnosing appendicitis because of the infrequent visualization of the appendix. In one study, US was able to detect the appendix in 29% of cases but did not visualize it in 71% of surgically proven cases in the second and third trimesters.[32] In another study where US was used to assess for appendicitis in pregnant patients, sensitivity and specificity was only 78% and 83%, respectively.[33]

The false-positive rate is also reported to be relatively high (18% for graded compression US vs 10% for CT).[33]

CT is an easily available alternative that can provide a quick diagnosis in cases of inconclusive US. Protocols for the evaluation of acute appendicitis in pregnant women are variable. Avoidance of intravenous contrast material in pregnancy is preferable when reasonable. CT has been shown to be highly sensitive (92%) and specific (99%), with a high negative predictive value (99%) for diagnosing appendicitis.[34] Imaging findings suggestive of acute appendicitis on unenhanced CT include a thickened appendix greater than 6 mm in diameter, and evidence of periappendiceal inflammation, including fat stranding, as well as presence of a phlegmon, fluid collection, or extraluminal air.[35,36] It is also valuable in giving an alternative diagnosis for right lower abdominal pain. The main concern regarding use of CT is radiation exposure to the developing fetus. The fetal radiation dose reported in the literature with multidetector-row CT using an appendix protocol is between 20 and 43 mGy, depending on the trimester of pregnancy.[37,38]

MR imaging, with its excellent soft-tissue contrast resolution and lack of ionizing radiation, is another option for investigating right lower quadrant pain in pregnancy. The initial field of view can include from the dome of the liver superiorly, through the symphysis pubis inferiorly. The overall MR imaging protocol for acute abdomen followed in the authors' department is summarized in **Box 1**.

As pregnancy progresses, the gravid uterus displaces and tilts the cecum anteriorly and outwardly out of the pelvis. A cecal tilt angle of at least 90° on sagittal MR images is predictive of the appendix being located in the right upper quadrant rather than its usual location within the right lower quadrant.[39] MR imaging features of a normal appendix include a diameter of less than 6 mm, an appendiceal wall thickness of less than 2 mm, low luminal signal intensity on T1-weighted and T2-weighted images, and no periappendiceal fat stranding or fluid (**Fig. 1**). Noncontrast MR findings of appendicitis are enlarged appendix with signs of periappendiceal inflammation with or without perforation (**Figs. 2 and 3**). The sensitivity, specificity, positive predictive value, and negative predictive value of MR imaging in the diagnosis of appendicitis are 90% to 100%, 93% to 98%, 61% to 82%, and 99% to 100%, respectively.[40–42] The routine incorporation of MR imaging into the clinical workup for suspicion of appendicitis in pregnant patients has been associated with a decrease in the negative laparotomy rate of 47%, without a significant change in the perforation rate.[40] A patient with a negative MR imaging examination in all likelihood does not need to undergo an emergent appendectomy.

Pancreaticobiliary Diseases

Gallbladder disease is a leading nonobstetric cause for hospitalization during pregnancy and in the first year postpartum.[2] Cholelithiasis occurs in up to 12% of pregnant women and is symptomatic in 0.1% to 0.3%.[43]

US remains the best initial modality to evaluate the liver and biliary system. Acute cholecystitis is

---

Box 1
MR imaging in acute abdomen in pregnancy

1. Written informed consent needed before scan

2. Use 1.5-T MR imaging

3. Supine position with phased-array coil to improve signal-to-noise ratio

4. No gadolinium given

   MR imaging sequences

   - Multiplanar single-shot fast spin-echo T2-weighted images of abdomen and pelvis
   - Axial single-shot fast spin-echo T2-weighted fat-suppressed images of abdomen and pelvis: increases ability to detect edema, inflammation, and free fluid
   - Axial unenhanced T1-weighted 3-dimensional spoiled gradient echo
   - Axial T1-weighted gradient dual echo in-phase and out-phase images
   - Axial bright-blood vascular sequence
   - Magnetic resonance cholangiopancreatography if biliary abnormality
   - Diffusion-weighted images

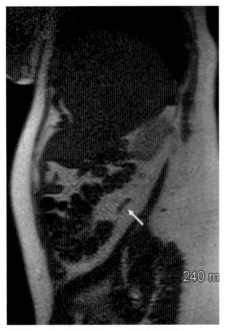

Fig. 1. Normal magnetic resonance (MR) imaging appearances of the appendix. Sagittal single-shot fast spin-echo (SSFSE) MR images through the abdomen in a pregnant patient. The normal appendix (*arrow*) is seen as a thin-walled, tubular structure within the pericecal region. Note the absence of luminal fluid and periappendiceal stranding. The location of the appendix is variable depending on the stage of pregnancy.

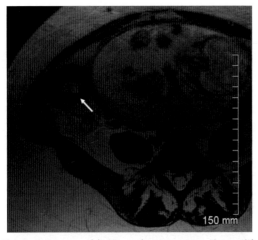

Fig. 2. A 32-year-old, 25-week pregnant patient with acute appendicitis, presenting with right lower quadrant pain and high white blood cell count. Axial T2-weighted SSFSE images demonstrate the inflamed, dilated, partially fluid-filled appendix (*arrow*) with a caliber of 15 mm, and markedly thickened wall. Appendectomy was confirmatory.

the most common acute complication of cholelithiasis. Acute cholecystitis is the second most common condition necessitating surgery during pregnancy, occurring in 1 in 1600 to 10,000 pregnancies.[44] Cholelithiasis with either positive sonographic Murphy sign or gallbladder wall thickening (>3 mm) has high positive predictive value for diagnosing cholecystitis (92.2% and 95.2%, respectively).[45] Secondary findings such as pericholecystic fluid and wall hyperemia may also be helpful (Fig. 4). However, sensitivity of US in the detection of common bile duct stones in the general population has been reported at only between 20% and 38%.[46] MR cholangiopancreatography (MRCP) can be used as a second-line imaging tool, complementing US. It can help in management decisions for pregnant patients with suspected choledocholithiasis or indeterminate intrahepatic biliary dilatation. At MR imaging, choledocholithiasis is best visualized on T2-weighted images as a dependent signal void in the common bile duct, with or without intrahepatic or extrahepatic biliary dilatation. Furthermore, MRCP may be particularly helpful in differentiating choledocholithiasis from intrahepatic cholestasis of pregnancy, because the clinical and biochemical presentation of these 2 entities overlap.[5] Potential complications of choledocholithiasis include cholecystitis, pancreatitis, and ascending cholangitis (Fig. 5).

Pancreatitis complicates 1 in 3333 pregnancies.[47] Pancreatitis most often occurs in the third trimester and is usually self-limiting. Typically it presents with acute abdominal pain radiating to the back, and elevations of pancreatic amylase/lipase levels. MR imaging can better evaluate the pancreatic edema, pancreatic ductal obstruction, and peripancreatic inflammation (Fig. 6). The pancreas is normally hyperintense on T1-weighted images, owing to high manganese content, but this may be lost in acute pancreatitis because of edema. MR imaging can serve as a useful alternative to endoscopic retrograde cholangiopancreatography (ERCP) by excluding biliary abnormality in patients with equivocal US findings for suspected choledocholithiasis. Recently the combination of MRCP, ERCP without radiation, and laparoscopic cholecystectomy have been shown to be a safe approach to definitive treatment of biliary-induced pancreatitis.[48] Complications of pancreatitis include abscess or pseudocyst formation, pancreatic necrosis, and splenic vein thrombosis. Diffusion-weighted imaging may show restriction of diffusion in the early edematous phase. Perinatal mortality is 3.6%, and maternal mortality is very low with improved management.[49]

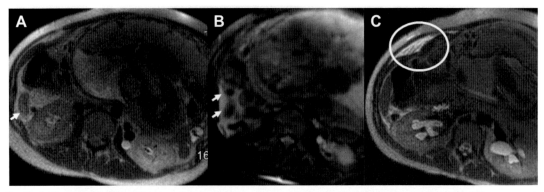

Fig. 3. A 17-year-old, 29-week pregnant girl with perforated appendicitis. The patient presented with severe sub-costal pain of 3 days' duration. Axial T2-weighted fat-suppressed (A) and Axial SSFSE images (B, C) demonstrate dilated inflamed appendix (*single arrow*) with fluid and stranding in periappendiceal fat (*double arrows*), as well as a collection in the abdominal wall (*circle*). Perforated appendicitis with abscess formation was confirmed surgically.

Hepatic Diseases

Three percent to 5% of all pregnancies are complicated by liver dysfunction.[50] A wide array of hepatic diseases can occur during pregnancy, including cirrhosis, hepatitis, infections, adenomas, primary sclerosing cholangitis (**Fig. 7**), Wilson disease, and autoimmune hepatitis. Hepatic diseases unique to pregnancy include HELLP (hemolysis, elevated liver enzymes, low platelets) syndrome and acute fatty liver of pregnancy.[50]

HELLP syndrome occurs in 4% to 12% of patients with severe pregnancy-induced hypertension.[51] HELLP syndrome can be associated with subcapsular or intraparenchymal hemorrhage (**Fig. 8**), hepatic rupture, and hepatic parenchymal infarction, and these findings can be seen in 1% of patients with HELLP.[50,52] The differential diagnosis of intrahepatic hematoma in pregnancy includes adenoma, trauma, or rupture of a hepatic artery pseudoaneurysm.[52]

Acute fatty liver of pregnancy is an acute condition usually occurring in the third trimester of pregnancy. A hyperechoic appearance of liver on US or an attenuation of fewer than 40 Houns-field units on noncontrast CT suggests steatosis. MR imaging with in-phase and out-phase imaging can demonstrate a drop in signal, suggesting intracytoplasmic fat deposition.[52]

Pregnancy leads to a hypercoagulable state and increases the risk of Budd-Chiari syndrome, which may occur secondary to hepatic venous or inferior vena cava occlusion. Clinically patients present with abdominal pain, ascites, and hepatomegaly. The clinical presentation and imaging findings may be variable depending on the stage of the disease. Imaging features may include venous occlusion with formation of intrahepatic and systemic venous collaterals, hepatic parenchymal heterogeneity, hepatomegaly, dysmorphic liver, and findings of portal hypertension (**Fig. 9**).[52] Thrombosis

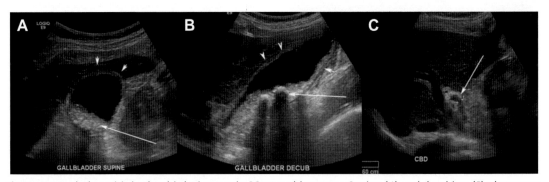

Fig. 4. Acute cholecystitis in the third trimester in 26-year-old woman. Supine (A) and decubitus (B) ultrasonography (US) showing dependent sludge with multiple calculi in the gallbladder (*long arrow in A and B*). The patient had a positive sonographic Murphy sign with diffuse wall thickening (*short arrow*) and pericholecystic edema (*arrowheads*). Additional findings included a mildly dilated common bile duct (*long arrow in C*) secondary to common bile duct stone (not shown here).

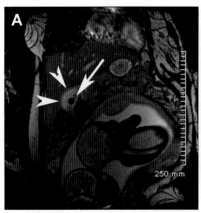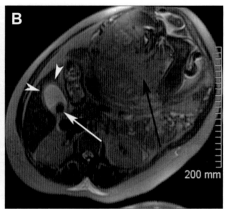

Fig. 5. (*A, B*) Acute cholecystitis in a 22-year-old pregnant patient at 32 weeks' gestation (*black arrow*). Coronal and axial T2-weighted SSFSE image shows cholelithiasis (*white arrow*) with an acutely inflamed gallbladder and wall edema (*arrowheads*).

of some or all of the hepatic veins can be identified sonographically with Doppler evaluation in cases of Budd-Chiari syndrome.

Gastrointestinal Diseases

Gastrointestinal causes of abdominal pain in pregnancy include bowel obstruction, diverticulitis (**Fig. 10**), and inflammatory bowel disease (IBD). Intestinal obstructions complicate as many as 1 in 1500 to 3000 pregnancies.[9,53] These obstructions most often occur in the third trimester, likely resulting from the mechanical effects of the enlarging gravid uterus on the bowel.[54] The maternal mortality rate can be as high as 6%, and the fetal mortality rate may exceed 25% among patients with bowel obstruction.[55] Adhesions account for 60% to 70% of small-bowel obstructions during pregnancy.[54] Other causes include volvulus, hernia, neoplasm, and intussusception. Intestinal obstruction classically presents with the triad of abdominal pain, emesis, and obstipation. The initial imaging approach is an abdominal series of radiographs, with both supine and upright views. If radiographs are inconclusive, additional imaging should not be withheld. A CT or MR imaging scan can show dilated, fluid-filled bowel loops with or without a transition zone (**Fig. 11**). Gangrenous changes in the form of lack of bowel enhancement, or pneumatosis with pneumoperitoneum are ominous signs if seen at imaging. Ultimately, evaluation by a surgeon should not be delayed once the diagnosis is suspected.

The incidence of ulcerative colitis in women younger than 40 years is 40 to 100 in 100,000, and that of Crohn disease is 2 to 4 in 100,000. The exacerbation of IBD during pregnancy may present with bloody diarrhea and crampy abdominal pain.[54] However, disease activity is mostly independent of pregnancy.[56] As in nonpregnant patients, key MR and CT imaging features include mural thickening, mural enhancement, high signal intensity in the bowel wall on T2-weighted images, a narrowed bowel lumen, perienteric inflammation, fibrofatty proliferation, and reactive adenopathy (**Fig. 12**). Complications of IBD include abscess (**Fig. 13**), fistula, sinus tract formation, acute bowel obstruction, and chronic bowel strictures, all of which can be readily detected with MR imaging. MR has excellent sensitivity and specificity, ranging from 88% to 98% and 78% to 100%, respectively, for the detection IBD-related imaging features.[57]

Fig. 6. A 27-year-old woman with acute abdominal pain and elevated lipase in second trimester. MR image of abdomen shows enlargement of pancreatic head with peripancreatic stranding and fluid (*long arrow*). There is pericholecystic fluid (*small arrow*) and extension of inflammation in the Morrison pouch (*circle*). These findings suggest acute pancreatitis. The patient was managed conservatively.

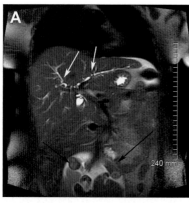
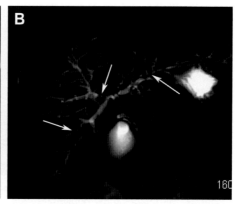

Fig. 7. A 28-year-old pregnant woman with unexplained elevated liver enzymes. MR imaging and MR cholangio-pancreatography (MRCP) were performed to exclude a common bile duct calculus. (*A*) Coronal T2-weighted SSFSE demonstrates areas of narrowing of the biliary tree (*white arrows*) in addition to the gravid uterus (*black arrows*) at the bottom of the image. 3-dimensional volume-rendered MRCP (*B*) demonstrates areas of stenosis (*arrows*) and dilation of the intrahepatic and extrahepatic bile ducts, consistent with primary sclerosing cholangitis. Subsequent to the pregnancy, the patient was diagnosed with ulcerative colitis as well.

Urinary Tract Diseases

Physiologic hydronephrosis is the most significant change in the urinary tract during pregnancy, occurring in about 90% of pregnant women by the third trimester.[4] Symptomatic hydronephrosis occurs in less than 3% of cases.[58] Perinatal outcome is very good, as more than 90% of cases will resolve with conservative treatment.

Obstructive hydronephrosis most commonly occurs as a result of renal calculi. Urolithiasis complicates 1:200 to 1:2000 pregnancies.[59] Presentation with pain is usually after the second trimester

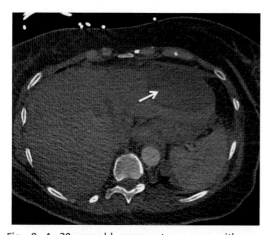

Fig. 8. A 30-year-old pregnant woman with pre-eclampsia, hemolysis, elevated liver enzymes, low platelets, and acute abdominal pain. Axial computed tomography (CT) image shows large subcapsular hematoma (*arrow*) in the left liver lobe. Follow-up CT after 6 weeks (not shown) showed reduction in size of hematoma on conservative management.

when ureteric dilatation is most marked. The diagnosis of obstructive uropathy is challenging during pregnancy, as differentiation between symptomatic urolithiasis and painful hydronephrosis is often difficult.

Sonography is the initial diagnostic test of choice, with accuracy improved by the use of color Doppler to look for Twinkling artifact, use of transvaginal imaging, delineation of ureteral jets (Doppler), and measurement of intrarenal resistance indices, although this latter technique has fallen out of favor.[60] The reported sensitivity, specificity, and accuracy of detecting calculi on US is 40%, 84%, and 53%.[61] However, negative ureteroscopy rates as high as 50% have been reported in pregnant patients when US alone is used.[62]

Low-dose noncontrast CT is a very sensitive (95%–100%) and specific (92%–100%) technique for patients with a negative sonogram and clinically suspected urolithiasis. The average reported fetal radiation dose is 0.7 rad.[63]

MR urography is an alternative imaging technique to CT that has shown excellent preliminary results. Single-shot T2-weighted sequences without and with fat saturation are often used. MR urography findings in physiologic hydronephrosis include extrinsic compression of the middle third of the ureter, lack of visible filling defects, and a collapsed ureter below the pelvic brim. Other MR imaging findings include renal enlargement and perinephric fluid (**Fig. 14**). When distal ureteric calculi are present, the MR urography appearance of a "double kink sign," with constriction at the pelvic brim and the vesicoureteral junction with a standing column of urine in the pelvic

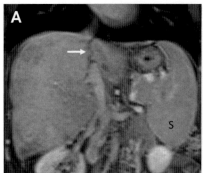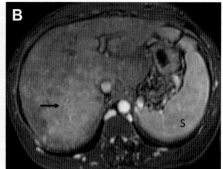

Fig. 9. (*A, B*) A 29-year-old pregnant woman with subacute to chronic changes of Budd-Chiari syndrome. Coronal and axial postcontrast MR images show nonvisualization of inferior vena cava (*white arrow*), heterogeneous hepatic parenchymal enhancement (*black arrow*), and splenomegaly (S). The patient was treated with anticoagulation.

ureter, has been described.[64] MR imaging is also particularly helpful in demonstrating complications of pyelonephritis, such as abscess formation. Diffusion-weighted imaging has been suggested to be useful in differentiating hydronephrosis and pyonephrosis. MR urography has several disadvantages when compared with noncontrast CT because of its poorer spatial resolution, prolonged imaging times, and inferior sensitivity for detecting calcifications and calculi in comparison with low-dose CT.[65] Overall, recent literature reveals that the positive predictive value of CT, MR imaging, and US is 96%, 80%, and 77%, respectively for the detection of urolithiasis during pregnancy.[66] Decisions on the optimal treatment of pregnant women with intractable flank pain must involve assessment of the risks and benefits of diagnostic and therapeutic intervention for the mother and fetus. Treatment includes aggressive hydration and analgesia, and antibiotics for concomitant infection. Renal calculi may pass spontaneously (64%–84%) during pregnancy, but may require stent placement or ureteroscopy in cases that are more complex.[4,67]

Acute pyelonephritis and cystitis may occur in 1% to 2% of pregnancies. Risk factors include nephrolithiasis, recurrent lower urinary tract infection, diabetes mellitus, sickle-cell anemia, and congenital ureteral abnormalities. *Escherichia coli* is the most common infecting organism. Urine and blood cultures should be obtained; however, the initial therapy is usually empiric. Renal US is performed in patients who fail to respond clinically within 3 days or who have recurrent infection. Complications of pyelonephritis are septicemia and renal abscess, and may be associated with premature labor and delivery.

Vascular

Asymptomatic gonadal vein dilatation is often physiologic but may rarely cause pain. Abdominal vascular complications during pregnancy include aneurysm rupture, aortic dissection (**Fig. 15**), and venous thrombosis (apart from Budd-Chiari syndrome discussed earlier). Pregnancy is a hypercoagulable state, with patients at increased risk for venous thromboses of the lower extremities, pelvis, liver (Budd-Chiari syndrome), mesenteric veins (**Fig. 16**), and gonadal veins. There is also increased risk of abdominal aortic, renal, and splenic artery aneurysm rupture.

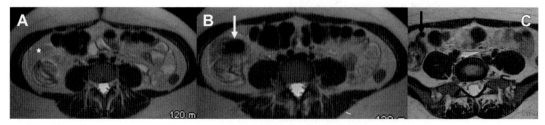

Fig. 10. A 25-year-old, 6-week pregnant woman with noncomplicated, acute right-sided diverticulitis. Axial SSFSE images (*A, B*) demonstrate an inflamed diverticulum (*white arrow in B*) arising from right hemicolon with inflammation in surrounding fat (*star in A*). A normal appendix is identified separately (*black arrow in C*).

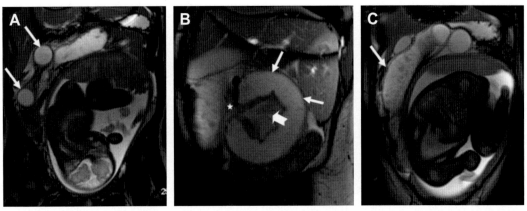

Fig. 11. A 29-year-old primigravida with closed-loop obstruction, presenting with severe abdominal pain. Coronal (*A, C*) and coronal oblique (*B*) steady-state free precession (SSFP) MR images demonstrate multiple dilated bowel loops (*arrows in A–C*) with C-shape of obstructed small-bowel loop (*arrows in B*) and 2 transition points converging to the same site (*star in B*). Note mesenteric congestion and ascites (*notched arrow in B*). Surgical findings confirmed closed-loop obstruction with ischemic bowel. Resection and end-to-end anastomosis were performed. The patient later underwent a normal vaginal delivery at term.

US can be used for evaluation of lower limb thrombus. Acute thrombus typically causes expansion of the lumen and identification of an echogenic thrombus. Noncontrast MR imaging can be effective tool in detecting suspected acute thrombosis in pregnancy (**Fig. 17**). On T1-weighted images, the venous thrombus can be of variable signal intensity, depending on the age of luminal blood products. The MR steady-state free precession sequence demonstrates a luminal thrombus as a low-signal-intensity filling defect, whereas normal vein is seen as high signal intensity with patent lumen. Venous thrombosis on T2-weighted images appears as lack of the normal low-signal-intensity flow void. However, images from these unenhanced MR imaging sequences should be interpreted with caution, as unenhanced sequences can be limited by flow-signal artifacts.[68]

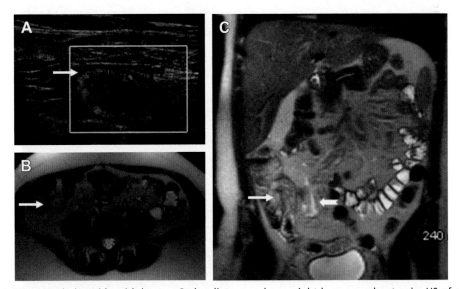

Fig. 12. A 32-year primigravida with known Crohn disease and new right lower quadrant pain. US of abdomen (*A*) reveals circumferential thickening of a small-bowel loop (*arrow*) within the right lower quadrant, with hyperemia on Doppler interrogation. Axial (*B*) and coronal (*C*) SSFSE MR images demonstrate thickened, edematous terminal ileum (*arrow*) with preserved mural stratification. Trace of free fluid is identified within the adjacent mesenteric fat (*notched arrow in C*). MR imaging is important to confirm the diagnosis and rule out complications that may adversely affect the clinical outcome.

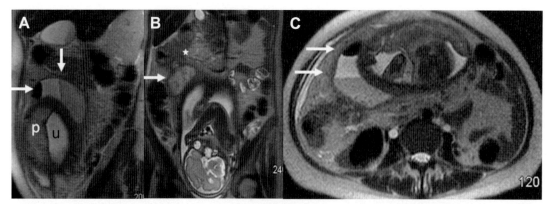

Fig. 13. A 21-year-old, third-trimester pregnant woman with known inflammatory bowel disease. Sagittal (*A*), coronal (*B*), and axial (*C*) SSFSE MR images demonstrate a fluid collection in the right lower abdomen (*arrow in B*) with air-fluid-debris levels within (*arrows in A and C*), suggestive of an abscess juxtaposed to the uterus. Note the presence of inflamed colon adjacent to the abscess (*star in B*). A normal appendix was identified separately. P, placenta; u, uterus. The abscess was drained using fluoroscopic guidance.

Trauma

Approximately 7% of pregnant women experience trauma during their gestation, with the greatest incidence occurring within the last trimester. Falls (52%) are the most common mechanism of injury, and 9.5% of all injuries during pregnancy are intentionally inflicted.[69] Overall, the fetal-loss rate in trauma is reported to be from 1% to 34%, depending on the severity and locations of the injuries.[70]

The gravid uterus displaces the liver and spleen against the ribs and elevates the bladder out of the pelvis, making these structures more prone to

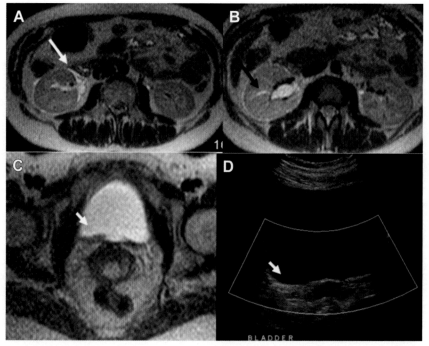

Fig. 14. A 32-year-old, 21-week pregnant woman with renal colic. Axial SSFSE images (*A–C*) demonstrate right perinephric stranding and fluid (*white arrow in A*). Note intrarenal edema (*black arrow in B*) within the parenchyma of right kidney. Also identified is edema of the right ureterovesical junction (*arrow in C*). The patient passed a calculus shortly after the MR imaging. Radiologic findings correlate with the patient's symptom of right renal colic. US of the urinary bladder (*D*) revealed absence of right ureteric jet (*arrow*).

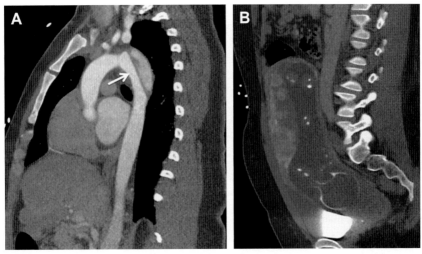

Fig. 15. (*A, B*) A 27-year-old woman with history of Marfan syndrome, presented with acute tearing chest pain at 27 weeks of gestation. The patient underwent CT angiography, which revealed focal dissection involving the aortic arch and proximal descending thoracic aorta (*arrow, A*) without extension into the abdominal aorta (*B*).

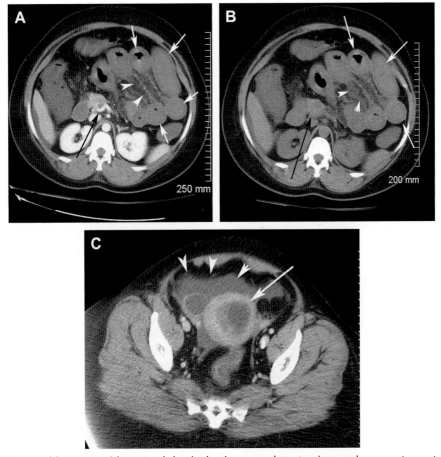

Fig. 16. A 22-year-old woman with acute abdominal pain, severe hypotension, and prearrest symptoms underwent CT with (*A*) and without (*B*) intravenous contrast. There is diffuse thickening of small-bowel loops (*white arrows in A and B*) and edema in the mesentery (*white arrowheads in A and B*). Postcontrast (*A*) there is a filling defect in the superior mesenteric vein (*black arrow in A and B*) and lack of enhancement of the thick small-bowel loops (*white arrows*). Axial image in the pelvis (*C*) reveals a 9-week pregnancy (*arrow*) and free fluid in the pelvis (*arrowheads*). The patient was diagnosed with acute ischemic bowel and had to undergo resection of the majority of the small bowel. She was subsequently found to have Factor V Leiden deficiency.

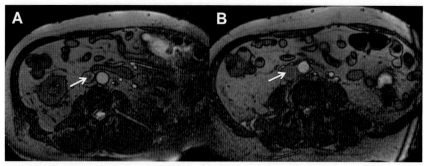

Fig. 17. A 28-year-old woman with known pulmonary embolism during her first trimester underwent noncontrast MR imaging to look for thrombus source. Axial noncontrast T2-weighted SSFP images (*A, B*) through the abdomen show hypointense filling defect (*white arrow*) within the inferior vena cava, suggestive of thrombosis.

injury.[71] Furthermore, the kidneys and spleen enlarge, making them more susceptible to injury (**Fig. 18**).[13] Complications associated with obstetric trauma include internal hemorrhage, placental abruption, uterine rupture, direct fetal injury or demise, and maternal injury or demise. The most common injury to the gravid uterus after blunt trauma is placental abruption. Splenic rupture is the most common cause of free intraperitoneal hemorrhage in pregnant patients.[6] In hemodynamically unstable pregnant women, a focused assessment with sonography for trauma (FAST) examination should be performed during the primary survey to assess for possible sources of bleeding. The specificity of FAST in pregnancy has been shown to be similar to that of nonpregnant patients, and positive findings in unstable patients warrant emergent operative evaluation.[72] However, FAST cannot detect retroperitoneal

hemorrhage, which is more likely in pregnant women because of the increased blood flow to the uterus.[73] CT is the test of choice for injured pregnant patients. When treating pregnant trauma victims, the initial focus should be on maternal resuscitation.[74]

Gynecologic

Gynecologic entities that cause abdominal and pelvic pain during pregnancy include infracting leiomyomas, ovarian torsion, adnexal masses, endometriosis, pelvic inflammatory disease, and ovarian edema. Here the focus is on imaging of red degeneration of fibroid and ovarian torsion.

During pregnancy, the physiologic enlargement of the uterus can alter the blood supply to fibroids, resulting in degeneration. When this occurs, patients may present with localized pain, tenderness, and fever. On MR imaging, a fibroid undergoing degeneration will demonstrate internal high signal intensity on T2-weighted images as a result of edema or presence of fluid attributable to necrosis. On T1-weighted images, the fibroid is usually of heterogeneous signal intensity, with central low signal intensity and foci of peripheral increased signal intensity secondary to internal hemorrhage (**Fig. 19**).

Ovarian torsion affects approximately 7% of known ovarian masses in pregnancy.[75] The prevalence of ovarian torsion during pregnancy is 1 in 1800.[44] Ovarian torsion occurs most often in the first trimester. Classically the ovary is enlarged and edematous, with small peripheral follicles. Ovarian stroma is seen as a central area of low echogenicity on US and as intermediate signal on T2-weighted MR images. Late torsion demonstrates increased signal intensity on T2-weighted images secondary to necrosis. Another specific imaging finding includes identification of a

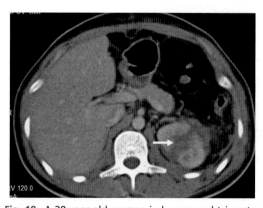

Fig. 18. A 28-year-old woman in her second trimester with a history of blunt trauma following a motor vehicle accident. There is linear grade 3 laceration (>1 cm deep) in the upper pole of the left kidney (*arrow*). Adjacent soft-tissue edema and thickening is also seen along the left lateral abdominal wall.

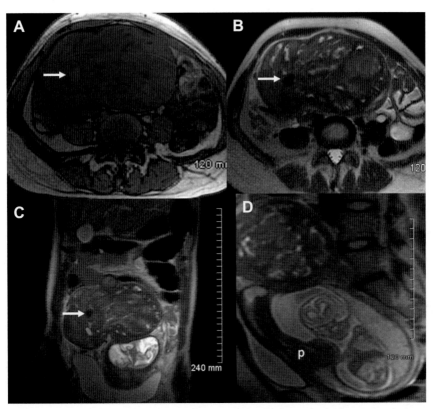

Fig. 19. A 26-year-old woman presented with acute severe abdominal pain in the late second trimester. Axial T1-weighted (*A*), axial (*B*), coronal (*C*), and sagittal (*D*) MR images show large lobulated gravid uterus with multiple uterine fibroids. The fibroids are heterogeneously hypointense on T1-weighted images and show T2-heterogeneous signal hyperintensity. The fibroid shows an area of hemorrhage (*white arrow*) appearing hyperintense on T1-weighted and hypointense on T2-weighted images. It contains a more recent bleeding component with T2-dephasing, suggesting acute hemorrhagic degeneration of fibroid. No relationship with the placenta (p) was seen.

thickened, twisted fallopian tube. On T1-weighted images, the signal intensity of the torted ovary varies according to the presence of internal blood products. Occasionally torsion is associated with an underlying mass, most commonly a teratoma (**Fig. 20**). Identification of intrauterine pregnancy is helpful in differentiating ovarian torsion from ectopic pregnancy.

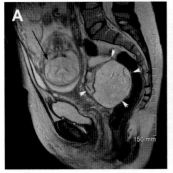
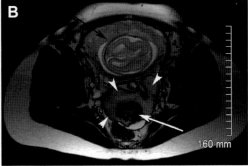

Fig. 20. A 27-year-old woman, approximately 20 weeks pregnant, presents with sudden onset of acute abdominal pain. The sagittal T2-weighted image (*A*) demonstrates a mass (*white arrowheads*) posterior to the gravid uterus (*black arrows*). This mass *arrowhead* was found to be midline on axial images (*B*). There is a heterogeneous low-signal-intensity structure within this mass, which represents the dermoid plug (*white arrow*) of a cystic teratoma. The pain was due to torsion of the long-standing dermoid. A midline position of the adnexal mass in association with severe and sudden onset of pain is a specific sign of torsion.

SUMMARY

Evaluation of abdominal pain in a pregnant patient is often challenging to clinicians and radiologists alike. Abdominal US followed by MR imaging are techniques of choice because of their safety profile for both mother and fetus. However, CT should be considered on a case-by-case basis if its diagnostic yield is expected to be high in problem solving. The principle of ALARA should be followed without compromising diagnostic accuracy. Obtaining informed written consent is an essential part of the imaging protocol. Maternal health is usually the first priority in management. A reliable and reproducible imaging protocol should be deployed when assessing a pregnant patient with an acute abdomen. Although there is no general consensus, this article provides the current up-to-date recommendations, protocols, and imaging appearance for the diagnosis of diverse causes of acute abdomen in pregnancy.

ACKNOWLEDGMENTS

Special thanks to Dr Vivek Virmani, Department of Medical Imaging, University of Ottawa, The Ottawa Hospital, Ottawa, Canada, for contributing to **Figs. 6** and **9**.

REFERENCES

1. Augustin G, Majerovic M. Non-obstetrical acute abdomen during pregnancy. Eur J Obstet Gynecol Reprod Biol 2007;131(1):4–12.
2. Ko CW. Risk factors for gallstone-related hospitalization during pregnancy and the postpartum. Am J Gastroenterol 2006;101:2263–8.
3. Baron TH, Ramirez B, Richter JE. Gastrointestinal motility disorders during pregnancy. Ann Intern Med 1993;118(5):366–75.
4. Fiadjoe P, Kannan K, Rane A. Maternal urological problems in pregnancy. Eur J Obstet Gynecol Reprod Biol 2010;152:13–7.
5. Hepburn IS, Schade RR. Pregnancy-associated liver disorders. Dig Dis Sci 2008;53(9):2334–58.
6. Wang PI, Chong ST, Kielar AZ, et al. Imaging of pregnant and lactating patients: part 1, evidence-based review and. AJR Am J Roentgenol 2012;198(4):778–84.
7. Brent RL. Saving lives and changing family histories: appropriate counseling of pregnant women and men and women of reproductive age, concerning the risk of diagnostic radiation exposures during and before pregnancy. Am J Obstet Gynecol 2009;200:4–24.
8. Koren G. Medication safety in pregnancy and breastfeeding. Philadelphia: McGraw Hill; 2007.
9. Kilpatrick CC, Monga M. Approach to the acute abdomen in pregnancy. Obstet Gynecol Clin North Am 2007;34(3):389–402, x.
10. ACOG Committee on Obstetric Practice. ACOG Committee opinion. Number 299, September 2004 (replaces No. 158, September 1995). Guidelines for diagnostic imaging during pregnancy. Obstet Gynecol 2004;104:647–51.
11. Williams PM, Fletcher S. Health effects of prenatal radiation exposure. Am Fam Physician 2010;82:488–93.
12. Angel E, Wellnitz CV, Goodsitt MM, et al. Radiation dose to the fetus for pregnant patients undergoing multidetector CT imaging: Monte Carlo simulations estimating fetal dose for a range of gestational age and patient size. Radiology 2008;249:220–7.
13. Pearlman MD, Tintinalli JE, Lorenz RP. Blunt trauma during pregnancy. N Engl J Med 1990;323(23):1609–13.
14. Protection of the patient in diagnostic radiology. A report of Committee 3 of the International Commission on Radiological Protection. Ann ICRP 1982;9:1–82.
15. Wagner LK, Huda W. When a pregnant woman with suspected appendicitis is referred for a CT scan, what should a radiologist do to minimize potential radiation risks? Pediatr Radiol 2004;34(7):589–90.
16. Brent RL. Counseling patients exposed to ionizing radiation during pregnancy. Rev Panam Salud Publica 2006;20:198–204.
17. Brent RL. The effect of embryonic and fetal exposure to x-ray, microwaves, and ultrasound: counseling the pregnant and nonpregnant patient about these risks. Semin Oncol 1989;16(5):347–68.
18. International Commission on Radiological Protection. Pregnancy and medical radiation. Ann ICRP 2000;30:iii–viii, 1–43.
19. Streffer C, Shore R, Konermann G, et al. Biological effects after prenatal irradiation (embryo and fetus). A report of the International Commission on Radiological Protection. Ann ICRP 2003;33:5–206.
20. De Wilde JP, Rivers AW, Price DL. A review of the current use of magnetic resonance imaging in pregnancy and safety implications for the fetus. Prog Biophys Mol Biol 2005;87:335–53.
21. Gowland PA, De Wilde J. Temperature increase in the fetus due to radio frequency exposure during magnetic resonance scanning. Phys Med Biol 2008;53:L15–8.
22. Kanal E, Barkovich AJ, Bell C, et al. ACR guidance document on MR safe practices: 2013. J Magn Reson Imaging 2013;37(3):501–30.
23. Hand JW, Li Y, Thomas EL, et al. Prediction of specific absorption rate in mother and fetus associated with MRI examinations during pregnancy. Magn Reson Med 2006;55(4):883–93.

24. Bottomley PA. Turning up the heat on MRI. J Am Coll Radiol 2008;5:853–5.

25. Widmark JM. Imaging-related medications: a class overview. Proc (Bayl Univ Med Cent) 2007;20(4):408–17.

26. Leyendecker JR, Gorengaut V, Brown JJ. MR imaging of maternal diseases of the abdomen and pelvis during pregnancy and the immediate postpartum period. Radiographics 2004;24(5):1301–16.

27. Pedrosa I, Levine D, Eyvazzadeh AD, et al. MR imaging evaluation of acute appendicitis in pregnancy. Radiology 2006;238:891–9.

28. Firstenberg MS, Malangoni MA. Gastrointestinal surgery during pregnancy. Gastroenterol Clin North Am 1998;27(1):73–88.

29. Doberneck RC. Appendectomy during pregnancy. Am Surg 1985;51(5):265–8.

30. Barloon TJ, Brown BP, Abu-Yousef MM, et al. Sonography of acute appendicitis in pregnancy. Abdom Imaging 1995;20(2):149–51.

31. Long SS, Long C, Lai H, et al. Imaging strategies for right lower quadrant pain in pregnancy. AJR Am J Roentgenol 2011;196(1):4–12.

32. Lehnert BE, Gross JA, Linnau KF, et al. Utility of ultrasound for evaluating the appendix during the second and third trimester of pregnancy. Emerg Radiol 2012;19(4):293–9.

33. van Randen A, Bipat S, Zwinderman AH, et al. Acute appendicitis: meta-analysis of diagnostic performance of CT and graded compression US related to prevalence of disease. Radiology 2008;249:97–106.

34. Lazarus E, Mayo-Smith WW, Mainiero MB, et al. CT in the evaluation of nontraumatic abdominal pain in pregnant women. Radiology 2007;244:784–90.

35. Ames Castro M, Shipp TD, Castro EE, et al. The use of helical computed tomography in pregnancy for the diagnosis of acute appendicitis. Am J Obstet Gynecol 2001;184:954–7.

36. Rao PM, Rhea JT, Novelline RA, et al. Helical CT technique for the diagnosis of appendicitis: prospective evaluation of a focused appendix CT examination. Radiology 1997;202(1):139–44.

37. Damilakis J, Perisinakis K, Voloudaki A, et al. Estimation of fetal radiation dose from computed tomography scanning in late pregnancy: depth-dose data from routine examinations. Invest Radiol 2000;35(9):527–33.

38. Hurwitz LM, Yoshizumi T, Reiman RE, et al. Radiation dose to the fetus from body MDCT during early gestation. AJR Am J Roentgenol 2006;186:871–6.

39. Lee KS, Rofsky NM, Pedrosa I. Localization of the appendix at MR imaging during pregnancy: utility of the cecal tilt angle. Radiology 2008;249:134–41.

40. Rapp EJ, Naim F, Kadivar K, et al. Integrating MR imaging into the clinical workup of pregnant patients suspected of having appendicitis is associated with a lower negative laparotomy rate: single-institution study. Radiology 2013;267(1):137–44.

41. Pedrosa I, Lafornara M, Pandharipande PV, et al. Pregnant patients suspected of having acute appendicitis: effect of MR imaging on negative laparotomy rate and appendiceal perforation rate. Radiology 2009;250:749–57.

42. Oto A, Ernst RD, Ghulmiyyah LM, et al. MR imaging in the triage of pregnant patients with acute abdominal and pelvic. Abdom Imaging 2009;34(2):243–50.

43. Ko CW, Beresford SA, Schulte SJ, et al. Incidence, natural history, and risk factors for biliary sludge and stones during pregnancy. Hepatology 2005;41(2):359–65.

44. Spalluto LB, Woodfield CA, DeBenedectis CM, et al. MR imaging evaluation of abdominal pain during pregnancy: appendicitis and other. Radiographics 2012;32(2):317–34.

45. Ralls PW, Colletti PM, Lapin SA, et al. Real-time sonography in suspected acute cholecystitis. Prospective evaluation of primary and secondary signs. Radiology 1985;155(3):767–71.

46. Oto A, Ernst R, Ghulmiyyah L, et al. The role of MR cholangiopancreatography in the evaluation of pregnant patients with acute pancreaticobiliary disease. Br J Radiol 2009;82:279–85.

47. Ramin KD, Ramsey PS. Disease of the gallbladder and pancreas in pregnancy. Obstet Gynecol Clin North Am 2001;28(3):571–80.

48. Polydorou A, Karapanos K, Vezakis A, et al. A multimodal approach to acute biliary pancreatitis during pregnancy: a case series. Surg Laparosc Endosc Percutan Tech 2012;22:429–32.

49. Eddy JJ, Gideonsen MD, Song JY, et al. Pancreatitis in pregnancy. Obstet Gynecol 2008;112:1075–81.

50. Mufti AR, Reau N. Liver disease in pregnancy. Clin Liver Dis 2012;16:247–69.

51. Rooholamini SA, Au AH, Hansen GC, et al. Imaging of pregnancy-related complications. Radiographics 1993;13(4):753–70.

52. Heller MT, Tublin ME, Hosseinzadeh K, et al. Imaging of hepatobiliary disorders complicating pregnancy. AJR Am J Roentgenol 2011;197:W528–36.

53. Parangi S, Levine D, Henry A, et al. Surgical gastrointestinal disorders during pregnancy. Am J Surg 2007;193:223–32.

54. Cappell MS, Friedel D. Abdominal pain during pregnancy. Gastroenterol Clin North Am 2003;32(1):1–58.

55. Perdue PW, Johnson HW Jr, Stafford PW. Intestinal obstruction complicating pregnancy. Am J Surg 1992;164(4):384–8.

56. Mogadam M, Korelitz BI, Ahmed SW, et al. The course of inflammatory bowel disease during pregnancy and postpartum. Am J Gastroenterol 1981; 75(4):265–9.

57. Mazziotti S, Ascenti G, Scribano E, et al. Guide to magnetic resonance in Crohn's disease: from common findings to the more rare complicances. Inflamm Bowel Dis 2011;17(5):1209–22.

58. Rasmussen PE, Nielsen FR. Hydronephrosis during pregnancy: a literature survey. Eur J Obstet Gynecol Reprod Biol 1988;27(3):249–59.

59. Charalambous S, Fotas A, Rizk DE. Urolithiasis in pregnancy. Int Urogynecol J Pelvic Floor Dysfunct 2009;20(9):1133–6.

60. Vallurupalli K, Atwell TD, Krambeck AE, et al. Pearls and pitfalls in sonographic imaging of symptomatic urolithiasis in pregnancy. Ultrasound Q 2013;29(1):51–9.

61. Viprakasit DP, Sawyer MD, Herrell SD, et al. Limitations of ultrasonography in the evaluation of urolithiasis: a correlation with computed tomography. J Endourol 2012;26(3):209–13.

62. Srirangam SJ, Hickerton B, Van Cleynenbreugel B. Management of urinary calculi in pregnancy: a review. J Endourol 2008;22(5):867–75.

63. White WM, Zite NB, Gash J, et al. Low-dose computed tomography for the evaluation of flank pain in the pregnant population. J Endourol 2007; 21(11):1255–60.

64. Spencer JA, Chahal R, Kelly A, et al. Evaluation of painful hydronephrosis in pregnancy: magnetic resonance urographic patterns in physiological dilatation versus calculous obstruction. J Urol 2004;171:256–60.

65. Silverman SG, Leyendecker JR, Amis ES Jr. What is the current role of CT urography and MR urography in the evaluation of the urinary tract? Radiology 2009;250:309–23.

66. White WM, Johnson EB, Zite NB, et al. Predictive value of current imaging modalities for the detection of urolithiasis during pregnancy: a multicenter, longitudinal study. J Urol 2013;189(3): 931–4.

67. Hoscan MB, Ekinci M, Tunckiran A, et al. Management of symptomatic ureteral calculi complicating pregnancy. Urology 2012;80(5):1011–4.

68. Nagayama M, Watanabe Y, Okumura A, et al. Fast MR imaging in obstetrics. Radiographics 2002; 22(3):563–80 [discussion: 580–2].

69. Tinker SC, Reefhuis J, Dellinger AM, et al. Epidemiology of maternal injuries during pregnancy in a population-based study, 1997-2005. J Womens Health (Larchmt) 2010;19(12):2211–8.

70. Sadro C, Bernstein MP, Kanal KM. Imaging of trauma: part 2, abdominal trauma and pregnancy—a radiologist's guide to doing what is best for the mother and baby. AJR Am J Roentgenol 2012;199:1207–19.

71. Grossman NB. Blunt trauma in pregnancy. Am Fam Physician 2004;70(7):1303–10.

72. Richards JR, Ormsby EL, Romo MV, et al. Blunt abdominal injury in the pregnant patient: detection with US. Radiology 2004;233:463–70.

73. Raja AS, Zabbo CP. Trauma in pregnancy. Emerg Med Clin North Am 2012;30(4):937–48.

74. Brown S, Mozurkewich E. Trauma during pregnancy. Obstet Gynecol Clin North Am 2013;40(1): 47–57.

75. Schmeler KM, Mayo-Smith WW, Peipert JF, et al. Adnexal masses in pregnancy: surgery compared with observation. Obstet Gynecol 2005; 105:1098–103.

Gestational Trophoblastic Disease

Alampady K.P. Shanbhogue, MD[a],*, Neeraj Lalwani, MD[b],
Christine O. Menias, MD[c]

KEYWORDS

- Hydatidiform mole • Choriocarcinoma • Magnetic resonance imaging

KEY POINTS

- With the advent of routine ultrasonographic examination in first trimester, most molar pregnancies now present with findings of early pregnancy failure rather than the classic "cluster of grapes" appearance. Ultrasonography has low sensitivity, but high positive predictive value, for the diagnosis of molar pregnancy.
- Pelvic magnetic resonance (MR) imaging can accurately depict the degree of uterine myometrial and extrauterine invasion in malignant gestational trophoblastic disease, and thus aids in the anatomic staging of disease.
- Imaging detection of persistent trophoblastic disease on pelvic MR imaging is determined by the extent of tumor burden as quantified by β–human chorionic gonadotropin (β-hCG) levels. Patients with low β-hCG levels (<500 mIU/mL) often have normal MR imaging findings.
- ^{18}F-Fluorodeoxyglucose positron emission tomography is useful in assessing viable tumor after chemotherapy, detecting occult chemoresistant lesions, differentiating viable from nonviable tumor lesions seen on computed tomography, and confirming complete treatment response after salvage therapy in placental-site trophoblastic tumor or recurrent/resistant gestational trophoblastic tumor.

INTRODUCTION

Gestational trophoblastic disease (GTD) encompasses a spectrum of disease arising from uncontrolled growth of placental trophoblastic tissue, with a spectrum of severity ranging from premalignant hydatidiform mole through malignant invasive mole, choriocarcinoma, placental-site trophoblastic tumor (PSTT), and the extremely rare epithelioid trophoblastic tumor. Early, accurate diagnosis of GTD is necessary to avoid morbidity associated with delayed diagnosis from multidrug chemotherapy and surgery. Most hydatidiform moles are benign, although a small percentage may persist as invasive moles or progress to choriocarcinoma and PSTT.

Pelvic ultrasonography is the initial investigation of choice, as it aids in excluding a normal pregnancy, detecting the molar pregnancy and, in some cases, assessing the local tumor extent. Routine use of antenatal ultrasonography in early pregnancy has brought forth a significant change in the most frequently encountered findings of molar pregnancy from the classic "cluster of grapes" or "snowstorm" appearance to that of missed abortion or failed pregnancy. Magnetic resonance (MR) imaging of the pelvis better delineates the extent of myometrial and extrauterine invasion in invasive mole and choriocarcinoma, and can serve as a problem-solving tool in select cases. The current cure rate of GTD exceeds

The authors have no conflicts of interest to declare.

[a] Department of Radiology, Beth Israel Medical Center, 16th Street and 1st Avenue, New York, NY 10003, USA;
[b] Department of Radiology, University of Washington, 325 9th Avenue, Seattle, WA 98104-2499, USA; [c] Mayo Clinic LL Radiology, 13400 East Shea Boulevard, Scottsdale, AZ 85259, USA
* Corresponding author.
E-mail address: shanbhoguekp@gmail.com

Radiol Clin N Am 51 (2013) 1023–1034
http://dx.doi.org/10.1016/j.rcl.2013.07.011

90%, attributable to routine surveillance using highly sensitive β subunit of human chorionic gonadotropin (β-hCG) and high chemosensitivity of the tumor.[1,2] Although surveillance with β-hCG can serve as an excellent surrogate tumor marker in early detection of disease, it does not indicate the site of recurrence or metastases. Imaging with computed tomography (CT) of the chest, abdomen, and pelvis, and CT or MR imaging of the brain thus play a crucial role in determining the site, and the number and extent of metastases, all of which are important prognostic indicators in the management of GTD.

EPIDEMIOLOGY

Hydatidiform mole, commonly referred to as molar pregnancy, accounts for 80% of all GTDs.[3] Hydatidiform mole is estimated to occur in 0.6 to 1.1 per 1000 pregnancies in North America.[4] Choriocarcinoma, on the other hand, is rare, with an estimated incidence of 1 in 20,000 to 40,000 pregnancies.[4] Approximately 50% of choriocarcinomas arise from molar pregnancies, 25% from term or preterm pregnancies, and the remainder from pregnancy termination.[5] Regional variations have been reported in the incidence of GTD, with an increased incidence in Asia in comparison with North America and Europe.[6,7] For instance, the incidence of hydatidiform mole and choriocarcinoma in southeast Asia is up to 2 per 1000 pregnancies and 9.2 per 40,000 pregnancies, respectively.[7,8] Choriocarcinoma is also reported to be more prevalent in American Indian and African women.[9] Overall, there has been significant decrease in the incidence of GTD over the last 3 decades, which can partially be attributed to improved socioeconomic conditions and dietary changes.[10,11] Some of the established risk factors for GTD include maternal age (both <20 years and >40 years), history of prior molar pregnancy, and history of oral contraceptive use.[7,12] For instance, the risk of subsequent molar pregnancy increases by 1% to 2% after diagnosis of 1 molar pregnancy and 15% to 20% after diagnosis of 2 molar pregnancies.[11] Choriocarcinoma is 1000 times more likely to occur after complete hydatidiform mole compared with other pregnancies.[9] Several other factors such as parity and spontaneous or induced abortions, maternal A and AB blood groups, maternal/paternal A0 or A blood groups, smoking, exposure to pesticides/herbicides, oncogenes, and tumor-suppressor genes have been variably attributed to increase the risk of GTD.[13] Patients with familial molar pregnancy tend to exhibit mutations in the NLRP7 gene at chromosome 19q13.3-13.4.[11]

HYDATIDIFORM MOLE

Hydatidiform mole is a benign but premalignant subtype of GTD originating from fertilization error. Hydatidiform mole is classified into 2 different subtypes, complete hydatidiform mole and partial or incomplete hydatidiform mole, based on the epidemiology, cytogenetics, pathology, natural history, and clinical presentation. Complete hydatidiform mole arises from fertilization of an ovum devoid of maternal chromosomes by a sperm, with subsequent of duplication of paternal DNA. The chromosome in a complete molar gestation is therefore solely paternally derived and has a 46,XX karyotype[14] also termed uniparental disomy. A small number of complete moles (<10%) may carry a 46,XY androgenetic karyotype arising from fertilization by 2 sperms.[15] Partial hydatidiform moles or partial molar pregnancies arise from fertilization of an otherwise healthy ovum by 2 sperms with resultant triploid 69,XXY karyotype.[16] Complete hydatidiform moles therefore do not have any fetal tissue, and partial hydatidiform moles may have an embryo that may survive up to the second trimester.

Clinically the two types of molar pregnancy differ in the mode of presentation, laboratory findings, and prognosis. Complete hydatidiform moles classically present with vaginal bleeding (84%), uterine enlargement (50%), and high levels of hCG (50%).[17,18] Incomplete or partial hydatidiform moles tend to present with signs and symptoms of missed or incomplete abortion, without an enlarged uterus or significantly elevated β-hCG levels.[17,18] Other less common manifestations of hydatidiform mole include anemia, toxemia of pregnancy, hyperemesis gravidarum, hyperthyroidism, and respiratory failure.[19] With the advent of routine early antenatal care, most molar pregnancies are diagnosed on pathologic evaluation after evacuation for early pregnancy failure, and only about one-half of all cases present with vaginal bleeding.[20] Pregnancy-induced hypertension or gestational hypertension in the first trimester of pregnancy is thought to be virtually diagnostic of hydatidiform mole. From a pathologic perspective, complete hydatidiform mole arises from villous trophoblasts and is characterized by trophoblastic hyperplasia, abnormal budding of villi with hydropic appearance, and abnormal villous blood vessels.[11] By contrast, villous hydrops and trophoblastic hyperplasia is typically patchy and focal in partial moles.[11]

Ultrasonography is the initial investigation of choice for the detection of hydatidiform mole. Clinical and laboratory abnormalities may favor a diagnosis of hydatidiform mole, and ultrasonography should be performed in all suspected cases to exclude a normal pregnancy and confirm this diagnosis. On ultrasonography, complete hydatidiform mole classically presents with an enlarged uterus with a heterogeneous endometrial cavity containing multiple small cystic spaces, creating a characteristic "snowstorm" and "cluster of grapes" appearance (Fig. 1). A normal fetus is not visible. Transvaginal ultrasonography may also show invasion of the myometrium, a finding that can predict the recurrence or residual disease after surgical evacuation. Partial mole classically presents with cystic changes to a lesser degree with an associated, usually abnormal fetus (Fig. 2). Although distinction of complete mole from partial mole is not always possible, cystic degeneration of an abnormal placenta in conjunction with the presence of an abnormal embryo and gestational sac is fairly characteristic of partial molar pregnancy.[21] Rarely, molar pregnancy may coexist with a normal gestation (twin molar pregnancy) (Fig. 3). With the advent of routine ultrasonography examination in first trimester, most molar pregnancies now present with findings of early pregnancy failure rather than the classic "cluster of grapes" appearance.[22] Overall, however, ultrasonography is not very sensitive or specific for detection of GTD and identifies less than 50% of all hydatidiform moles.[22,23] Sebire and colleagues[24] reported that ultrasonography accurately detected molar pregnancy in only 34% of 155 pathologically proven molar pregnancies. However, 83% of sonographically suspected cases of molar pregnancy were histopathologically proved (53 out of 63), indicating a high positive predictive value. Overall, the accuracy of ultrasonography for the diagnosis of complete mole was 58% and for partial mole 17%. Benson and colleagues[25] were able to accurately sonographically diagnose 71% (17 of 24) of cases of complete

hydatidiform mole in the first trimester. In the largest series of more than 1000 patients with molar pregnancy, the reported sensitivity, specificity, positive predictive value, and negative predictive value of ultrasonography were 44%, 74%, 88%, and 23%, respectively.[22,23] Therefore, ultrasonography can miss the diagnosis in more than 50% of cases and can give rise to a false diagnosis of molar pregnancy in more than 10% of nonmolar pregnancy losses. Overall, the accuracy of ultrasonography in the detection of complete mole is better than that for partial mole, and increases after the 16th week of gestation. It is also prudent that correlation with serum β-hCG is necessary to distinguish missed abortion from molar pregnancy, and this should be used routinely in first-trimester scanning.[26] Multidetector-row CT (MDCT) findings of molar pregnancy recapitulate the sonographic findings, and manifestation with a distended "fluid-filled" endometrial cavity with areas of abnormal enhancement is characteristic of hydatidiform mole in the setting of abnormally high hCG levels (Fig. 4). MDCT may also show myometrial invasion, as seen in invasive moles (see later discussion). MR imaging can serve as a problem-solving tool in doubtful cases, but is not usually indicated for diagnosis of molar pregnancy. The endometrial cavity typically appears expanded with a heterogeneously high T2 signal intensity, with multiple cystic spaces representing the hydropic villi. These features correlate with the classic multicystic appearance of the endometrium on ultrasonography described as the "cluster of grapes". Noninvasive molar pregnancies demonstrate a normal hypointense myometrial layer surrounding the endometrial cystic changes.[27,28]

The reported incidence of gestational trophoblastic neoplasm (GTN) after evacuation of complete hydatidiform mole ranges from 18% to

A   **B**

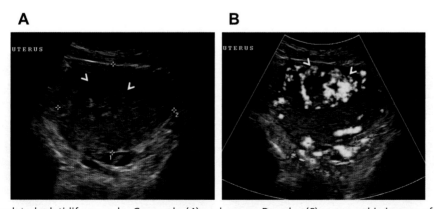

Fig. 1. Complete hydatidiform mole. Gray-scale (A) and power Doppler (B) sonographic images of the uterus demonstrate multiple cystic spaces within the endometrial cavity with increased vascularity (*arrowheads*) in a 22-year-old woman with significantly elevated β-hCG levels. No fetus or gestational sac is seen.

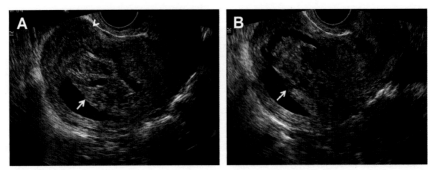

Fig. 2. (*A, B*) Partial hydatidiform mole in a 23-year-old woman with significantly elevated β-hCG levels. Gray-scale sonographic images of the uterus demonstrate cystic changes within the placenta (*arrowhead* in *A*), and an abnormal nonviable fetus (*arrows* in *A* and *B*).

29%, and that of partial hydatidiform mole ranges from 0% to 11%.[9,19] After evacuation, local uterine invasion can be seen in up to 15% of cases of complete hydatidiform mole and in 3% to 5% of partial hydatidiform moles.[9,19] Metastasis is seen in up to 5% of postmolar GTNs that develop after evacuation of complete hydatidiform mole.[9,17,18] An estimated 25% to 40% of patients with complete hydatidiform mole develop theca lutein cysts with ovarian enlargement of more than 6 cm.[29–31] These cysts appear as large, usually bilateral, multicystic ovarian masses that can be seen on ultrasonography, CT, or MR imaging (**Fig. 5**).

MALIGNANT NEOPLASMS

Malignant GTD labeled as GTN include invasive mole, choriocarcinoma, PSTT, and the extremely rare epithelioid trophoblastic tumor. Choriocarcinomas are tumors that arise from villous trophoblast, and PSTTs arise from the interstitial trophoblast.[11] Histologically both subtypes demonstrate malignant epithelial architecture; however, areas of necrosis and hemorrhage are more commonly seen in choriocarcinoma.[32] Similar to

choriocarcinoma, PSTTs can arise from any type of pregnancy and produce β-hCG, but to a lesser extent.[32] Moreover, PSTT exhibits a much more indolent growth pattern with a tendency for lymphatic metastases. It is a rare neoplasm and accounts for less than 1% of all GTD. Epithelioid trophoblastic tumors are extremely rare variants of PSTTs and have been shown to present several years after term delivery. Occasionally, choriocarcinoma remains confined to the substance of the placenta (intraplacental choriocarcinoma). These are thought to be a source of metastatic disease after term pregnancies, including the so-called neonatal choriocarcinoma.[33]

Clinical manifestations of malignant GTD or gestational trophoblastic neoplasia depend on the stage at the time of the diagnosis, including the location and extent of metastases. Whereas seizures, headache, or hemiparesis may be the presenting symptom in patients with brain metastases, hemoptysis, dyspnea, and chest pain indicate pulmonary metastases. Gynecologic symptoms such as vaginal bleeding and pelvic pain may not be seen in a substantial number of patients and, thus, the diagnosis can be missed.

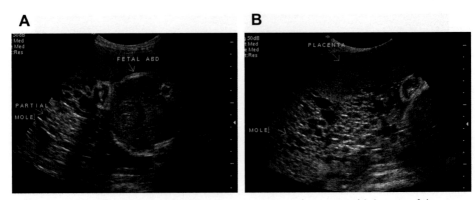

Fig. 3. (*A, B*) Partial hydatidiform mole with twin pregnancy. Gray-scale sonographic images of the uterus demonstrate cystic changes within the placenta; a normal fetus is seen.

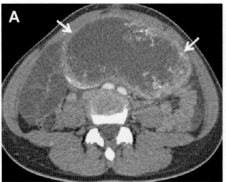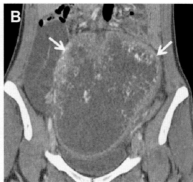

Fig. 4. Complete hydatidiform mole in a 22-year-old woman who presented with rapidly increasing abdominal girth. Qualitative serum hCG was negative. Axial (*A*) and coronal reformatted (*B*) contrast-enhanced CT of the abdomen shows an enlarged uterus with abnormal heterogeneous enhancement of the endometrium as well as multiple small cystic spaces, typical of molar pregnancy (*arrows*). Enlargement of both ovaries was also seen, resulting from increased estrogen levels. There is no evidence of myometrial extension or extrauterine disease. Quantitative β-hCG was more than 1 million IU/L. Dilatation and curettage was performed, with findings consistent with those of complete hydatidiform mole.

However, the presence of an enlarged uterus, irregular bleeding, and persistence of bilateral enlarged ovaries after evacuation of a molar pregnancy should raise the suspicion for postmolar GTN. Some of the criteria used by the Federation of Gynecologists and Obstetricians (FIGO) guidelines for the diagnosis of postmolar GTN include demonstration of a persistently elevated β-hCG over a 2- to 3-week period, histologic diagnosis of choriocarcinoma, documentation of metastases, and persistence of β-hCG 6 months after evacuation of molar pregnancy.[9,34]

On ultrasonography, choriocarcinoma manifests as heterogeneous endometrial masses with varying echogenicity related to the extent of necrosis and hemorrhage. These masses are markedly hypervascular on Doppler interrogation, and may demonstrate myometrial or parametrial invasion. Extension through the myometrium may

also be demonstrated in invasive mole and is not specific to choriocarcinoma. Accurate measurement of uterine size is also essential, as the uterine size is an independent prognostic factor incorporated in the FIGO risk-stratification system.[35] Certain Doppler parameters such as the uterine artery pulsatility index (PI) have been more commonly used in patients with persistent trophoblastic disease, and predict the response to chemotherapy. Agarwal and colleagues,[36] in their prospective study in 239 patients with GTN treated with methotrexate, demonstrated that the uterine artery PI can function as a measure of tumor vascularity, and thus can serve as an independent marker to predict tumor response to chemotherapy. Median uterine artery PI was lower in methotrexate-resistant patients, and a PI of 1 or less predicted methotrexate resistance independent of the FIGO staging/scoring system. For instance, in FIGO score 6 GTN, the risk of methotrexate resistance was 20% in patients with PI<1 vs 100% in patients without PI>1. Lower PI likely reflects more intense tumor neovascularity, thus accounting for poorer response to methotrexate therapy.

MDCT of the chest, abdomen, and pelvis is usually performed for the detection of metastases. The primary uterine mass of GTD manifests as heterogeneously hypervascular mass with or without myometrial or extrauterine invasion (**Figs. 6–8**). CT may also aid in the differentiation of residual molar pregnancy from postmolar GTN (**Fig. 9**). MR imaging is used as a problem-solving tool in equivocal cases and allows detection of local invasion or distant metastases, thereby enabling risk stratification and guiding further management.

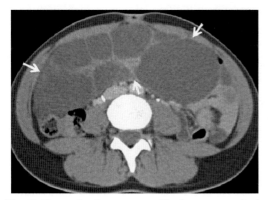

Fig. 5. Theca lutein cysts manifesting as massively enlarged ovary with multiple cysts (*arrows*).

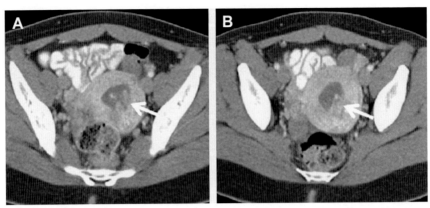

Fig. 6. Invasive mole after evacuation of a complete molar pregnancy in a 17-year-old girl with persistent vaginal bleeding and elevated β-hCG. Axial contrast-enhanced CT images (*A, B*) demonstrate residual endometrial trophoblastic tissue containing multiple cystic spaces and an enhancing component, also extending into the myometrium of the posterior uterine wall (*arrow*), which signifies an invasive component. The patient underwent repeat dilatation and curettage (D&C) and received chemotherapy, and her β-hCG level returned to normal.

MR imaging is rarely required in the diagnosis of choriocarcinoma.[37] Given its excellent contrast resolution and multiplanar capability, MR imaging is preferred over MDCT and ultrasonography for the demonstration of local extent, and can accurately depict the degree of uterine myometrial invasion.[28,38] Invasive mole appears as an infiltrating endometrial lesion that disrupts the junctional zone (as evident on T2-weighted images) invading into or through the myometrium, with cystic areas as well as intensely enhancing solid components (**Fig. 10**).[39] Choriocarcinoma typically presents as heterogeneous endometrial or myometrial mass with areas of necrosis, hemorrhage, and solid enhancing components within the tumor.[40] The signal intensity on T2-weighted images is usually heterogeneously hyperintense, and invasion through the myometrium and extrauterine invasion is also readily detectable on MR imaging.[39] MR imaging may also aid in quantifying the tumor vascularity, and aids in disease staging.[27] However, it should be noted that findings on MR imaging are largely determined by the extent of tumor burden as quantified by β-hCG. Consequently, normal MR imaging findings in a patient with low β-hCG levels (<500 mIU/mL) does not exclude the diagnosis of persistent trophoblastic disease.[38] Following successful chemotherapy, normalization of uterine appearance has been shown to occur within about 6 to 9 months.[41] Intralesional hemorrhage and necrosis can occur after treatment.[41] Persistent uterine vascular malformation has been reported to occur in up to 15% of patients after complete tumor

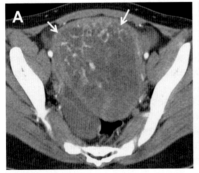
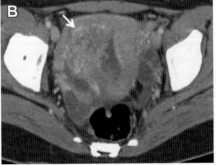
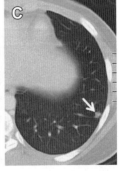

Fig. 7. Postmolar choriocarcinoma with myometrial invasion and lung metastases. A 14-year-old girl presented with irregular vaginal bleeding and an abnormally high β-hCG level (622,136 IU/L). Axial contrast-enhanced CT (*A*) shows a distended endometrial cavity with multiple enhancing septae and nonenhancing cystic components, consistent with molar pregnancy (*arrows*). D&C was performed, which confirmed the diagnosis. One month after D&C she had persistently elevated β-hCG (29,538 IU/L). Axial contrast-enhanced CT 1 month after D&C (*B, C*) shows a heterogeneously enhancing myometrial mass (*arrow in B*) with metastases to the lung (*arrow in C*).

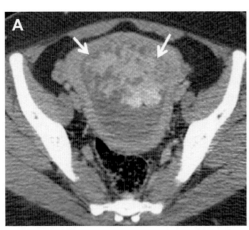
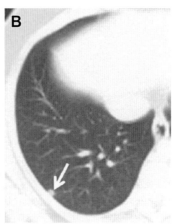

Fig. 8. Choriocarcinoma with lung metastases. A 23-year-old woman with history of 3 prior molar pregnancies presented with abnormally high serum β-hCG and vaginal bleeding. Axial contrast-enhanced CT of the pelvis (A) shows an abnormal heterogeneously enhancing mass within the endometrial cavity (arrows). No myometrial invasion is seen. Axial CT of the chest (B) shows multiple pulmonary nodules consistent with metastases (arrow in B).

response.[27] Placental-site trophoblastic disease manifests with an enlarged uterus containing heterogeneously hyperechoic myometrial mass with cystic change and increased flow on Doppler interrogation.[27,42,43] MR imaging appearances also vary, ranging from hypervascular to hypovascular mass lesions (Fig. 11).[27] Imaging features are therefore nonspecific and do not differentiate this entity from choriocarcinoma or invasive mole.

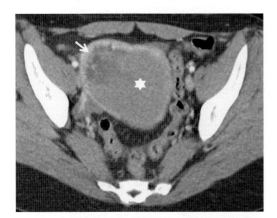

Fig. 9. Residual noninvasive hydatidiform mole in a 23-year-old woman 1 month after D&C for complete mole. Axial contrast-enhanced CT of the pelvis demonstrates high-density contents within the endometrial cavity, consistent with hematometra (asterisk). A sliver of cystic-appearing tissue with mild heterogeneous enhancement is seen in the endometrial cavity peripherally, in the region of the right cornu and at the fundus (arrow). The underlying myometrium is normal, without evidence of invasion. The patient was treated with chemotherapy, and postchemotherapy serum β-hCG declined to zero.

Metastasis occurs in 10% to 19% of GTNs and is primarily hematogenous.[27,44] The lung is the most common site (76%–87%) followed by the liver (10%), brain (10%), kidney, gastrointestinal tract, and spleen.[27,44–47] The vagina is the second most common site of metastasis (30%), but this occurs through contiguous spread rather than hematogenously.[46–48] MDCT of the chest, abdomen, and pelvis is usually performed for metastatic workup. Although CT is more sensitive than chest radiography for detection of pulmonary metastases, with detection of up to 40% of radiographically occult lesions, the clinical significance of these additional lesions has not been established.[49–51] It has also been shown that several pulmonary nodules may persist at the end of successful chemotherapy, and routine follow-up of these nodules does not affect clinical outcome.[49] Given this finding, chest radiography is the recommended initial imaging modality by FIGO in the staging of malignant GTD, both at baseline and after completion of chemotherapy. Pulmonary metastases from choriocarcinoma typically manifest as single or multiple nodules, which are hypervascular and rarely cavitate. Intralesional hemorrhage may be seen, which may manifest as pleural effusion or areas of consolidation. Metastases in the liver, spleen, and gastrointestinal tract also are hypervascular and tend to bleed. ^{18}F-Fluorodeoxyglucose positron emission tomography (FDG PET) imaging has been shown to be potentially useful in select patients with GTNs by superior demonstration of tumor extent and metastases, and assessment of tumor response to therapy in high-risk gestational trophoblastic tumors (GTTs). Given that FDG PET is a functional imaging

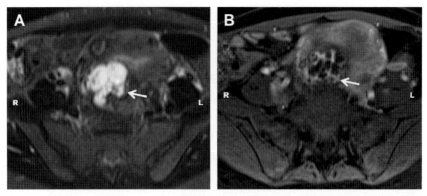

Fig. 10. Invasive mole in a 37-year-old woman who presented with persistently elevated β-hCG 1 month after D&C for complete mole. Axial T2-weighted (A) and T1-weighted gadolinium-enhanced (B) MR images demonstrate a heterogeneous lesion seen in the uterine fundus invading the myometrium, with multiple T2-hyperintense cystic foci, heterogeneous enhancing septae, and multiple nonenhancing cystic spaces (arrow).

technique, it is able to detect occult chemoresistant lesions, differentiate false-positive lesions on CT from true metastases, locate viable tumor after chemotherapy, and confirm complete treatment response after salvage therapy in PSTT or recurrent/resistant GTN.[52]

MANAGEMENT

The unique epidemiology, tumor biology, and chemosensitivity of GTNs allow for an accurate noninvasive diagnosis without histologic examination, even in patients with metastases. Treatment is initiated once the imaging and clinical diagnosis is established. Molar pregnancies are treated with suction curettage followed by blunt curettage of the uterine cavity.[53] Intraoperative ultrasonography has been used as a guide to reduce the risk of uterine perforation.[11] Medical termination is rarely used in partial mole, and carries a risk of persistent trophoblastic disease.[54] In twin pregnancies with one living fetus, current recommendations allow

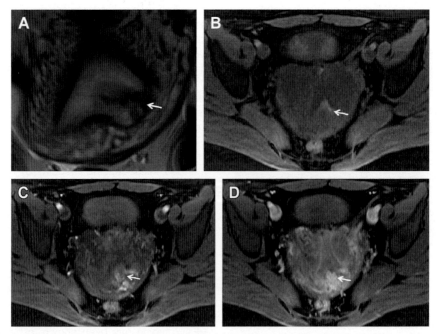

Fig. 11. Placental-site trophoblastic tumor in a 34-year-old woman who developed persistent abnormal uterine bleeding after cesarean section. Coronal T2-weighted MR images of the pelvis demonstrate a polypoid lesion in the left cornu (arrow) that is hypointense on T2-weighted image (A), isointense on T1-weighted image (B), and enhances intensely after gadolinium administration (C, D). The uterus was also mildly enlarged. Serum hCG measured 36.6 IU/L (normal 0–5 IU/L). Hysteroscopic resection and histopathologic analysis was consistent with placental-site trophoblastic tumor. Total abdominal hysterectomy was performed.

Table 1
International Federation of Gynecology and Obstetrics (FIGO) anatomic staging system

Stage	
I	Disease confined to the uterus
II	Gestational trophoblastic neoplasm (GTN) extends outside of the uterus, but is limited to the genital structures (adnexa, vagina, broad ligament)
III	GTN extends to the lungs, with or without known genital tract involvement
IV	All other metastatic sites

age, antecedent pregnancy, interval from antecedent pregnancy, β-hCG concentration, number and site of metastases, size of tumor mass, and history of prior chemotherapy.[11] Placental-site trophoblastic disease, however, is staged: stage I disease is confined to the uterus; stage II disease extends to the genital tract; stage III disease is pulmonary metastases ± extension into the genital tract; and stage IV disease is systemic metastatic disease involving the liver, kidney, spleen, and brain.[11]

Single-agent chemotherapy is the treatment of choice for low-risk disease (score of 0–6). More than 95% of patients developing choriocarcinoma following molar pregnancy belong to this category. Methotrexate or dactinomycin therapy has shown to induce remission in 50% to 90% of these patients.[11] The role of dilatation and curettage in low-risk stage I disease is controversial and may not be necessary.[57,58] Multidrug chemotherapy is necessary for all high-risk disease (FIGO score ≥7).[53] Overall, 80% to 85% of molar pregnancies follow a benign course without local recurrences or metastases; 15% to 20% are invasive; and only around 3% to 5% develop postmolar GTN with metastatic lesions. Both primary and recurrent malignant trophoblastic diseases generally have a good prognosis, with an overall cure rate of more than 90%. The advent of multiagent chemotherapy has enabled a 5-year survival rate of 100% for low-risk GTT and 94% for high-risk GTT.[56] With routine β-hCG surveillance, it is now possible to detect relapse at an early stage. Consequently, cure rates of up to 100% (for low-risk disease) and 84% (for high-risk disease) can be achieved even in patients with relapse.[59] Surgery and radiotherapy are also used in some high-risk patients. PSTTs are usually chemoresistant and hence are treated with a

continuation of pregnancy. It has been shown that risk of malignant sequelae does not depend on the time of evacuation of the molar pregnancy.[1,55] Following initial uterine evacuation, surveillance is done by obtaining weekly serum β-hCG levels until 3 negative levels, followed by monthly β-hCG levels for 6 months to detect recurrence or malignancy.[53] Pregnancy is avoided for 12 months, and early screening ultrasonography is recommended in all subsequent pregnancies given a 1% to 2% risk of recurrence in subsequent pregnancy. Surveillance with serum quantitative β-hCG levels should also be obtained 6 weeks and 12 weeks after any future child birth.[53,56]

Management of invasive mole and choriocarcinoma primarily involves chemotherapy. The FIGO scoring system is used to assess prognosis, predict response to therapy, and guide appropriate management strategy in GTN (**Tables 1** and **2**).[35] It is mandatory for all physicians treating GTN to use this system to allow better comparison of data. Scoring is based on 8 prognostic factors:

Table 2
FIGO scoring system modified from the World Health Organization scoring system

	Scores			
	0	**1**	**2**	**4**
Age	<40	≥40	—	—
Antecedent pregnancy	Mole	Abortion	Term	—
Interval in months from index pregnancy	<4	4–6	7–12	>12
Pretreatment serum β-hCG (IU/L)	$<10^3$	10^3–10^4	10^4–10^5	$>10^5$
Largest tumor size (including uterus)	<3	3–4 cm	≥5 cm	—
Site of metastases	Lung	Spleen, kidney	Gastrointestinal	Liver, brain
No. of metastases	—	1–4	5–8	>8
Previous failed chemotherapy	—	—	Single drug	≥2 drugs

combination of multidrug chemotherapy and surgery, which involves hysterectomy and lymph node dissection. The survival rate for PSTT and epithelioid trophoblastic tumor ranges from 100% for nonmetastatic disease to 50% to 60% for metastatic disease.[56] Long-term survival has also been reported to depend on the site of metastases. Patients with both brain and liver metastases have poorer results (5-year survival 10%) than isolated hepatic metastases (5-year survival 70%).[60,61] Successful pregnancy has been reported in more than 80% of women who undergo chemotherapy.[62] However, women should be advised to avoid pregnancy for up to 12 months after completion of chemotherapy to reduce potential teratogenic effects on the fetus.[11] This approach also enables accurate detection and differentiation of disease relapse from a normal pregnancy. Theca lutein cysts, which often coexist with GTD, may take several months to regress after evacuation of uterine contents.

SUMMARY

GTD is a relatively uncommon, almost completely curable pregnancy-related disorder encompassing a spectrum of disease ranging from benign, premalignant hydatidiform mole to malignant choriocarcinoma. Most hydatidiform moles are now detected early in the antenatal period, and may be mislabeled sonographically as miscarriages or anembryonic pregnancy. Ultrasonography plays a crucial role in excluding a normal pregnancy and establishing the diagnosis of molar pregnancy in women with disproportionately high β-hCG levels. Imaging also plays a quintessential role in the diagnosis, staging, and risk stratification in malignant GTD, including precise localization of metastases as well as determination of the site of disease relapse in patients with elevated β-hCG following chemotherapy or surgery. FDG PET can be used to detect viable tumor after chemotherapy, and may aid in surgical planning for chemoresistant viable residual or recurrent disease.

REFERENCES

1. Seckl MJ, Dhillon T, Dancey G, et al. Increased gestational age at evacuation of a complete hydatidiform mole: does it correlate with increased risk of requiring chemotherapy? J Reprod Med 2004; 49:527–30.
2. Seckl MJ, Gillmore R, Foskett M, et al. Routine terminations of pregnancy—should we screen for gestational trophoblastic neoplasia? Lancet 2004; 364:705–7.
3. Sebire NJ, Foskett M, Fisher RA, et al. Risk of partial and complete hydatidiform molar pregnancy in relation to maternal age. BJOG 2002;109:99–102.
4. Semer DA, Macfee MS. Gestational trophoblastic disease: epidemiology. Semin Oncol 1995;22: 109–12.
5. Soper JT, Mutch DG, Schink JC. Diagnosis and treatment of gestational trophoblastic disease: ACOG practice bulletin no. 53. Gynecol Oncol 2004;93:575–85.
6. Bracken MB. Incidence and aetiology of hydatidiform mole: an epidemiological review. Br J Obstet Gynaecol 1987;94:1123–35.
7. Palmer JR. Advances in the epidemiology of gestational trophoblastic disease. J Reprod Med 1994; 39:155–62.
8. Atrash HK, Hogue CJ, Grimes DA. Epidemiology of hydatidiform mole during early gestation. Am J Obstet Gynecol 1986;154:906–9.
9. Goldstein DP, Berkowitz RS. Current management of gestational trophoblastic neoplasia. Hematol Oncol Clin North Am 2012;26:111–31.
10. Smith HO, Qualls CR, Prairie BA, et al. Trends in gestational choriocarcinoma: a 27-year perspective. Obstet Gynecol 2003;102:978–87.
11. Seckl MJ, Sebire NJ, Berkowitz RS. Gestational trophoblastic disease. Lancet 2010;376:717–29.
12. Buckley JD, Henderson BE, Morrow CP, et al. Case-control study of gestational choriocarcinoma. Cancer Res 1988;48:1004–10.
13. Altieri A, Franceschi S, Ferlay J, et al. Epidemiology and aetiology of gestational trophoblastic diseases. Lancet Oncol 2003;4:670–8.
14. Fisher RA, Newlands ES. Gestational trophoblastic disease. Molecular and genetic studies. J Reprod Med 1998;43:87–97.
15. Pattillo RA, Sasaki S, Katayama KP, et al. Genesis of 46,XY hydatidiform mole. Am J Obstet Gynecol 1981;141:104–5.
16. Lawler SD, Fisher RA, Dent J. A prospective genetic study of complete and partial hydatidiform moles. Am J Obstet Gynecol 1991;164:1270–7.
17. Berkowitz RS, Goldstein DP. Chorionic tumors. N Engl J Med 1996;335:1740–8.
18. Goldstein DP, Berkowitz RS. Current management of complete and partial molar pregnancy. J Reprod Med 1994;39:139–46.
19. Berkowitz RS, Goldstein DP. Clinical practice. Molar pregnancy. N Engl J Med 2009;360:1639–45.
20. Gemer O, Segal S, Kopmar A, et al. The current clinical presentation of complete molar pregnancy. Arch Gynecol Obstet 2000;264:33–4.
21. Naumoff P, Szulman AE, Weinstein B, et al. Ultrasonography of partial hydatidiform mole. Radiology 1981;140:467–70.
22. Fowler DJ, Lindsay I, Seckl MJ, et al. Routine pre-evacuation ultrasound diagnosis of hydatidiform

mole: experience of more than 1000 cases from a regional referral center. Ultrasound Obstet Gynecol 2006;27:56–60.

23. Kirk E, Papageorghiou AT, Condous G, et al. The accuracy of first trimester ultrasound in the diagnosis of hydatidiform mole. Ultrasound Obstet Gynecol 2007;29:70–5.

24. Sebire NJ, Rees H, Paradinas F, et al. The diagnostic implications of routine ultrasound examination in histologically confirmed early molar pregnancies. Ultrasound Obstet Gynecol 2001;18:662–5.

25. Benson CB, Genest DR, Bernstein MR, et al. Sonographic appearance of first trimester complete hydatidiform moles. Ultrasound Obstet Gynecol 2000;16:188–91.

26. Romero R, Horgan JG, Kohorn EI, et al. New criteria for the diagnosis of gestational trophoblastic disease. Obstet Gynecol 1985;66:553–8.

27. Allen SD, Lim AK, Seckl MJ, et al. Radiology of gestational trophoblastic neoplasia. Clin Radiol 2006;61:301–13.

28. Levine D. Obstetric MRI. J Magn Reson Imaging 2006;24:1–15.

29. Berkowitz RS, Im SS, Bernstein MR, et al. Gestational trophoblastic disease. Subsequent pregnancy outcome, including repeat molar pregnancy. J Reprod Med 1998;43:81–6.

30. Santos-Ramos R, Forney JP, Schwarz BE. Sonographic findings and clinical correlations in molar pregnancy. Obstet Gynecol 1980;56:186–92.

31. Wagner BJ, Woodward PJ, Dickey GE. From the archives of the AFIP. Gestational trophoblastic disease: radiologic-pathologic correlation. Radiographics 1996;16:131–48.

32. Baergen RN, Rutgers JL, Young RH, et al. Placental site trophoblastic tumor: a study of 55 cases and review of the literature emphasizing factors of prognostic significance. Gynecol Oncol 2006;100:511–20.

33. Sebire NJ, Lindsay I, Fisher RA, et al. Intraplacental choriocarcinoma: experience from a tertiary referral center and relationship with infantile choriocarcinoma. Fetal Pediatr Pathol 2005;24:21–9.

34. Kohorn EI. Negotiating a staging and risk factor scoring system for gestational trophoblastic neoplasia. A progress report. J Reprod Med 2002;47:445–50.

35. FIGO Committee on Gynecologic Oncology. Current FIGO staging for cancer of the vagina, fallopian tube, ovary, and gestational trophoblastic neoplasia. Int J Gynaecol Obstet 2009;105:3–4.

36. Agarwal R, Harding V, Short D, et al. Uterine artery pulsatility index: a predictor of methotrexate resistance in gestational trophoblastic neoplasia. Br J Cancer 2012;106:1089–94.

37. Green CL, Angtuaco TL, Shah HR, et al. Gestational trophoblastic disease: a spectrum of radiologic diagnosis. Radiographics 1996;16:1371–84.

38. Barton JW, McCarthy SM, Kohorn EI, et al. Pelvic MR imaging findings in gestational trophoblastic disease, incomplete abortion, and ectopic pregnancy: are they specific? Radiology 1993;186:163–8.

39. Nagayama M, Watanabe Y, Okumura A, et al. Fast MR imaging in obstetrics. Radiographics 2002;22: 563–80 [discussion: 580–2].

40. Leyendecker JR, Gorengaut V, Brown JJ. MR imaging of maternal diseases of the abdomen and pelvis during pregnancy and the immediate postpartum period. Radiographics 2004;24:1301–16.

41. Hricak H, Demas BE, Braga CA, et al. Gestational trophoblastic neoplasm of the uterus: MR assessment. Radiology 1986;161:11–6.

42. Sakamoto C, Oikawa K, Kashimura M, et al. Sonographic appearance of placental site trophoblastic tumor. J Ultrasound Med 1990;9:533–5.

43. Sumi Y, Ozaki Y, Shindoh N, et al. Placental site trophoblastic tumor: imaging findings. Radiat Med 1999;17:427–30.

44. Kumar J, Ilancheran A, Ratnam SS. Pulmonary metastases in gestational trophoblastic disease: a review of 97 cases. Br J Obstet Gynaecol 1988;95: 70–4.

45. Soper JT. Identification and management of high-risk gestational trophoblastic disease. Semin Oncol 1995;22:172–84.

46. Berkowitz RS, Goldstein DP. Pathogenesis of gestational trophoblastic neoplasms. Pathobiol Annu 1981;11:391–411.

47. May T, Goldstein DP, Berkowitz RS. Current chemotherapeutic management of patients with gestational trophoblastic neoplasia. Chemother Res Pract 2011;2011:806256.

48. Masselli G, Gualdi G. MR imaging of the placenta: what a radiologist should know. Abdom Imaging 2013;38(3):573–87.

49. Powles T, Savage P, Short D, et al. Residual lung lesions after completion of chemotherapy for gestational trophoblastic neoplasia: should we operate? Br J Cancer 2006;94:51–4.

50. Gamer EI, Garrett A, Goldstein DP, et al. Significance of chest computed tomography findings in the evaluation and treatment of persistent gestational trophoblastic neoplasia. J Reprod Med 2004;49:411–4.

51. Mutch DG, Soper JT, Baker ME, et al. Role of computed axial tomography of the chest in staging patients with nonmetastatic gestational trophoblastic disease. Obstet Gynecol 1986;68:348–52.

52. Chang TC, Yen TC, Li YT, et al. The role of ^{18}F-fluorodeoxyglucose positron emission tomography in gestational trophoblastic tumours: a pilot study. Eur J Nucl Med Mol Imaging 2006;33:156–63.

53. Gerulath AH, Ehlen TG, Bessette P, et al. Gestational trophoblastic disease. J Obstet Gynaecol Can 2002;24:434–46.

54. Newlands ES. Presentation and management of persistent gestational trophoblastic disease and gestational trophoblastic tumours. London: Chapman and Hall; 1997.

55. Sebire NJ, Foskett M, Paradinas FJ, et al. Outcome of twin pregnancies with complete hydatidiform mole and healthy co-twin. Lancet 2002;359:2165–6.

56. Lurain JR. Gestational trophoblastic disease II: classification and management of gestational trophoblastic neoplasia. Am J Obstet Gynecol 2011;204:11–8.

57. Pezeshki M, Hancock BW, Silcocks P, et al. The role of repeat uterine evacuation in the management of persistent gestational trophoblastic disease. Gynecol Oncol 2004;95:423–9.

58. van Trommel NE, Massuger LF, Verheijen RH, et al. The curative effect of a second curettage in persistent trophoblastic disease: a retrospective cohort survey. Gynecol Oncol 2005;99:6–13.

59. Powles T, Savage PM, Stebbing J, et al. A comparison of patients with relapsed and chemorefractory gestational trophoblastic neoplasia. Br J Cancer 2007;96:732–7.

60. Bower M, Newlands ES, Holden L, et al. EMA/CO for high-risk gestational trophoblastic tumors: results from a cohort of 272 patients. J Clin Oncol 1997;15:2636–43.

61. Crawford RA, Newlands E, Rustin GJ, et al. Gestational trophoblastic disease with liver metastases: the Charing Cross experience. Br J Obstet Gynaecol 1997;104:105–9.

62. Woolas RP, Bower M, Newlands ES, et al. Influence of chemotherapy for gestational trophoblastic disease on subsequent pregnancy outcome. Br J Obstet Gynaecol 1998;105:1032–5.

Three-dimensional Volumetric Sonography in Gynecology
An Overview of Clinical Applications

Linda Armstrong, DO, Arthur Fleischer, MD*,
Rochelle Andreotti, MD

KEYWORDS

• 3D pelvic sonography • Uterine anomalies • IUD localization

KEY POINTS

- Three-dimensional (3D) sonography of the uterus is a method that allows reconstruction of the coronal plane, which better evaluates uterine disorders and their relationships to the endometrial canal.
- Approximately 9% of all women with infertility are affected by uterine anomalies.
- 3D sonography can help establish intrauterine device positioning, even when it normal on two-dimensional images.
- 3D sonography is a cost-effective and quick way to evaluate a variety of pelvic disorders.

INTRODUCTION

Three-dimensional (3D) pelvic sonography has become a problem-solving technique in evaluation of a variety of gynecologic disorders such as uterine anomalies, endometrial disorders, fibroids, intrauterine device (IUD) localization, adnexal masses, and tubal disorders. It should be used as a standard imaging protocol in the evaluation of most of these disorders. It can add significant clinical information to that obtained by two-dimensional (2D) imaging, and it can also be used selectively for evaluation of adnexal masses. This article provides examples of clinical applications.

3D sonographic imaging of the female organs allows rapid acquisition of ultrasound images with the ability to display volume-rendered images of the uterus, ovaries, and adnexa. It has the potential to decrease operator dependency compared with 2D imaging because volume acquisitions should contain all of the anatomic information, which can subsequently be reviewed and manipulated by a different operator in various planes. Any desired plane can be obtained from the volume of data that is acquired, stored, and reformatted. Volumetric imaging has the potential to improve patient management. It requires selective evaluation of the acquired volume and may be limited by accessibility to optimal scan planes for image acquisition.

In the evaluation of the uterus, the most useful plane that can be obtained with 3D transvaginal sonography (TVS) is the coronal view of the uterus and adnexa. This plane cannot routinely be acquired by standard 2D acquisitions. The outline and internal contour can be reconstructed to show the shape of the uterus and endometrium, which includes the fundal contour and uterine cornua as well as the contiguity of adnexal disorders involving the fallopian tube. These images can be used to better detect uterine disorders, including the evaluation of uterine anomalies, presence and position of endometrial polyps and uterine leiomyomas, IUD positioning, and evaluation of adnexal or endometrial masses. The coronal plane may also be used to confirm the contiguity of adnexal structures that represent the fallopian

Department of Radiology, Vanderbilt University Medical Center, 1161 Medical Center Drive, Medical Center North, Suite CCC-1121, Nashville, TN 37232, USA
* Corresponding author.
E-mail address: arthur.fleischer@vanderbilt.edu

Radiol Clin N Am 51 (2013) 1035–1047
http://dx.doi.org/10.1016/j.rcl.2013.07.005

tube. In contrast, in the evaluation of the pelvic floor, the most useful view is the axial plane, which cannot be acquired using 2D imaging but can be reconstructed using 3D volume manipulations. These 3D-rendered images may also allow the patient and the ordering physicians to better understand the imaging findings and assist with intraoperative planning.[1]

Other major contributions of 3D imaging include Doppler evaluation within 3D volumes, improved anatomic evaluation of the pelvic organs, and more accurate volume measurements to better assess therapy. Vessels and volume of flow can be localized within an area of interest.[2] 3D imaging allows the vascularity within a volume to be quantitated. Volume measurements can be made from the original data set. The volume can also be analyzed with power Doppler.[3] 2D imaging depends on the operator to obtain appropriate images and can miss important findings or anatomy. Volume imaging can be reviewed at a later time, even if it was not originally perceived by the primary operator or if the patient is no longer available. The images can be reviewed and discussed at a later time. 2D sonography has limited depiction of the anatomy in the coronal plane. 3D ultrasound allows the assessment of the coronal plane, which is valuable in assessing the external contour, uterine anomalies, evaluation of uterine polyps or leiomyomas, and assessment of IUD placement. Exact anatomic relationships can also be reconstructed and recorded.

NORMAL ANATOMY/IMAGING TECHNIQUE

At present, sonographic acquisition can be obtained via a transabdominal or transvaginal approach. However, the transvaginal approach has become the most useful for reconstruction of the coronal plane with 3D imaging. This view was not previously obtainable with 2D ultrasound via the transvaginal approach. Most standard imaging protocols obtain 2D images first, with images being obtained if an abnormality is detected or suspected. A pitfall of relying on 2D images before obtaining 3D images is that the primary operator may not perceive an abnormality on the 2D images. Some uterine anomalies may not be perceived on 2D imaging, and could be missed if 3D imaging is not performed.

The transvaginal probe with 3D capability has automated sector capability. The operator holds the transducer in place while the probe sweeps across the obtained volume. The images are electronically stored. 3D images are then processed and modified, and can then be displayed in multiple planes and orientations. The data can be displayed on the screen as sagittal, coronal, and axial planes. The operator can view or manipulate the displayed images in one plane, and the same manipulations apply to the other planes. The operator can manipulate these displays to show the uterine cavity, serosal contour, or in inverse mode. The uterine cavity can be better delineated to show polyps or leiomyomas. The serosal contour can be shown when there is a question of congenital uterine anomalies. The myometrium can be windowed to better show the intramural leiomyomas and their relationship to one another. The inverse mode, which changes a hypoechoic structure to an echogenic structure, can show the inside of a volume as a cast.[4] This feature is helpful in showing a dilated fallopian tube. These images are obtained in addition to selected 2D transvaginal and transabdominal images of the uterus and adnexa. Once displayed on the screen, the data can be manipulated with the following steps to obtain the coronal plane. The coronal plane is most important for the uterus, but it can be manipulated to gather information in any plane. If other planes are desired, they can also be obtained in a similar fashion.

1. Place a reference point within the midportion of the endometrium on the sagittal plane.
2. Rotate the image to align the long axis of the endometrium parallel with a horizontal line.
3. Place the reference point within the midportion of the endometrium, again on the transverse plane.
4. Rotate the transverse plane image to align the long axis of the endometrium parallel with a horizontal line.
5. The midportion of the coronal plane should be properly aligned when displayed.
6. Window and level the image to best display the contrast between the endometrium and myometrium.
7. The fourth quadrant shows the surface-rendered image.

IMAGING FINDINGS/PATHOLOGY

The coronal view of the uterus is one of the most important benefits of 3D sonography. 2D sonography was once limited with this view because it was obscured by the bony pelvis and limited by the port of entry of the probe. 3D sonography can reconstruct this plane to better display normal anatomy and affords better depiction of abnormal anatomy. The uterine cavity and outline of the serosal surface can be reconstructed as well. This reconstruction allows diagnosis or confirmation of suspected uterine or endometrial findings, which is especially beneficial to confirm the location of IUDs, fibroids, and endometrial polyps.

UTERINE ANOMALIES

Uterine anomalies may be associated with the inability to achieve pregnancy. In addition, there is a higher proportion of issues of infertility in the first trimester and pregnancy loss in the second trimester in patients with known uterine anomalies compared with patients with a normal uterus.[5] These müllerian anomalies are seen in approximately 5% of all women, with approximately 8% of all women with infertility being affected.[6] Other studies have estimated that higher numbers of women with infertility are affected.

Uterine anomalies are related to müllerian duct development, fusion, and septal resorption defects. If one of the müllerian ducts fails to develop or develops incompletely, a unicornuate uterus develops. About 65% of these are associated with rudimentary horns. This condition leads to failure of development of half the uterus. On sagittal 2D imaging, this can be mistaken for a normal uterus (**Fig. 1**A). 3D sonography assists in delineating the central uterine cavity and outer serosal contour (see **Fig. 1**B 3D for a transvaginal image in the coronal plane).

In failure of fusion of the müllerian ducts, uterine didelphys or bicornuate uterus can develop. In uterine didelphys, 2 uteri and cervices develop and the uterine horns are widely separated. This condition can be confused with a bicornuate uterus. With a bicornuate uterus, there is incomplete fusion of the fundal uterine horns leaving intervening myometrium from the fundus to the cervix. However, there is a distinct fundal cleft that is greater than 1.0 cm, as shown on the coronal image.

Uterine septate malformations are more common than bicornuate malformations. This condition results from failure of resorption of the uterovaginal septa (the outer contour of the uterus has already fused at this point), which usually leaves a smooth outer contour. There can be a fundal cleft of less than 1.0 cm. The fundal contour is usually smooth or convex (**Fig. 2**). These women have the highest risk of reproductive complications. This anomaly can be mistaken for bicornuate uterus on 2D sonography. It is important to differentiate these two uterine entities because septate uteri can be treated with hysteroscopic resection of the septum, and bicornuate uteri are not treated. An arcuate uterus shows a single uterine cavity with identification of a small cleft at the fundal myometrium that is greater than 1.5 cm. The outer uterine contour is convex or flat, and can easily be missed on 2D sonography (**Fig. 3**).

For diagnosis of certain uterine anomalies, careful attention during 2D imaging through the transverse sections shows a double endometrial/myometrial echo. This imaging is best performed during the secretory phase of the menstrual cycle, when the endometrium is thickest. The double endometrium can be evaluated within the midportion of the uterus. 3D evaluation of septate and bicornuate uterus is useful. For arcuate and unicornuate uterine malformations, 3D sonography is necessary because these may not always be seen on 2D imaging.

Accurate diagnosis of uterine anomalies is most essential in those patients with infertility and recurrent spontaneous abortions. Women with bicornuate and unicornuate uteri have increased risk of miscarriage, preterm birth, and fetal malpresentation. Women with arcuate uteri have a higher proportion of preterm labor and second trimester loss compared with those with normal uteri.[7,8] The specific differentiation between the septate uterus and bicornuate uterus has proved challenging in the past, which is especially important in their implications for infertility. Septate uterus has a higher risk of spontaneous abortion and infertility and can be treated surgically with good success. The septate uterus is the most common uterine anomaly, whereas a bicornuate uterus usually requires no surgery.[7,8] 3D

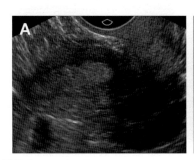
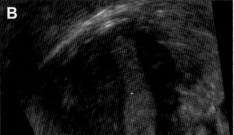

Fig. 1. (*A*, *B*) Unicornuate uterus.

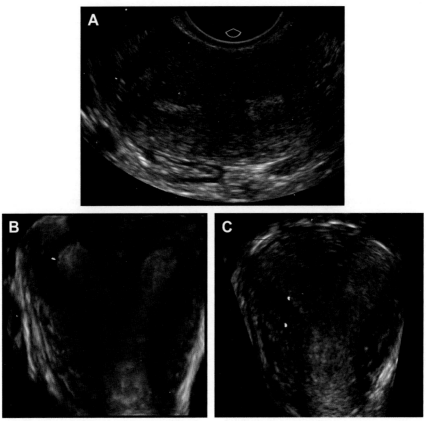

Fig. 2. (*A–C*) Septate uterus: 2 islands of endometrium are seen, suggesting a uterine anomaly on 2D imaging. 3D imaging (*B* and *C*) confirms that there is no fundal serosal surface indentation.

sonography can differentiate between these entities. It is particularly invaluable in unicornuate uterus, which often appears normal on 2D imaging. 3D sonography also helps in uterine anomalies with a rudimentary horn, which can become a potential site for ectopic pregnancy.

In the past, uterine anomalies were often investigated by routine 2D sonography or contrast hysterosalpingography. These modalities can be limited in evaluation of the outer serosal contour. Furthermore, hysterosalpingography involves radiation and the presence of a radiologist or

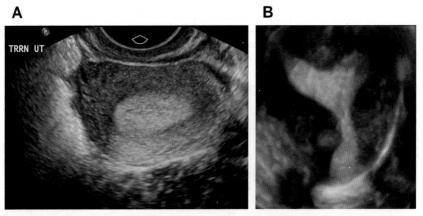

Fig. 3. (*A*, *B*) Arcuate uterus: this appears normal on transverse imaging. (*B*) 3D sonographic images show an arcuate-configuration uterus. A submucosal polyp is also better delineated on the right side.

gynecologist. The development of 2D saline infusion hysterosonography (SIS) allowed evaluation of the inner uterine cavity, but was also limited in evaluation of the outer contour of the uterus, which involves a sterile saline solution that is instilled into the uterine cavity before multiple images are subsequently obtained. With 3D sonography, the outer contour and inner cavity can be assessed in a quick sweep. More investigations are showing that 3D sonography is more accurate than laparoscopy or magnetic resonance (MR) imaging.[8,9] MR imaging is limited when the uterus is retroflexed and when there is adjacent bowel peristalsis. MR imaging is more expensive and time consuming. Several investigators report that the accuracy of 3D sonography is similar to surgical findings but without the morbidity and cost of surgery.[9–11]

LEIOMYOMAS

Evaluation of the endometrium and myometrium for leiomyomas is important for clinical management. They can be a significant source of morbidity caused by pelvic pain, mass effect, and bleeding. Leiomyomas are the most common uterine neoplasm. Leiomyomas are usually described in terms of their location because their location can affect their treatment. Subserosal leiomyomas project from the intraperitoneal surface and into the pelvis. Intramural leiomyomas are confined to the myometrium and submucosal leiomyomas project from the myometrium into the endometrium (**Fig. 4**).

Leiomyomas present with a variable sonographic appearance depending on their relative composition of smooth muscle and connective tissue. They tend to be hypoechoic, often with areas of increased attenuation or acoustic shadowing. They can calcify once they outgrow their blood supply and degenerate. On color Doppler imaging, they usually have a peripheral distribution of vessels.

The distinction between submucosal and intramural leiomyomas can prove challenging on 2D imaging because multiple leiomyomas can cause artifacts that obscure the borders of other leiomyomas. It can also be challenging on 2D imaging, especially when multiple leiomyomas are present, to assess the location of each mass and their proximity to one another. 3D imaging allows a better depiction of the uterine cavity to better assess the location of the leiomyomas, submucosal or intramural components, and location compared with

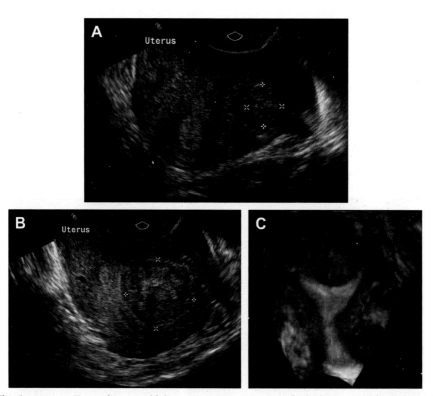

Fig. 4. (*A–C*) Leiomyomas. Two submucosal leiomyomas are seen, one of which is central fundal and the other is seen near the left cornua. Their relationship to each other and the endometrium is better delineated on 3D sonography.

other leiomyomas. 3D imaging allows an exact depiction of the location of the leiomyoma to the endometrium and their relative sizes.

The relative vascularity of leiomyomas can often be better assessed with 3D imaging before and after embolization. Detecting ovarian collaterals before possible uterine artery embolization is important because embolization can sometimes negatively affect ovarian function. Hypervascular fibroids tend to respond to treatment better than isovascular or hypovascular fibroids. It can also be used to assess for completeness of embolization after a procedure and assess for uterine and ovarian collaterals before embolization,[12] which is important for possible myomectomy, embolization, or ablation of submucosal leiomyomas for preservation of fertility. A thick endometrium plays an important role in assessing the uterine cavity because it presents a contrast with the adjacent myometrium. With a thin endometrium, particularly in patients who are postmenopausal or have had prior ablation, it can be challenging to assess the location of leiomyomas and reformat the 3D imaging.

POLYPS/ADHESIONS

The coronal plane of 3D imaging is a useful adjunct to 2D imaging for the delineation of the location and number of endometrial polyps. Polyps are common benign endometrial lesions seen mainly in perimenopausal and menopausal women. Polyps have a nonspecific appearance on sonogram but often appear as a focal, round, echogenic mass that projects within the endometrial lumen, and they can also present as endometrial thickening. They can contain punctate cysts that represent glandular elements. A prominent feeding artery can be seen on color Doppler extending into the pedicle (**Figs. 5** and **6**).

Once one polyp is detected, there is a 20% chance of other polyps being present.[13] Polyps can often be obscured by a thickened, heterogenous endometrium. Sonohysterograms can be used to assess for polyps because the saline outlines the borders of the polyps. The two modalities can be complementary because 3D imaging allows precise and reliable localization of polyps and fibroids within the uterine cavity with sonohysterography. The endometrial cavity outline can be assessed for additional polyps. La Torre and colleagues[14] showed that 3D sonography combined with saline sonohysterography detected all polyps in their series. Specificity of 3D imaging alone had a specificity of 89% versus 70% with 2D imaging and 100% with 3D SIS. Sylvestre and colleagues[15] showed high sensitivity and specificity with 3D sonohysterography in the detection of polyps, concluding that hysteroscopy could be avoided if this examination is normal.

ADHESIONS

Endometrial adhesions can be suspected in patients in whom focal narrowing of the normal endometrial thickness is seen. They can also present as echogenic bands that bridge the uterine cavity. If the bands are thick and fibrotic, they can blend into the endometrium. These bands can be seen as Asherman syndrome after a clinical history of infertility, pregnancy loss, menstrual abnormalities, or cyclic pelvic pain. These bands are conventionally assessed with sonohysterography or hysterosalpingography. 3D sonography allows visualization of the exact size of the uterine cavity, and allows a better evaluation of any areas of possible distortion (**Fig. 7**). The cavity can sometimes be of normal size. The bands can be better visualized on 3D sonogram, and the severity can be better characterized for treatment.[16,17]

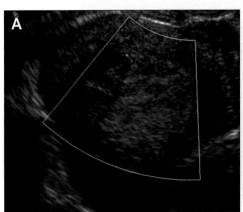
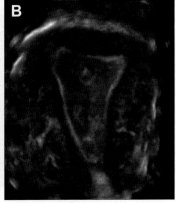

Fig. 5. (*A, B*) A prominent feeding vessel is seen on color Doppler imaging associated with an ill-defined hypoechoic area within the endometrium. On 3D sonography, more polyps are seen.

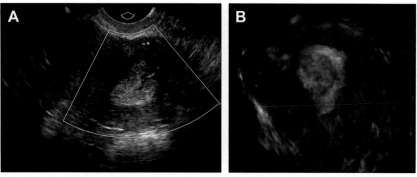

Fig. 6. (*A, B*) A large polyp is seen on 2D imaging within the endometrial canal, with a prominent feeding vessel. 3D images show the polyp as a large filling defect within the endometrial canal.

IUD PLACEMENT AND INTRATUBAL DEVICES

IUD is an increasingly prevalent and effective form of birth control. Most are T shaped and many have a metallic portion. Almost all are hyperechoic with associated extensive shadowing, which can limit evaluation on 2D imaging. The shadowing can sometimes be confused for the IUD. 2D sonography can sometimes mistakenly show normal placement of an IUD that is low lying or partially embedded into the myometrium (**Fig. 8**).

There is a significantly higher proportion of patients with pelvic pain and/or bleeding with abnormally located IUDs compared with those with normally positioned IUDs.[18]

When assessing IUD placement, the operator should review all the images to ensure that the shadow from the IUD arms and shaft are not incorrectly mistaken for the IUD. The main longitudinal axis of the IUD should align with the uterine cavity. The top of the T portion should extend horizontally through the fundal part of the endometrium. There are instances in which the IUD may appear normal on the sagittal and transverse images, but 3D sonography can show malpositioning (**Fig. 9**).

The IUD is considered abnormal in position if any part of it extends past the endometrial cavity or into the myometrium or cervix. Some patients have a small endometrial cavity or anatomic variant that causes abnormal IUD positioning. 3D transvaginal sonography allows precise determination of the amount of myometrial embedment. Pregnancy with an IUD can occur and is associated with ectopic pregnancy because the device prevents normal endometrial implantation. The 3D images can help locate the IUD in relation to an intrauterine gestation (**Fig. 10**).

Sonography can also assess the location of Essure devices. These devices are a permanent form of contraceptive. They are seen sonographically as echogenic metallic coils extending from the cornual portion of the endometrium into the proximal tubes (**Fig. 11**). These devices can also be depicted in a reconstructed coronal image.

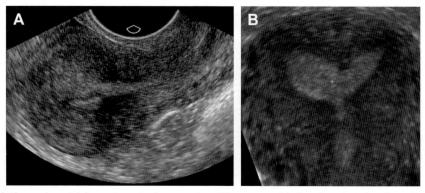

Fig. 7. (*A, B*) The endometrial canal can look normal on 2D sonographic imaging, but the distortion within the mid and lower canal is best seen on the 3D coronal images. The distortion was caused by adhesions.

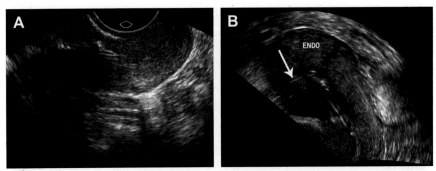

Fig. 8. (A, B) Malpositioned IUD seen partly within the cervix on the sagittal imaging. 3D imaging confirms the low position with the arms deployed into the myometrium (*arrow*).

POLYCYSTIC OVARIAN DISEASE

Criteria for polycystic ovarian syndrome were standardized in 2003 by the Rotterdam Consensus Conference, which established 2D sonography criteria for the evaluation of polycystic ovarian syndrome when 2 of 3 criteria were documented (in the absence of other endocrinopathy): chronic anovulation, hyperandrogenism, pelvic sonogram showing greater than or equal to 12 follicles measuring 2 to 9 mm in diameter, or ovarian volume greater than or equal to 10 mL. Battaglia and colleagues[18] found that ovaries in patients with polycystic ovarian syndrome had a higher stromal volume than the normal controls, which facilitated follicular count. Some studies have shown that ovarian stromal echogenicity is increased in polycystic ovarian syndrome, which is a criterion that can be difficult to compare reliably. Other studies have shown that polycystic ovaries have more pronounced vascularity. 3D sonography affords accurate depiction of follicles and stromal volume. 3D imaging can often more accurately depict overall vascularity.

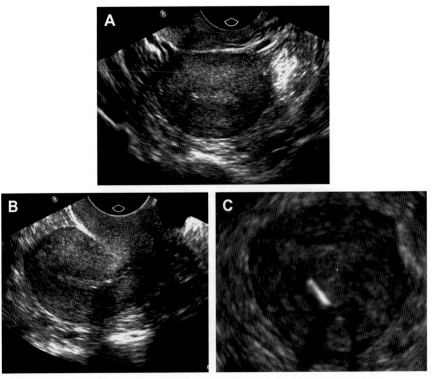

Fig. 9. (A–C) This malpositioned IUD was to the right within the endometrium, and the arms were not deployed. This IUD was best seen on 3D imaging (C).

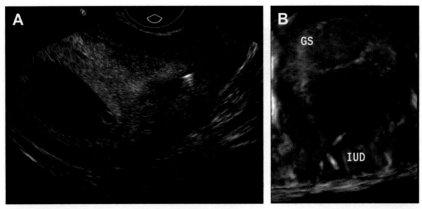

Fig. 10. (*A, B*) This IUD is seen within the lower uterine segment and cervix. A gestational sac is seen within the uterus. The 3D imaging shows the relationship of the IUD and gestational sac. The IUD is in the endocervical canal.

Pelvic Floor

3D transperineal sonography of tape and mesh implants

Many women are affected by pelvic floor disorders, which manifest as stress incontinence, fecal incontinence, and prolapse of pelvic organs. Transperineal sonography (TPS) can evaluate the pelvic floor dynamically. It can also be used to evaluate location of suburethral tensionless vaginal tape (TVT), whereas MR imaging has difficulty depicting the device. TPS can detect recurrence of cystocele, enterocele, or rectal prolapse. It can also detect herniation around the mesh, retraction of the mesh, and dislodgement of the mesh. 3D TPS provides direct visualization of the pelvic floor structures relative to the urethra, vagina, and rectum (**Fig. 12**A), particularly within the axial plane in which the urethra, vagina, and rectum/anus are depicted. The major muscles of the pelvic floor can be evaluated with real-time imaging, which is of particular benefit when evaluating TVT as well (see **Fig. 12**B, C).[19]

Adnexa

Adnexal masses

3D sonography has also contributed to evaluation of the adnexa. It can be used to assess spatial relationships, evaluate walls of structures for possible papillary projections, and to calculate volumes. Tumor vascularity within the volume can be better assessed. 3D evaluation can allow better depiction of the morphology of ovarian masses, including papillary excrescences, septa, solid components, and mixed echogenicity (**Fig. 13**). 3D angiography allows independent operators to review the vascularity of tumors (**Fig. 14**).

Kalmantis and colleagues[3] found that irregular and randomly branching dispersed vessels were associated with ovarian malignancy on evaluation with 3D sonography. They found that 3D sonography helped in obtaining detailed characterization of ovarian masses and had higher diagnostic accuracy in differentiating malignant from benign ovarian tumors. In particular, 3D sonography is superior for showing papillary projections,

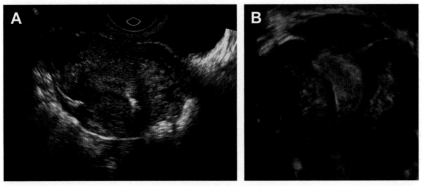

Fig. 11. (*A, B*) Essure devices are seen as linear echogenic structures projecting from the cornual endometrium into the tubes.

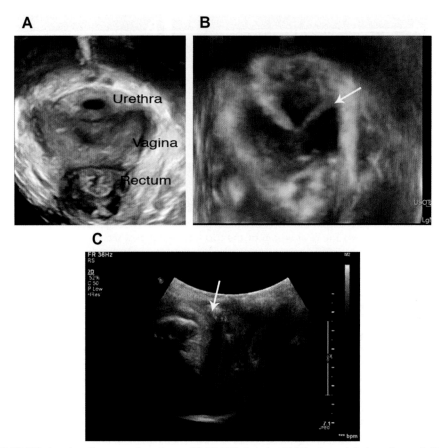

Fig. 12. (*A*) 3D TPS showing the normal anatomy. (*B*) 3D TPS showing TVT in the axial plane (*arrow*). (*C*) 2D image of TVT in the sagittal plane (*arrow*). ([*A*] *Courtesy of* B. Benacceraf, MD.)

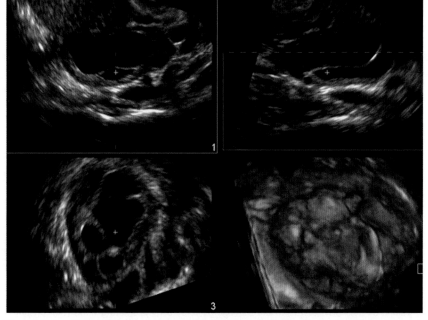

Fig. 13. Multiloculated cystic ovary, better seen on 3D ultrasound (3). Papillary excrescences are excluded.

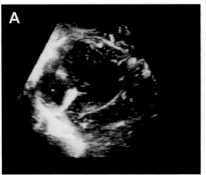 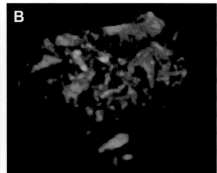

Fig. 14. (*A, B*) 3D power Doppler of a papillary serous carcinoma shows a prominent feeding artery and neovascularity. Abnormal branching pattern of the vessels is seen in this malignant polyp (*B*).

showing irregular walls of cysts, and evaluating septae.

3D power Doppler (PD) can also be performed on adnexal masses. The 3D probe can be used on a region of interest to estimate vascular indices such as the vascularization index (VI), flow index (FI), and vascularization-flow index (VFI). The VI is a percentage of color voxels in the studied volume that represent the blood vessel within the tissue. The FI is the average color value of all color vessels, and represents the blood vessels within the tissue. The VFI is the average color value of all gray and color vessels, representing blood flow and vascularization or perfusion. Alcázar and colleagues[20] sampled suspicious areas within tumors, particularly in cystic/solid tumors. 3D PD-derived indices were significantly higher in malignant tumors. FI was significantly higher in malignant tumors and there were no differences in the VI and VFI. Other investigators have also found FI, VI, and VFI to be increased in malignant tumors. 3D PD can be performed of a larger area, but data may be misled by voxels coming from nontissue areas in the volume as well as from artifacts or noise in cystic areas.

These images and indices can help the clinician to decide on the proper management of the adnexal masses. They may have the capability to reduce false-positives and change operative management, which could affect morbidity because a lymph node dissection could be performed along with a different surgical path in patients with suspected malignancy.

TUBAL DISORDERS

Tubal structures such as a hydrosalpinx can appear as a row of cysts on normal 2D imaging. With 3D imaging, connections between the supposed multiple cysts can show a dilated tube and allow a correct diagnosis (Fig. 15). These connections can be traced back to the cornua of the uterus, and intraluminal endosalpingeal folds can be better depicted.

The tube can then be displayed in multiple planes to give an accurate diagnosis. An inverse mode can also show the tube well in cases in which the tube does not fit a single plane. Other tubal disorders, such as a tubo-ovarian abscess, can also be better depicted with 3D sonography,

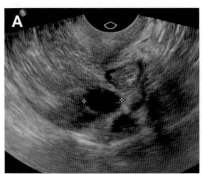 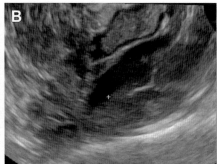

Fig. 15. (*A, B*) Hydrosalpinx. Transverse image through the adnexa shows a cystic-appearing structure. 3D sonography shows a tube with endosalpingeal folds, consistent with a hydrosalpinx.

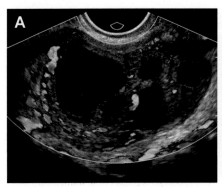 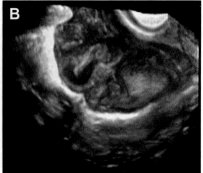

Fig. 16. (*A, B*) Tubo-ovarian abscess. The tubal nature is better seen on 3D sonography. This patient also presented with leukocytosis and fevers.

which clearly shows the tubal nature, whereas in other circumstances it could be confused for an ovarian mass (**Fig. 16**).

PITFALLS AND VARIANTS

The faster the speed of the volume acquisition, the lower the resolution of the images, and this affects the quality and appearance of the images. The large amount of data acquired from 3D imaging requires many data to be retrieved or archived, which can be slower and more cumbersome for older picture archive and communication system. 3D imaging requires more user input than 2D imaging because the data must be manipulated after being obtained. Artifacts in 3D sonography can sometimes be difficult to recognize. These artifacts can be confusing and compounded within a volume.[1] It is important to review the images from which the volume has been obtained in order to recognize these artifacts. If the data are manipulated with inappropriate settings, artifacts can be created, which can alter the diagnosis. The data manipulation can be difficult when inexperienced users are trying to acquire images too quickly.

SUMMARY

3D sonography can significantly improve on the diagnostic ability of 2D sonography of the pelvic organs. 3D sonography has become a problem-solving technique in the evaluation of a variety of gynecologic disorders involving the uterus, adnexa, and pelvic floor. It allows an accurate depiction of the uterine cavity and outline of the uterus in the coronal plane, which is difficult to visualize on 2D imaging. It is possible that volumetric techniques may shorten examination times, thereby improving patient throughput. Future improvements in 3D TVS may involve matrix array

transducers and afford live 3D or four-dimensional imaging.

Other modalities such as MR imaging are limited because of cost, patient size, time, and artifact from adjacent bowel peristalsis. Computed tomography is also costly, has the added risk of radiation and intravenous contrast reaction, and is also more expensive than ultrasound. 3D sonography is less expensive, is convenient, and does not have the risk of radiation or potential nephrotoxicity from contrast that other imaging modalities have. It is a cost-effective tool to assess the pelvic organs.

REFERENCES

1. Benacerraf BR, Benson CB, Abuhamad AZ, et al. Three and 4 dimensional ultrasound in obstetrics and gynecology: proceedings of the American Institute of Ultrasound in Medicine Consensus Conference. J Ultrasound Med 2005;24:1587–97, 2.
2. Jokubkiene L, Sladkevicius P, Rovas L, et al. Assessment of changes in volume and vascularity of the ovaries during the normal menstrual cycle using three dimensional power Doppler ultrasound. Hum Reprod 2006;216:2661–8.
3. Kalmantis K, Rodolakis A, Daskalakis G, et al. Characterization of ovarian tumors and staging ovarian cancer with 3-dimensional power Doppler angiography: correlation with pathologic findings. Int J Gynecol Cancer 2013;23(3):469–74.
4. Flesicher AC, Toy EC, Lee W, et al. Sonography in obstetrics and gynecology: principles and practice. New York: McGraw Hill; 2011.
5. Woelfer B, Salim R, Banerjee S, et al. Reproductive outcomes in women with congenital uterine anomalies detected by three dimensional ultrasound screening. Obstet Gynecol 2001;98:1099–103.
6. Chan YY, Jayaprakasan K, Zamora J, et al. The prevalence of congenital uterine anomalies in unselected and high-risk populations: a systematic review. Hum Reprod Update 2011;17(6):761–71.

7. Chan YY, Jayaprakasan K, Tan A, et al. Reproductive outcomes in women with congenital uterine anomalies: a systematic review. Ultrasound Obstet Gynecol 2011;38(4):371–82.

8. Bocca SM, Abuhamad AZ. Use of 3-dimensional sonography to assess uterine anomalies. J Ultrasound Med 2013;32(1):1–6.

9. Faivre E, Fernandez H, Deffieux X, et al. Accuracy of three-dimensional ultrasonography in differential diagnosis of septate and bicornuate uterus compared with office hysteroscopy and pelvic magnetic resonance imaging. J Minim Invasive Gynecol 2012; 19(1):101–6.

10. Ludwin A, Pityński K, Ludwin I, et al. Two- and three-dimensional ultrasonography and sonohysterography versus hysteroscopy with laparoscopy in the differential diagnosis of septate, bicornuate, and arcuate uteri. J Minim Invasive Gynecol 2013; 20(1):90–9.

11. Deutch T, Bocca S, Oehninger S, et al. Magnetic resonance imaging versus three-dimensional transvaginal ultrasound for the diagnosis of mullerian anomalies. Fertil Steril 2006;86(Suppl):S308.15.

12. Muniz CJ, Fleischer AC, Donnelly EF, et al. Three-dimensional color Doppler sonography and uterine artery arteriography of fibroids: assessment of changes in vascularity before and after embolization. J Ultrasound Med 2002;21(2):129–33.

13. Rumack CM, Wilson SR, Charboneau JW, et al. Diagnostic ultrasound. New York: Elsevier; 2011.

14. La Torre R, De Felice C, De Angelis C, et al. Transvaginal sonographic evaluation of endometrial polyps: a comparison with two dimensional and three dimensional contrast sonography. Clin Exp Obstet Gynecol 1999;26(3–4):171–3.

15. Sylvestre C, Child TJ, Tulandi T, et al. A prospective study to evaluate the efficacy of two- and three-dimensional sonohysterography in women with intrauterine lesions. Fertil Steril 2003;79(5):1222–5.

16. Knopman J, Copperman AB. Value of 3D ultrasound in the management of suspected Asherman's syndrome. J Reprod Med 2007;52(11):1016–22.

17. Benacerraf BR, Shipp TD, Bromley B. Three-dimensional ultrasound detection of abnormally located intrauterine contraceptive devices which are a source of pelvic pain and abnormal bleeding. Ultrasound Obstet Gynecol 2009;34(1):110–5.

18. Battaglia C, Battaglia B, Morotti E, et al. Two- and three-dimensional sonographic and color Doppler techniques for diagnosis of polycystic ovary syndrome. The stromal/ovarian volume ratio as a new diagnostic criterion. J Ultrasound Med 2012;31(7):1015–24.

19. Fleischer AC, Harvey SM, Kurita SC, et al. Two-/three-dimensional transperineal sonography of complicated tape and mesh implants. Ultrasound Q 2012;28(4):243–9.

20. Alcázar JL, Iturra A, Sedda F, et al. Three-dimensional volume off-line analysis as compared to real-time ultrasound for assessing adnexal masses. Eur J Obstet Gynecol Reprod Biol 2012;161(1):92–5.

Role of Interventional Procedures in Obstetrics/ Gynecology

Jorge Lopera, MD[a],*, Rajeev Suri, MD[a],
Ghazwan M. Kroma, MD[a], Andres Garza-Berlanga, MD[a],
John Thomas, MD[b]

KEYWORDS

- Uterine fibroid • Uterine leiomyomata • Uterine artery embolization • Postpartum hemorrhage
- Pelvic congestion syndrome • Fallopian tube recanalization • Transcervical sterilization

KEY POINTS

- In uterine fibroid embolization (UFE), knowledge of the potential ovarian-uterine anastomoses is important because they provide collateral blood flow that may result in the failure of the UFE or ovarian nontarget embolization.
- Uterine artery embolization is an alternative treatment of postpartum hemorrhage with bleeding control in the order of 80% to 90% and in which the uterus and patient fertility can be preserved.
- Diagnosis of pelvic congestion syndrome on routine sonographic or computed tomography/ magnetic resonance imaging is often missed, because venous distension may not be prominent in the supine and non-Valsalva position.
- Fallopian tube recanalization allows couples to have unlimited attempts to conceive naturally and avoids the risks (multiple pregnancies, ovarian hyperstimulation syndrome), and high cost of in vitro fertilization.

INTRODUCTION

Interventional radiology plays an important role in the management of many conditions of the female reproductive tract. This article reviews current techniques and outcomes of uterine artery embolization (UAE) for the management of symptomatic fibroids and for the often life-threatening bleeding conditions during pregnancy and delivery. It also reviews the role of endovascular treatment of pelvic congestion syndrome and the often underused fluoroscopy-guided fallopian tube (FT) interventions.

UTERINE FIBROID EMBOLIZATION
Introduction

Uterine fibroids are the most common tumor found in women. Approximately 25% of premenopausal women have fibroids,[1] whereas the overall prevalence of these tumors could be as high as 77%.[2] The incidence of fibroids in African American women is 3 times that of White women.[3] These benign tumors are hormone dependent, often increasing in size during pregnancy and decreasing in size after menopause.[4]

Author Contributions: Uterine fibroid embolization, G.M. Kroma; postpartum hemorrhage, A. Garza-Berlanga; pelvic congestion syndrome, R. Suri; fallopian tube interventions, J. Lopera; images, J. Thomas; editing, J. Lopera.
[a] Department of Radiology, UT Health Science Center at San Antonio, 7703 Floyd Curl Drive, San Antonio, TX 78229, USA; [b] Methodist Hospital, 7700 Floyd Curl Drive, San Antonio, TX 78229, USA
* Corresponding author.
E-mail address: lopera@uthscsa.edu

Radiol Clin N Am 51 (2013) 1049–1066
http://dx.doi.org/10.1016/j.rcl.2013.07.008
0033-8389/13/$ – see front matter © 2013 Elsevier Inc. All rights reserved.

The presence of symptomatic fibroids is the commonest indication for hysterectomy, accounting for approximately one-third of those performed.[5] As an alternative, myomectomy can be done in some cases to preserve the ability to conceive. Medical treatment of the uterine fibroids using a gonadotropin-releasing hormone analogues, has been also used in some cases; however, its effect to reduce the fibroid size is reversible. The first pelvic embolization specifically for the treatment of symptomatic uterine fibroids was performed in France by Ravina and colleagues,[6] initially as a treatment preceding myomectomy to reduce blood loss, and the investigators discovered that many of the patients cancelled their surgery because of almost complete disappearance of their symptoms.

At present, uterine fibroid embolization (UFE) is well-established minimal invasive treatment of symptomatic uterine fibroids.

Diagnosis

The location of the fibroid is classified as subserosal, submucosal, or intramural and is probably more important than size in causing the symptoms (**Fig. 1**).[7] Prolonged and intensive cyclical menstrual bleeding is the most frequent clinical presentation of submucosal fibroids. Bulk symptoms are usually caused by subserosal fibroids that compress the nearby pelvic structures, resulting in the associated symptoms of pain, urinary frequency, and constipation. Uterine fibroids may

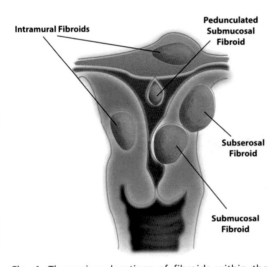

Fig. 1. The various locations of fibroids within the uterus. Submucosal fibroids indent into the uterine cavity. They may also be almost entirely within the cavity. Intramural fibroids are located within the wall of the uterus. Subserosal fibroids extend from the surface of the uterus.

affect fertility,[8] usually because of a submucosal fibroid distorting the endometrial cavity.[9]

Magnetic resonance (MR) imaging is the preferred method for accurately characterizing pelvic masses. Fibroids are typically well-defined masses of low signal intensity compared with the myometrium on T2-weighted (T2W) images and isointense to the myometrium on T1-weighted (T1W) images (**Fig. 2**).[10,11]

MR imaging is also used both to predict and to assess the response of fibroids to UFE. Fibroids that show high signal on T1W images before embolization are likely to have a poor response to UFE because they may already have outgrown their blood supply and undergone hemorrhagic necrosis. High signal on T2W images before embolization has been shown to be a predictor of good response.[12] The vascularity of a fibroid shown by gadolinium enhancement is also a predictor of good response to UFE (**Fig. 3**). Post-UFE fibroids typically show high signal on T1W images because of hemorrhagic necrosis (**Fig. 4**).

Anatomic note

In approximately 10% of women, the blood to the uterine fundus is supplied by the ovarian arteries. The ovarian artery may, rarely, supply blood to most of or the entire uterus. In 40% of women, the ovarian artery solely supplies the ovary, whereas there is a shared supply with the uterine artery in 30% of women (**Fig. 5**). In 10% of patients, the uterine artery is the main supply to the ovaries. Knowledge of these ovarian-uterine anastomoses is important because they provide collateral blood flow that may result in the failure of the UFE or ovarian nontarget embolization.

Patient selection

The typical patient is a premenopausal woman with prolonged regular bleeding during menses without bleeding between periods (menorrhagia). Irregular or intermenstrual bleeding (menometrorrhagia) should raise the suspicion of other disorders and an endometrial biopsy is essential to exclude endometrial carcinoma. The initial diagnosis is confirmed by MR imaging, which also allows the differentiation of the fibroids from other pathologic conditions (endometrial carcinoma, leiomyosarcoma, adenomyosis, and endometrial polyp). Patient desire to conceive should be discussed before the procedure. Despite reports of pregnancies following UFE,[13] prospective studies are needed to determine the effect of UFE on the ability of women to conceive. In addition, the small risk of early menopause as a result of UFE should be discussed with the patient. It is more likely to occur in women in their mid-40s

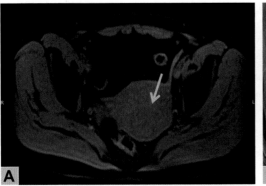
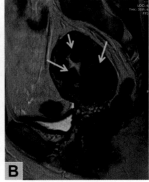

Fig. 2. MR imaging of the uterine fibroids. (*A*) Axial T1-weighted image showing intramural lesion (*arrow*) that is isointense to the uterus. (*B*) Sagittal T2-weighted image showing multiple hypointense intramural and pedunculated submucosal fibroids (*arrows*).

or older patients who are already nearing menopause.

Technique

Different techniques have been described to access the uterine arteries.[14–17] Because of extensive intrauterine collateral flow, bilateral Uterine Artery Embolization (UAE) is necessary to achieve fibroid infarction.[16,18] Catheterization is typically performed by the right common femoral artery approach with the use of Cobra catheter. Some practitioners use coaxial microcatheters to access the uterine artery to reduce the potential for spasm. Ipsilateral catheterization is commonly performed using the Waltman loop technique.[19] Others use the Roberts catheter (Cook Inc, Bloomington, IN), which is specifically designed for UFE with a long, reversed secondary curve. Some interventionalists[20] advocate using a bilateral femoral approach to reduce the radiation dose to the ovaries by simultaneously injecting the embolic agent into both uterine arteries.

Embolic material

The median size of the arteries in the perifibroid plexus is approximately 500 μm.[21] For that reason, most investigators use particles larger than 350 μm. Earlier reports described the use of polyvinyl alcohol (PVA) particles as the embolic agent. The main drawback of these particles is their propensity to aggregate in the syringe or catheter, causing catheter blockage or potentially proximal occlusions. At present, Embosphere (Biosphere Medical, Rockland, MA) particles have gained popularity. Their main advantage compared with PVA is a hydrophilic feature that prevents aggregation and facilitates delivery of the particles. The end point of the embolization generally depends on the embolization material and personal experience of the operator. As a rule, the Embospheres propagate deeper than PVA because of the elastic features of the particle. For this reason, most researchers recommend a less aggressive approach to embolization than with the use of PVA. Moderate flow is maintained to the uterine vessels while achieving a pruned-tree appearance

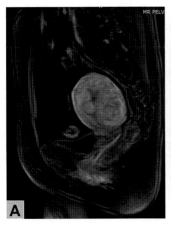
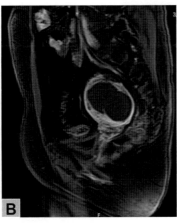

Fig. 3. MR imaging sagittal images after gadolinium enhancement. (*A*) Enhancing intramural fibroids. (*B*) Lack of enhancement after UFE indicating good response.

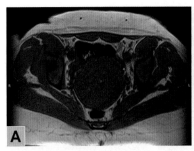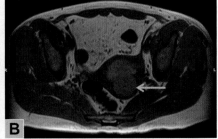

Fig. 4. Axial T1-weighted images of the pelvis. (*A*) Isointense intramural fibroid. (*B*) After UFE with hyperintense fibroid (*arrow*) indicating good response with hemorrhagic necrosis.

to the fibroids (**Fig. 6**). This approach is in contrast with the stagnant flow that is usually achieved with PVA.[12,22,23]

Postprocedure care

Postembolization syndrome with severe pain, fever, and an increase in the white blood count occurs in as many as 34% of patients.[12] Periprocedural pain control is of the utmost importance because it represents the major morbidity of the procedure. Pain generally starts early after the embolization and reaches the highest severity 24 to 48 hours after embolization. Most pain protocols use a combination of opioids and nonsteroidal antiinflammatory analgesics (nonsteroidal antiinflammatory drugs [NSAIDs]). The addition of superior hypogastric nerve block has been shown to enhance pain control, enabling the procedure to be offered with minimum pain on a routine outpatient basis.[24] Excessive use of narcotic can result in nausea and constipation, which can be managed by antiemetic and laxative as needed.

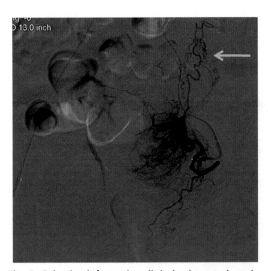

Fig. 5. Selective left uterine digital subtracted angiographic image showing vascular fibroid with uterine to ovarian anastomosis (*arrow*).

Routine use of antibiotics after UFE is not supported by most studies.

Results

The technical success rate of the procedure is high: 84% to 100%.[12,15,25–30] Difficulties in accessing the uterine artery or arterial spasm are the main causes of failure. The fibroids and uterus decrease in size following the embolization (**Fig. 7**). Overall shrinkage of the dominant fibroid is 40% to 70%, and of the uterus is 40% to 60%.[25,31] The overall clinical response of UFE is close to 90%. Menorrhagia is the most common indication for UFE and has the best response rate (81% to 100%).[12,22] For bulk-related symptoms, the success rate is 61% to 100%. Lack of response to embolization may be caused by perfusion to the fibroids by ovarian collaterals. In cases of an enlarged ovarian artery, selective embolization may be performed if definite fibroid supply is shown.[32,33] Ovarian embolization may increase the risk of ovarian failure. The effect of the UFE on fertility is still under investigation and, because of the risk of ovarian failure and possible hysterectomy, we generally do not recommend UFE for patients who desire pregnancy when surgical and medical options are available.

Complications

UFE has a low overall complication rate. Four deaths related to UFE are known among more than 15,000 cases.[34–36] Two are from pulmonary embolus and 2 from infection. This rate compares favorably with the mortality for hysterectomy performed for benign disease, which is 1 in 1600 operations.[37] Complications related to the catheterization are rare, with less than 1% reported throughout most studies. Fibroid expulsion is an uncommon event after UFE, with up to a 5% rate in 2 large studies.[16,29] The intrauterine necrotic fibroid tissue may become infected and cause significant morbidity. Patients may expel the necrotic tissue but often require gynecologic

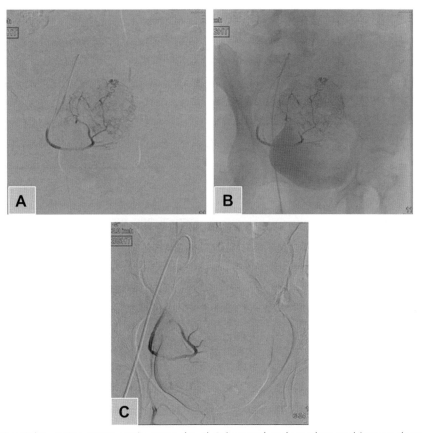

Fig. 6. Selective right uterine artery angiograms. (*A, B*) Subtracted and unsubtracted images showing vascular fibroid. (*C*) Pruned-tree appearance to the fibroid after UFE.

assistance. There is also a risk of hysterectomy if the debris cannot be removed or if the patient becomes septic. Infection is another complication that is related directly to ischemia of the fibroids or uterus. Endometritis and pyometra are responsible for most postembolization hysterectomies. Many patients experience amenorrhea for 1 or 2 months after UFE. Most have their periods

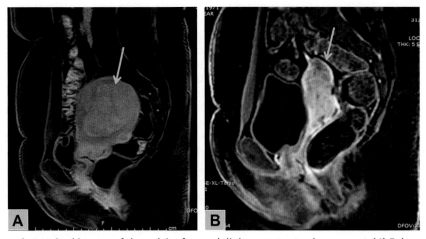

Fig. 7. MR imaging sagittal images of the pelvis after gadolinium contrast enhancement. (*A*) Enlarge uterus with large enhancing intramural fibroid (*arrow*). (*B*) The uterus and the fibroid are significantly decreased in size 4 months after UFE (*arrow*).

resume. However, a few go on to permanent amenorrhea; in most studies the incidence is less than 5% of cases.[12,31,38] The cause is probably nontarget embolization; however, other causes are possible, such as radiation to the ovaries.

Summary

UFE has become a commonly used procedure for the treatment of uterine fibroids. Symptom relief and sustained improvement in quality of life was proved in multiple randomized trials. UFE is a minimally invasive procedure to treat uterine fibroids with comparable results with surgery with less morbidity and faster recovery time.

UAE FOR TREATMENT OF POSTPARTUM HEMORRHAGE

Postpartum hemorrhage (PPH) remains a common health problem. The reported incidence varies between 1% and 10%. However, it remains the main cause of pregnancy-related maternal death worldwide.[39] Delayed recognition and insufficient management are important factors that contribute to the morbidity and mortality. UAE has a role in the treatment of PPH and should be available to these patients early in the proper setting.[40,41] The American College of Obstetricians and Gynecologists defines PPH as (1) postpartum hemorrhage of more than 500 mL if the delivery was vaginal, (2) postpartum hemorrhage of more than 1000 mL if the delivery was by cesarean section (C-section), (3) a decrease of more than 10% of the hematocrit caused by the delivery, (4) blood products transfusions required during the delivery or puerperium. In real life, the estimate of blood loss volume is difficult. The diagnosis is frequently performed subjectively based on the experience of the physician attending the delivery. It is important to note that only 500 to 1000 mL of blood loss is required to make the diagnosis of PPH and promptly start management, which is important because significant blood loss is usually determined by the development of signs and symptoms of hypovolemia: tachycardia, pallor, tachypnea, hypotension, anxiety, and weakness. However, these clinical changes usually do not develop until a patient has lost more than 2000 mL.[42] Once PPH diagnosis has been acknowledged, prompt and adequate management should be initiated. There are multiple possible causes to be considered for proper management when dealing with PPH. An easy way to remember the most common ones is by using the 4-Ts mnemonic.

The 4 Ts	
Tone	Uterine atony
Tissue	Retained products of conception Placental abnormalities (ie, placenta accreta) Ectopic (ie, cervical implantation) Vascular malformation Tumors
Thrombin	Coagulopathy
Trauma	Lacerations

The first measures are guided to diagnose, correct, and treat the most common causes of PPH. These measures should include a pelvic examination, correction of coagulopathy and blood products transfusions, oxytocin and uterine packing. If these measures fail to control PPH, further interventions need to be considered without delay.[41] Hysterectomy is the most radical and efficient treatment of persistent PPH; however, the patient becomes sterile.

UAE is an alternative treatment with success rates for bleeding control in the order of 80% to 90% and in which the uterus and patient fertility can be preserved.[43–46] UAE for treatment of PPH developed during the 1980s.[47] The technique was already in use for the treatment of bleeding pelvic tumors and cases of pelvic trauma when it started being applied for situations of PPH.

Technique

The technique is similar to UFE: bilateral selective and subselective catheterization of the internal iliacs and uterine arteries is performed in a sequential manner. If the operator is unable to select the uterine artery, embolization of the anterior iliac branch is acceptable. Most of the time the angiograms in patients with PPH fail to reveal contrast extravasation or injured vessels, but bilateral UAE should still be performed empirically. The appearance of the uterine artery in PPH is variable. Well-developed large arteries to small spastic arteries might be encountered. They usually have some degree of cephalic displacement of the arterial trajectory by the enlarged uterus (**Fig. 8**). Multiple embolic materials can be used. Gelatin sponge is probably the most commonly used agent because of its availability, distal embolization, and temporary occlusion effect. Polyvinyl alcohol and other synthetic particles are also used; however, although the occlusion level and delivery are better controlled, the occlusion effect is more permanent, which may be a problem for future reproduction.

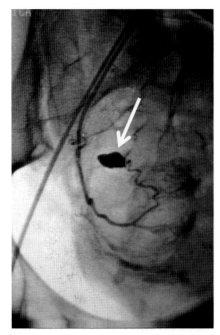

Fig. 8. Selective right uterine arteriogram in a patient with persistent postpartum hemorrhage shows pseudoaneurysm of the right uterine artery with active extravasation (*arrow*). It is uncommon to be able to identify the arterial injury as in this case. Usually bilateral UAE is done empirically in this clinical setting.

Other surgical options that conserve the uterus include applying compressive sutures to the uterus and systematic pelvic devascularization by surgical vascular ligations. Surgical arterial ligation has limited success rates, ranging from 40% to 60%, because of the rich arterial collateral network of the pelvis,[48–50] which is also why also proximal endovascular arterial coil embolization by itself is considered suboptimal (equivalent to surgical ligation). Endovascular techniques have also been used as adjuvant measures in the management of a few high-risk pregnancy situations, such as patients with abnormal placental position (previa) or insertion (accreta, percreta, or increta). In patients with placenta accreta, forcible manual removal of the placenta during delivery commonly results in massive hemorrhage and emergency hysterectomies. Although there is no consensus on how to manage these patients, current endovascular techniques have proved to be of significant benefit in the treatment. The most common management of placenta accreta is currently for the obstetrician to leave the placenta in place after the C-section delivery, and perform a hysterectomy with the placenta still attached.[51] However, the hysterectomy procedure is still associated with high blood volume losses. Transcatheter techniques have been successfully used to decrease blood losses in these patients and can even help conserve the uterus (**Fig. 9**). In the late 1990s, Dubois and colleagues[52] described a technique in which noninflated occlusion balloon catheters were positioned in the hypogastric arteries before the delivery/hysterectomy procedure. Then, during the hysterectomy procedure, the balloon catheters could be inflated to occlude the arteries and also to perform UAE if needed.[52,53] The clinical data on this technique are limited and controversial, but newer techniques were followed with better results, particularly a staged delivery approach in which UAE is performed after the C-section and the hysterectomy procedure is delayed, usually for about a week.[53,54] The hysterectomy blood volume losses are significantly reduced in the reported series. There are also descriptions of conservative techniques in which the uterus is devascularized after C-section, the placenta and uterus are left in place, and the patients are monitored with ultrasound or hysteroscopy until the placenta is resorbed.[55] These conservative techniques have good success rates, with preserved fertility resulting in term pregnancies, but with a high incidence of placenta accreta (6 of 21 term pregnancies).

Patients with ectopic cervical pregnancies typically abort spontaneously within the first trimester

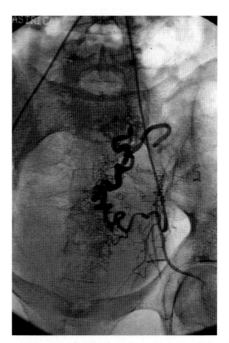

Fig. 9. Patient with placenta accreta. Patient decided for staged conservative management. Selective arteriogram before UAE with the catheter tip at the left uterine artery shows a well-developed uterine artery and tortuous corkscrew vessels supplying the uterus and placenta.

of gestation with transvaginal hemorrhage volumes that can require blood transfusions and hysterectomy. Timely and accurate diagnosis of the ectopic cervical pregnancy allows implementation of interventions that can reduce bleeding, transfusions, and prevent hysterectomy. Treatment with methotrexate has limited success.[56–59] It frequently needs to be followed by hysteroscopic resection of the ectopic gestational sac. The obstetrician uses techniques like curettage, cervical cerclage, and Foley catheter tamponade to control the hemorrhage but, despite these measures, there is a risk of significant procedural blood losses. Adjuvant UAE before the sac resection has been used to help reduce and control the procedural hemorrhage volumes (**Fig. 10**).[60,61]

Summary

Postpartum hemorrhage is a common and serious condition that carries high mortality and morbidity, with frequent need for hysterectomy. Endovascular techniques can be life saving and have been used successfully in cases of postpartum bleeding, and in selected cases of placental insertion abnormalities and ectopic cervical pregnancies, with the added advantage of preservation of the uterus and future fertility.

ENDOVASCULAR TREATMENT OF PELVIC CONGESTION SYNDROME

Pelvic congestion syndrome (PCS) is characterized by chronic noncyclic pelvic pain of greater than 6 months' duration secondary to pelvic venous insufficiency (PVI) and associated pelvic venous distention.[62] Although as many as 39%

of women experience chronic pelvic pain at some time in their lives, diagnostic work-up in one-third of these patients does not reveal any obvious cause and PCS is often overlooked in the differential diagnosis. Although pelvic varices have been described since 1857, the association of PCS with chronic pelvic pain was not described until 1949.[63]

Clinical Presentation

Affected patients usually present in their late 20s and 30s with chronic lower backache, pelvic pain, and fullness/heaviness in the lower pelvis, vulvar region, and upper thighs. The pain is typically exacerbated with prolonged standing, strenuous activity, and menses, and may be associated with dyspareunia and prolonged postcoital pain. Symptoms generally worsen at the end of the day and may improve with lying down. Physical findings that support the diagnosis include ovarian point tenderness and varicosities in the vulvar, pudendal, and thigh regions. The combination of ovarian point tenderness and postcoital pelvic ache is reported to be 94% sensitive and 77% specific for diagnosing PCS.[64]

Etiopathogenesis

The multifactorial causes of PCS include factors such as primary or acquired valvular insufficiency in the ovarian veins, venous outflow obstruction, and hormonally mediated vasomotor dysfunction. Valvular insufficiency caused by incompetent valves is most common in multiparous women because of the chronic venous distension that occurs during pregnancy. Venous outflow

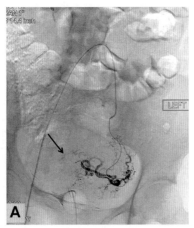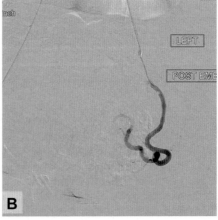

Fig. 10. Patient with a cervical ectopic pregnancy in the first trimester. UAE performed before the resection to decrease procedural blood loss. (*A*) Selective left uterine arteriogram shows enlarged uterine artery with tortuous vessels supplying the uterus and gestational sac area of the cervix (*arrow*). (*B*) Arteriogram after UAE shows pruning of left uterine artery. Embolization of the right uterine artery was then performed.

obstruction caused by variant renal vein anatomy and mesoaortic compression of the left renal vein may also cause PVI.

PCS is caused by retrograde flow through incompetent gonadal and pelvic veins, often associated with pelvic varicosities.

Ovarian venous anatomy

The left ovarian vein typically drains into the left renal vein; the left ovarian vein may also communicate with the portal vein (via the inferior mesenteric vein) and internal iliac veins. The right ovarian vein empties directly into the inferior vena cava. Upper limit of normal diameters for ovarian veins is 5 mm, with the left usually larger than the right. Multiple main trunks of the ovarian veins may also exist: up to 40% on the left and 25% on the right.

Diagnosis

Diagnosis of PCS on routine sonographic or computed tomography (CT)/MR imaging is often missed, because most imaging is performed in the supine position and venous distension may not be prominent in the supine and non-Valsalva positions. Findings of PCS on sonography include tortuous pelvic veins with a diameter of more than 5 mm, slow ($\leq$3 cm/s) or reversed (caudal) flow in the ovarian vein, dilated tortuous arcuate veins in the myometrium that communicate with bilateral pelvic varicosities, and polycystic changes of the ovaries. CT and MR imaging show similar findings and can be performed with the Valsalva maneuver to improve sensitivity (**Fig. 11**). In a study of 131 patients with confirmed diagnosis of PCS, the sensitivities of MR imaging,

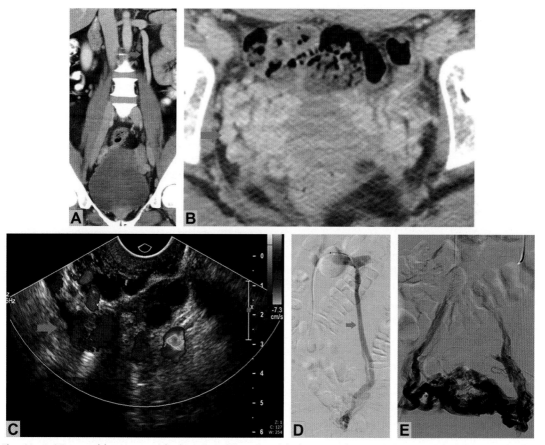

Fig. 11. A 27-year-old woman with chronic pelvic pain with dysmenorrhea and dyspareunia. (*A*) Coronal reformatted image from contrast-enhanced abdominal CT showing dilated left ovarian vein (*arrow*) measuring 8 mm in diameter and draining into the left renal vein. (*B*) Axial image from contrast-enhanced pelvic CT showing tortuous dilated pelvic varicosities (*arrow*) extending into the parametrium. (*C*) Transvaginal ultrasound for the left adnexal region showing dilated tortuous arcuate veins in the pelvis (*arrow*) that communicate with bilateral pelvic varicosities measuring 8 to 10 mm in diameter. (*D, E*) Selective left ovarian venography (via femoral venous approach catheter placed in left renal vein) remains the gold standard for diagnosis. The left ovarian vein (*arrow*) measures 8 mm in diameter with retrograde ovarian venous flow, and bilateral tortuous pelvic varicosities associated with delayed or stagnant clearance of injected contrast material.

ultrasound, and CT were 58.6%, 20%, and 12.5% respectively.[65]

Selective ovarian venography remains the gold standard for imaging-based diagnosis. Diagnostic findings of PCS in symptomatic patients include an ovarian vein diameter of more than 6 mm, retrograde ovarian or pelvic venous flow, presence of several tortuous collateral pelvic venous pathways, and delayed or stagnant clearance of injected contrast material. Dynamic flow information can also be obtained by performing the venogram with Valsalva and in the reverse Trendelenburg position.

Treatment

Treatment options for patients with PCS include medical management with hormonal suppression and analgesics, ligation of the ovarian veins, hysterectomy and oophorectomy, and transcatheter embolization. Medical treatment includes hormone analogues for ovarian suppression and increasing venous contraction (medroxyprogesterone acetate; gonadotropin receptor agonist), analgesics (NSAIDs), and psychotherapy. Studies have reported short-term relief up to 3 months after hormonal analogues, with no long-term residual benefit.[66] Surgical options including ligation of the ovarian veins and hysterectomy with and without bilateral salpingo-oophorectomy, have higher associated postsurgical morbidity, and although they give moderate relief, they are still associated with recurrence or residual pain in 30% of patients at 1-year follow-up.[67] Percutaneous endovascular pelvic vein embolization was introduced in 1993[68] and has evolved and improved technologically over the last 2 decades. Pelvic variceal embolization now offers an effective, minimally invasive therapeutic option for PCS with greater than 95% technical success rate and relief of symptoms in 68% to 100% of patients.[62]

Technique

The technique of transcatheter pelvic variceal embolization involves access to the ovarian and internal iliac veins from the jugular or femoral venous approach. A Cobra or reverse-curve catheter is used to select the left renal vein and maneuvered into the left gonadal vein. After confirmation of the number of gonadal veins/tributaries and opacification of pelvic varices, embolization of the gonadal veins and varices is performed to eliminate the hydrostatic pressure from PVI. The utero-ovarian venous plexus is selected and embolic treatment is performed with foamed sclerosant (sodium tetradecyl sulfate) or liquid embolic material (n-butyl cyanoacrylate), avoiding nontarget embolization. The main left gonadal vein

is then coil embolized to a level approximately 3 cm from the left renal vein. The right gonadal vein is then accessed with a reverse-curve catheter, and embolization is similarly repeated (Fig. 12). Because collateral communication exists between the ovarian and internal iliac veins, bilateral internal iliac veins are evaluated for variceal opacification after selective internal iliac balloon catheter inflation. The varices are selected with a microcatheter and similarly embolized with sclerosants and liquid embolic agents. Coils are avoided in the internal iliac veins because of increased potential of coil migration from the capacious internal iliac veins. The gonadal vein and internal iliac embolization can be performed together or staged (3-week to 6-week interval) depending on performer and patient preference (Fig. 13).

Clinical success has been reported in 70% to 100% of patients who underwent therapeutic embolization for PCS, with no negative effects on menstrual cycle or fertility. In one of the largest series, involving 127 patients who underwent pelvic embolization (126 ovarian and 108 internal iliac embolization), Kim and colleagues[65] showed that 83% of patients had significant relief of pain on long-term follow-up (mean follow-up of 45 months), with no major complications and no significant change in menses, fertility, or hormone levels. In another study with 56 patients who underwent variceal embolization (56 ovarian and 43 internal iliac) and were followed up to an average of 22.1 months, significant/partial relief of pain symptoms was seen in 96%.[69] A direct comparison of hysterectomy and bilateral oophorectomy (n = 32) versus venous embolization (n = 52) for patients with PCS was performed by Chung and Huh,[70] showing variceal embolization to be more effective than hysterectomy based on analysis of pain scores.

Complications that have been described after embolization are generally less than 4% and include gonadal vein perforation, nontarget embolization (ie, pulmonary coil embolization), cardiac arrhythmias, ovarian vein thrombophlebitis, and recurrence of varices.[71]

Summary

PCS is a recognized cause of chronic pelvic pain and can now be better diagnosed with ultrasound, CT/MR imaging, and venography. Although more investigation is needed to discern the best treatment option for PCS, transcatheter embolization is an established therapy for the treatment of pelvic congestion syndrome with great technical and clinical success rates, low associated morbidity, and preserved ovarian function and fertility.

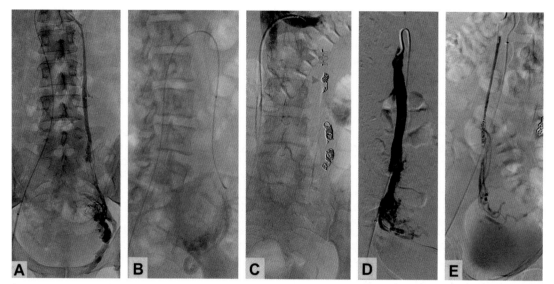

Fig. 12. A 24-year-old woman with chronic pelvic pain and postcoital discomfort undergoing transcatheter pelvic variceal embolization via bilateral ovarian veins. (*A*) Via the femoral venous access sheath, access to the left renal vein and then left ovarian vein was obtained using a 5-Fr Cobra catheter. Angiogram revealed single left ovarian vein, its 2 tributaries, and opacification of pelvic varices. (*B*) A microcatheter was advanced into the pelvic varices and superselective embolization was performed with foamed sclerosant (3% sodium tetradecyl sulfate) avoiding nontarget embolization (*arrow*). (*C*) Main left ovarian vein and its principal tributaries were embolized with coils (*arrowhead*) and Amplatzer plug (*arrow*), to a level approximately 3 cm from the left renal vein. Postembolization left renal angiogram does not show any opacification of the ovarian vein or pelvic varices. (*D, E*) The right ovarian vein arising from the inferior vena cava was accessed with a reverse-curve catheter, and embolization was similarly performed with coils and foamy sclerosant.

FALLOPIAN TUBE INTERVENTIONS
FT Recanalization

It has been estimated that tubal disease is the cause of up to a third of subfertility in women, with 10% to 25% of the occlusions located in the proximal tubes.[72,73] FT recanalization is accepted as an alternative to more invasive and costly infertility treatments and it is recommended by the American Society for Reproductive Medicine for patients with infertility in which hysterosalpingogram (HSG) shows proximal tubal occlusion.[74,75] Although the success rates for FT recanalization are acceptable and the cost is significant less than other fertility treatments, such as in vitro fertilization (IVF) and microsurgical tubocornual anastomosis, the technique is probably underused

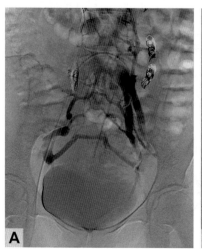

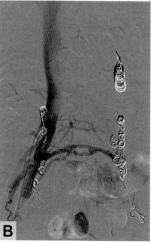

Fig. 13. A 24-year-old woman with chronic pelvic pain and postcoital discomfort undergoing transcatheter pelvic variceal embolization via bilateral internal iliac veins 6 weeks later (staged). (*A, B*) Because collateral communication exists between the ovarian and internal iliac veins, bilateral internal iliac veins were selectively catheterized and selective angiograms revealed dilated tortuous varices. These varices were selectively embolized with foamy sclerosant (3% sodium tetradecyl sulfate) avoiding nontarget embolization.

given the tendency of many fertility specialist to favor IVF.[72] FT recanalization allows couples to have unlimited attempts to conceive naturally and avoids the risks of IVF, including multiple pregnancies and ovarian hyperstimulation syndrome.[74]

The HSG remains an important radiologic procedure in the investigation of infertility; however, the false-positive rates to diagnose occlusion of the FT can vary from 16% to 40%.[73] In a significant proportion of patients an apparent proximal tubal occlusion is found to be patent in selective salpingography (SSG) or during laparoscopy.[73] The main reasons for false-positives are the lack of adequate distention during contrast injection or the presence of a temporal blockage caused by mucus or spasm.[73,76] SSG has been used to distinguish between a true occlusion and other conditions that may simulate occlusion in HSG. SSG also is used to provide recanalization of proximal fallopian tubes. The fluoroscopic technique of FT recanalization was pioneered by Amy Thurmond in the 1980s.[77,78]

Technique

The procedure is usually scheduled during the follicular menstrual phase between menstrual cycle days 6 and 11. Patients are asked to abstain from any unprotected sexual activity from the date of their last periods. In addition to contrast allergy, pregnancy and active pelvic infection are contraindications to the procedure.

Most women are apprehensive, so a careful, slow manipulation avoiding any sudden and forceful movement is important to avoid pain; slow injection of contrast is also recommended to prevent cramping and spasm. The use of prophylactic antibiotics is recommended by many, especially in patients with a history of previous pelvic infection or hydrosalpinx. Doxycycline100 mg orally twice daily for 5 days, ideally starting 2 days before the procedure, is the most common regimen.[74,75] Small doses of intravenous sedation and pain medication may be given, especially if the patient is apprehensive. The patient is positioned on the fluoroscopic table with the aid of leg supporters, a warmed plastic speculum is placed, and the cervix is identified and cleansed with iodine solution. Different devices are available to perform recanalization. A balloon sheath combination (Radiographic Tubal Assessment Set, Cook, Bloomington, IN) allows passage of devices through a hemostatic valve, whereas the inflated balloon provides traction and seal. The Thurmond-Rösch Hysterocath set (Cook, Bloomington, IN) has an acorn tip that engages the external cervical os and allows the introduction of catheters up to 9.0 Fr. A movable cup adjusts in length and provides an efficient seal to the cervix. The use of a tenaculum is more economical, but tends to be associated with more pain, so topical lidocaine spray can be useful. After adequate seal at the cervix is obtained, diluted 30% to 50% water-soluble contrast is injected for initial HSG. Once tubal occlusion is confirmed, SSG is performed with a curved 5-Fr catheter that is lodged at the ostium. The occlusion is then recanalized either using a coaxially placed 3-Fr microcatheter with the use of 0.46-mm to 0.36-mm microwires or with careful use of a 0.89-mm hydrophilic wire (Fig. 14).[79]

Results

FT recanalization has a high technical success rate (71%–92%). Main technical challenges are related to the variations of the position of the uterus, and many can be corrected with adequate traction of the cervix.[74] Catheters with different angulations may be required in cases of tortuous cornu. Potential causes of failure include congenital malformations of the uterus, presence of large leiomyomas, or polyps. Complete occlusions from infection, previous surgery, or endometriosis may be impossible to recanalize. Pregnancy rates vary in different series. Higher success rates (60%) are reported in patients without risk factors for distal FT disease. The average rate in most series is 30%.[74,80] Reocclusion of the FT is possible (25%) but it can be treated with repeat recanalization. Patients with previous surgical tubal repair and those with multifocal tubal disease have the worst prognoses.

Complications

Serious complications are rare. Mild uterine cramping and vaginal bleeding for up to 3 days are common and self-limited. The incidence of tubal perforation is less than 4%.[74] Adnexal infection is rare. Ectopic pregnancy is a well-known risk occurring in up to 3% of patients. Patients are advised to see their gynecologists as soon as they suspect they may be pregnant. Radiation to the gonads has been a particular concern. The dose to the ovaries has been calculated to be less than 1 rad (10 mGy), with an average dose of 2.7 mGy, and a patient effective dose of 1.2 mSv.[81,82] Performing the recanalization immediately after the diagnostic HSG reduces the radiation dose and the cost of a second procedure.[80,83]

Transcervical Sterilization

Worldwide, the most common method of sterilization is tubal ligation via laparoscopy or minilaparotomy. These procedures, although simple, are invasive and can be associated with infection

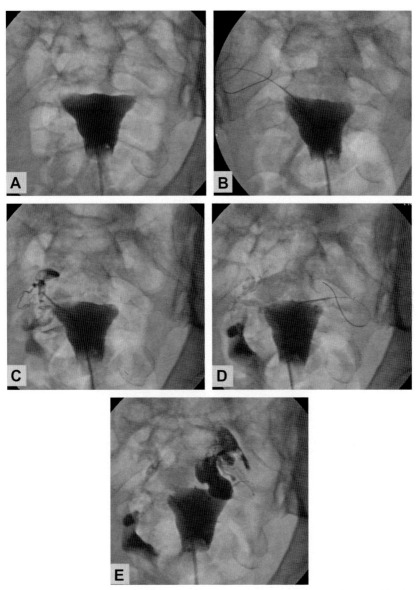

Fig. 14. (*A*) HSG in a 24-year-old woman who is unable to get pregnant shows occlusion of both FTs. (*B*) Radiograph shows recanalization of the right FT using a hydrophilic wire. (*C*) Right SSG shows patent right FT with spillage of contrast into the peritoneal cavity. (*D*) Radiograph shows recanalization of the left FT. (*E*) SSG shows patent left FT.

of the surgical incision, and some patients require general anesthesia.[84] Transcervical sterilization does not need to be performed in an operating room, requires less anesthesia, has a shorter recovery period, and it is more cost-effective. Multiple attempts to obtain sterilization by selective blockage of the tubes have been reported, with many successful experimental studies in animals, but few making it into clinical practice. With the advent of newer devices and improvement in hysteroscopy, these techniques are again gaining popularity.

Occlusion of the long and thin FT can be achieved in multiple ways. Chemical agents/thermal injuries create inflammatory changes and sclerosis that eventually occlude the lumen of the tube. Chemical agents include caustics such as ethanol, tetracycline, and quinacrine. These agents are easy to apply and inexpensive but the potential of spillage into the peritoneum has limited their clinical application. At present, quinacrine is used in many developing countries; it is applied into the uterine cavity in the form of a pellet or direct tubal instillation, with a sterilization rate of

98% to 99%.[85] Despite its 30-year safety data, the lack of US Food and Drug Administration approval and the need for repeat application has limited its use in developed countries. Liquid agents that produce a combination of mechanical and chemical occlusion, such as ethylene vinyl alcohol copolymer,[86] methylcyanoacrylate,[87] and n-butyl-2-cyanoacrylate,[88] are showing promising results in animals, but many of these new liquid agents are expensive.

Mechanical devices produce a direct blockage and later a tissue reaction that results in permanent occlusion of the tubes. Multiple versions have been described, including devices made of nylon, silicone plugs, and metallic coils. Many have failed because of migration and inconsistent occlusion.[89–91] At present, 2 devices are used in clinical practice in the United States. The Essure device (Conceptus Inc, San Carlos, CA) is a hybrid device made of a coil with polyethylene terephthalate woven fibers. The device measures 4 cm in length and 2 mm in diameter when expanded. The device is usually placed under hysteroscopy guidance, with a success rate of around 84%.[92] Fluoroscopic placement has also been described and it is highly effective (**Fig. 15**).[93] The sterilization rate is close to 100%.[92] Less than 50% of the inner coil of the device should be in the uterine cavity.[94] Placement of the device too proximally can result in device expulsion, with rates ranging from 0.6% to 3%.[94,95] In contrast, coils placed too peripherally can migrate into the peritoneum, potentially creating peritoneal adhesions that may result in small bowel obstruction. Removal is recommended.[96] Perforation of the tube can be seen in the HSG and is probably a complication during initial insertion. Three months after placement, HSG is performed to confirm tubal occlusion (**Fig. 16**). The Essure is highly effective but misinterpretation of the confirmatory HSG has resulted in undesired pregnancies.[97] Adequate distention of the cornual portion should be achieved during the HSG to rule out tubal patency. Because the microinserts are metallic, they are seen well in plain films and CT scans. In ultrasound, the portion inside the uterus

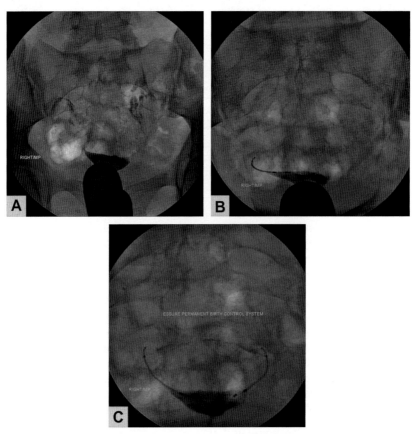

Fig. 15. Fluoroscopic placement of Essure. (*A*) HSG shows patent FT bilaterally. (*B*) Radiograph shows the device advanced into the right FT. Proximal radiopaque marker should ideally be at the ostium or slightly protruding into the uterine cavity. (*C*) Spot radiograph after placement of bilateral devices.

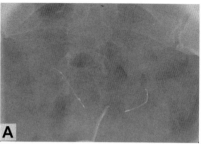
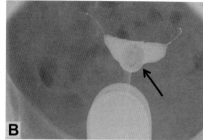

Fig. 16. HSG to confirm tubal occlusion 3 months after Essure placement. (*A*) Radiograph shows bilateral devices. (*B*) HSG shows occlusion of both FTs. Note inflated balloon for HSG (*arrow*).

is clearly seen but the tubular part is usually not seen because it is surrounded by intestinal loops.[94,98] The Essure has also been used to produce proximal occlusion of hydrosalpinges before IVF, as an alternative to salpingectomy.[99]

The Adiana System (Hologic, Inc, Bedford, MA) is a dual method that first creates thermal damage of the endosalpinx using a bipolar radiofrequency generator, then subsequent tissue growth by fibroblast into the holes of a small cylindrical shaped silicone tube results in tubal occlusion. The device is radiolucent and cannot be seen in imaging.[94] Confirmatory HSG after 3 months is also required, because excessive pressure during HSG can result in accidental dislodgement. The sterilization rates with this device seem similar to rates with other contraception methods.[100]

In addition, thermal techniques such as lasers, radiofrequency ablation, and electrosurgery also result in eventual sclerosis of the tubes. Some of the thermal techniques have been abandoned because of serious complications caused by the close proximity of the FT to the intestine. Newer techniques using lower energy probes show promise but are not currently used widely.[101]

Summary

FT recanalization is a simple procedure with high technical success that can be performed in many patients with proximal FT occlusion as an alternative to IVF. Transcervical FT occlusion is reemerging as an alternative to surgical ligation for permanent sterilization.

REFERENCES

1. Buttram VC Jr, Reiter RC. Uterine leiomyomata: etiology, symptomatology, and management. Fertil Steril 1981;36:433–45.
2. Pelage JP, Walker WJ, Le Dref O, et al. Treatment of uterine fibroids [letter]. Lancet 2001;357:1530.
3. Kjerulff KH, Langenberg P, Seidman JD, et al. Uterine leiomyomas. Racial differences in severity, symptoms and age at diagnosis. J Reprod Med 1996;41:483–90.
4. Rein MS, Barbieri RL, Friedman AJ. Progesterone: a critical role in the pathogenesis of uterine myomas. Am J Obstet Gynecol 1995;172:14–8.
5. Wallach EE, Vlahos NF. Uterine myomas: an overview of development, clinical features and management. Obstet Gynecol 2004;104:393–406.
6. Ravina JH, Merland JJ, Herbreteau D, et al. Preoperative embolization of uterine fibroma. Preliminary results (10 cases). Presse Med 1994;23:1540.
7. Stewart EA. Uterine fibroids. Lancet 2001;367: 293–8.
8. Stovall DW, Parrish SB, Van Voorhis BJ, et al. Uterine leiomyomas reduce the efficacy of assisted reproduction cycles: results of a matched follow-up study. Hum Reprod 1998;13:192–7.
9. Eldar-Geva T, Meagher S, Healy DL, et al. Effect of intramural, subserosal, and submucosal uterine fibroids on the outcome of assisted reproductive technology treatment. Fertil Steril 1998;70:687–91.
10. Murase E, Siegelman ES, Outwater EK, et al. Uterine leiomyomas: histopathologic features, MR imaging findings, differential diagnosis and treatment. Radiographics 1999;19:1179–97.
11. Ueda H, Togashi K, Konishi I, et al. Unusual appearances of uterine leiomyomas: MR imaging findings and their histopathologic backgrounds. Radiographics 1999;19:131–5.
12. Burn PR, McCall JM, Chinn RJ, et al. Uterine fibroleiomyoma: MR imaging appearance before and after embolization of uterine arteries. Radiology 2000;214:729–34.
13. Ravina JH, Vigneron NC, Aymard A, et al. Pregnancy after embolization of uterine myoma: report of 12 cases. Fertil Steril 2000;73:1241–3.
14. Goodwin SC, McLucas B, Lee M, et al. Uterine artery embolization for the treatment of uterine leiomyomata midterm results. J Vasc Interv Radiol 1999;10:1159–65.
15. Spies JB, Ascher SA, Roth AR, et al. Uterine artery embolization for leiomyomata. Obstet Gynecol 2001;98:29–34.

16. Pelage JP, Le Dref O, Jacob D, et al. Selective arterial embolization of the uterine arteries in the management of intractable post-partum hemorrhage. Acta Obstet Gynecol Scand 1999;78:698–703.

17. Hutchins FL Jr, Worthington-Kirsch R, Berkowitz RP. Selective uterine artery embolization as primary treatment for symptomatic leiomyomata uteri. J Am Assoc Gynecol Laparosc 1999;6:279–84.

18. McLucas B, Reed RA, Goodwin S, et al. Outcomes following unilateral uterine artery embolization. Br J Radiol 2002;75:122–6.

19. Waltman AC, Courey WR, Athanasoulis C, et al. Technique for left gastric artery catheterization. Radiology 1973;109:732–4.

20. Nikolic B, Spies JB, Campbell L, et al. Uterine artery embolization: reduced radiation with refined technique. J Vasc Interv Radiol 2001;12:39–44.

21. Pelage JP, Laurent A, Bonneau M, et al. Arterial blood supply to the uterus in nonpregnant sheep: a pertinent model for clinical practice? Invest Radiol 2001;36:721–5.

22. Siskin GP, Stainken BF, Dowling K, et al. Outpatient uterine artery embolization for symptomatic uterine fibroids: experience in 49 patients. J Vasc Interv Radiol 2000;11:305–11.

23. Hurst BS, Stackhouse DJ, Matthews ML, et al. Uterine artery embolization for symptomatic uterine myomas. Fertil Steril 2000;74:855–69.

24. Brunereau L, Herbreteau D, Gallas S, et al. Uterine artery embolization in the primary treatment of uterine leiomyomas: technical features and prospective follow-up with clinical and sonographic examinations in 58 patients. AJR Am J Roentgenol 2000;175:1267–72.

25. Katsumori T, Nakajima K, Mihara T, et al. Uterine artery embolization using gelatin sponge particles alone for symptomatic uterine fibroids: midterm results. AJR Am J Roentgenol 2002;178:135–9.

26. Rasuli P, Jolly EE, Hammond I, et al. Superior hypogastric nerve block for pain control in outpatient uterine artery embolization. J Vasc Interv Radiol 2004;15:1423–9.

27. Walker WJ, Pelage JP. Uterine fibroid embolization: results in 400 women with imaging follow-up [abstract]. J Vasc Interv Radiol 2002;13 (Suppl 2):s18.

28. McLucas B, Adler L, Perrella R. Uterine fibroid embolization: nonsurgical treatment for symptomatic fibroids. J Am Coll Surg 2001;192:95–105.

29. Ravina JH, Aymard A, Ciraru-Vigneron N, et al. Arterial embolization of uterine myoma: results apropos of 286 cases. J Gynecol Obstet Biol Reprod (Paris) 2000;29:272–5 [in French].

30. Andersen PE, Lund N, Justesen P, et al. Uterine artery embolization of symptomatic uterine fibroids. Initial success and short-term results. Acta Radiol 2001;42:234–8.

31. Spies JB, Scialli AR, Jha RC, et al. Initial results from uterine fibroid embolization for symptomatic leiomyomata. J Vasc Interv Radiol 1999;10:1149–57.

32. Binkert CA, Andrews RT, Kaufman JA. Utility of nonselective abdominal aortography in demonstrating ovarian artery collaterals in patients undergoing uterine artery embolization for fibroids. J Vasc Interv Radiol 2001;12:841–5.

33. Andrews RT, Bromley PJ, Pfister ME. Successful embolization of collaterals from the ovarian artery during uterine artery embolization for fibroids: a case report. J Vasc Interv Radiol 2000;11:607–10.

34. Vashisht A, Studd J, Carey A, et al. Fatal septicaemia after fibroid embolization. Lancet 1999;354:307–8.

35. Lanocita R, Frigerio LF, Patelli G, et al. A fatal complication of percutaneous transcatheter embolization for the treatment of uterine fibroids. Presented at the SMIT/CIMIT 11th Annual Scientific Meeting. Boston (MA), September 16–18, 1999.

36. Walker WJ, Pelage JP, Sutton C. Fibroid embolization. Clin Radiol 2002;57:325–31.

37. Wingo PA, Huezo CM, Rubin GL, et al. The mortality risk associated with hysterectomy. Am J Obstet Gynecol 1985;152:803–8.

38. Pelage JP, Le Dref O, Soyer P, et al. Arterial anatomy of the female genital tract: variations and relevance to transcatheter embolization of the uterus. AJR Am J Roentgenol 1999;172:989–94.

39. Chang J, Elam-Evans LD, Berg CJ, et al. Pregnancy-related mortality surveillance – United States, 1991–1999. MMWR Surveill Summ 2003;52(SS02):1–8.

40. Banovac F, Lin R, Shah D, et al. Angiographic and interventional options in obstetric and gynecologic emergencies. Obstet Gynecol Clin North Am 2007;34(3):599–616.

41. Varatharajan L, Chandraharan E, Sutton J, et al. Outcome of the management of massive postpartum hemorrhage using the algorithm "HEMOSTASIS". Int J Gynaecol Obstet 2011;113(2):152–4.

42. Pacagnella RC, Souza JP, Durocher J, et al. A systematic review of the relationship between blood loss and clinical signs. PLoS One 2013;8(3):e57594.

43. Kirby JM, Kachura JR, Rajan DK, et al. Arterial embolization for primary postpartum hemorrhage. J Vasc Interv Radiol 2009;20(8):1036–45.

44. Ganguli S, Stecker MS, Pyne D, et al. Uterine artery embolization in the treatment of postpartum uterine hemorrhage. J Vasc Interv Radiol 2011;22:169–76.

45. Stancato-Pasik A, Mitty HA, Richard HM 3rd, et al. Obstetric embolotherapy: effect on menses and pregnancy. Radiology 1997;204(3):791–3.

46. Vedantham S, Goodwin SC, McLucas B, et al. Uterine artery embolization: an underused method of controlling pelvic hemorrhage. Am J Obstet Gynecol 1997;176:938–48.

47. Brown BJ, Heaston DK, Poulson AM, et al. Uncontrollable postpartum bleeding: a new approach to hemostasis through angiographic arterial embolization. Obstet Gynecol 1979;54(3):361–5.

48. Tamizian O, Arulkumaran S. The surgical management of post-partum haemorrhage. Best Pract Res Clin Obstet Gynaecol 2002;16(1):81–98.

49. Clark SL, Phelan JP, Yeh SY, et al. Hypogastric artery ligation for obstetric hemorrhage. Obstet Gynecol 1985;66(3):353–6.

50. Joshi VM, Otiv SR, Majumder R, et al. Internal iliac artery ligation for arresting postpartum hemorrhage. BJOG 2007;114(3):356–61.

51. Oyelese Y, Smulian JC. Placenta previa, placenta accreta, and vasa previa. Obstet Gynecol 2006; 107(4):927–41.

52. Dubois J, Garel L, Grignon A, et al. Placenta percreta: balloon occlusion and embolization of the internal iliac arteries to reduce intraoperative blood losses. Am J Obstet Gynecol 1997;176(3):723–6.

53. Sumigama S, Itakura A, Ota T, et al. Placenta previa increta/percreta in Japan: a retrospective study of ultrasound findings, management and clinical course. J Obstet Gynaecol Res 2007; 33(5):606–11.

54. Angstmann T, Gard G, Harrington T, et al. Surgical management of placenta accreta: a cohort series and suggested approach. Am J Obstet Gynecol 2010;202:38.e1–9.

55. Sentilhes L, Ambroselli C, Kayem G, et al. Maternal outcome after conservative treatment of placenta accrete. Obstet Gynecol 2010;115(3):526–34.

56. Marston LM, Dotters DJ, Katz VL. Methotrexate and angiographic embolization for conservative treatment of cervical pregnancy. South Med J 1996; 89:246–8.

57. Corsan GH, Karacan M, Qasim S, et al. Identification of hormonal parameters for successful systemic single dose methotrexate therapy in ectopic pregnancy. Hum Reprod 1995;10:2719–22.

58. Bai SW, Lee JS, Park JH, et al. Failed methotrexate treatment of cervical pregnancy–predictive factors. J Reprod Med 2002;47:483–8.

59. Song MJ, Moon MH, Kim JA, et al. Serial transvaginal sonographic findings of cervical ectopic pregnancy treated with high-dose methotrexate. J Ultrasound Med 2009;28:55–61.

60. Meyerovitz MF, Lobel SM, Harrington DP, et al. Preoperative uterine artery embolization in cervical pregnancy. J Vasc Interv Radiol 1991;2:95–7.

61. Frates MC, Benson CB, Doubilet PM, et al. Cervical ectopic pregnancy: results of conservative treatment. Radiology 1994;191:773–5.

62. Black CM, Thorpe K, Venbrux A, et al. Research reporting standards for endovascular treatment of pelvic venous insufficiency. J Vasc Interv Radiol 2010;21:796–803.

63. Taylor HC. Vascular congestion and hyperemia; their effects on structure and function in the female reproductive system. Am J Obstet Gynecol 1949; 57:637–53.

64. Beard RW, Reginal PW, Wadsworth J. Clinical features of women with chronic lower abdominal pain and pelvic congestion. Br J Obstet Gynaecol 1988;95:153–61.

65. Kim HS, Malhotra AD, Lee ML, et al. Embolotherapy for pelvic congestion syndrome: long-term results. J Vasc Interv Radiol 2006;17:289–97.

66. Soysal ME, Soysal S, Vicdan K, et al. A randomized controlled trial of goserelin and medroxyprogesterone acetate in the treatment of pelvic congestion. Hum Reprod 2001;16:931–9.

67. Carter J. Surgical treatment for chronic pelvic pain. JSLS 1998;2:129–39.

68. Edwards RD, Robertson JR, MacLean AB, et al. Case report: pelvic pain syndrome–successful treatment of a case by ovarian vein embolization. Clin Radiol 1993;47:429–31.

69. Venbrux AC, Chang AH, Kim HS, et al. Pelvic congestion syndrome (pelvic venous incompetence): impact of ovarian and internal iliac vein embolotherapy on menstrual cycle and chronic pelvic pain. J Vasc Interv Radiol 2002;13: 171–8.

70. Chung MH, Huh CY. Comparison of treatments for pelvic congestion syndrome. Tohoku J Exp Med 2003;201:131–8.

71. Ganeshan A, Upponi S, Hon L, et al. Chronic pelvic pain due to pelvic congestion syndrome: the role of diagnostic and interventional radiology. Cardiovasc Intervent Radiol 2007;30:1105–11.

72. Dun EC, Nezhat CH. Tubal factor infertility: diagnosis and management in the era of assisted reproductive technology. Obstet Gynecol Clin North Am 2012;39(4):551–66.

73. Coughlan C, Li TC. An update on surgical management of tubal disease and infertility. Obst Gynecol Reprod Med 2011;21(10):273–80.

74. Thurmond AS. Fallopian tube catheterization. Semin Intervent Radiol 2008;25:425–31.

75. Steinkeler JA, Woodfield CA, Lazarus E, et al. Female infertility: a systematic approach to radiologic imaging and diagnosis. Radiographics 2009;29(5):1353–70.

76. Simpson WL Jr, Beitia LG, Mester J. Hysterosalpingography: a reemerging study. Radiographics 2006;26:419–31.

77. Thurmond AS, Novy MJ, Uchida BT, et al. Fallopian tube obstruction: selective salpingography and recanalization. Radiology 1987;163:511–4.

78. Thurmond AS, Rosch J. Nonsurgical fallopian tube recanalization for treatment of infertility. Radiology 1990;174:572–3.

79. Sowa M, Shimamoto T, Nakano R, et al. Diagnosis and treatment of proximal tubal obstruction by fluoroscopic transcervical fallopian tube catheterization. Hum Reprod 1993;8:1711–8.

80. Cobellis L, Argano F, Castaldi MA, et al. Selective salpingography: preliminary experience of an office operative option for proximal tubal recanalization. Eur J Obstet Gynecol Reprod Biol 2012;163(1):62–6.

81. Hedgpeth PL, Thurmond AS, Fry R, et al. Radiographic fallopian tube recanalization: absorbed ovarian radiation dose. Radiology 1991;180:121–2.

82. Perisinakis K, Damilakis J, Grammatikakis J, et al. Radiogenic risks from hysterosalpingography. Eur Radiol 2003;13(7):1522–8.

83. Mallarini G, Saba L. Role and application of hysterosalpingography and fallopian tube recanalization. Minerva Ginecol 2010;62(6):541–9.

84. Abbott J. Transcervical sterilization. Curr Opin Obstet Gynecol 2007;19:325–30.

85. Kessel E. 100,000 quinacrine sterilizations. Adv Contracept 1996;12:69–76.

86. Abdala N, Levitin A, Dawson A, et al. Use of ethylene vinyl alcohol copolymer for tubal sterilization by selective catheterization in rabbits. J Vasc Interv Radiol 2001;12:979–84.

87. Berkey GS, Nelson R, Zuckerman AM, et al. Sterilization with methylcyano-acrylate induced fallopian tube occlusion and a nonsurgical transvaginal approach in rabbits. J Vasc Interv Radiol 1995;6:669–74.

88. Pelage JP, Herbreteau D, Paillon JF, et al. Selective salpingography and fallopian tubal occlusion with n-butyl-2-cyanoacrylate: report of two cases. Radiology 1998;207:809–12.

89. Loffer FD. Hysteroscopic sterilization with the use of formed-in-place silicone plugs. Am J Obstet Gynecol 1984;149:261–70.

90. Castaño PM, Adekunle L. Transcervical sterilization. Semin Reprod Med 2010;28(2):103–9.

91. Post JH, Cardella JF, Wilson RP, et al. Experimental nonsurgical transcervical sterilization with a custom-designed platinum microcoil. J Vasc Interv Radiol 1997;8:113–8.

92. Nichols M, Carter JF, Fylstra DL, et al, Essure system US Post-Approval Study Group. A comparative study of hysteroscopic sterilization performed in office versus a hospital operating room. J Minim Invasive Gynecol 2006;13:447–50.

93. McSwain H, Shaw C, Hall L. Placement of the Essure permanent birth control device with fluoroscopic guidance: a novel method for tubal sterilization. J Vasc Interv Radiol 2005;16:1007–12.

94. Guelfguat M, Gruenberg TR, Dipoce J, et al. Imaging of mechanical tubal occlusion devices and potential complications. Radiographics 2012;32:1659–73.

95. Miño M, Arjona JE, Cordón J, et al. Success rate and patient satisfaction with the Essure sterilisation in an outpatient setting: a prospective study of 857 women. BJOG 2007;114(6):763–6.

96. Belotte J, Shavell VI, Awonuga AO, et al. Small bowel obstruction subsequent to Essure microinsert sterilization: a case report. Fertil Steril 2011;96(1):e4–6.

97. Cleary TP, Tepper NK, Cwiak C, et al. Pregnancies after hysteroscopic sterilization: a systematic review. Contraception 2013;87(5):539–48.

98. Weston G, Bowditch J. Office ultrasound should be the first-line investigation for confirmation of correct ESSURE placement. Aust N Z J Obstet Gynaecol 2005;45:312–5.

99. Galen DI, Khan N, Richter KS. Essure multicenter off-label treatment for hydrosalpinx before in vitro fertilization. J Minim Invasive Gynecol 2011;18(3):338–42.

100. Anderson TL, Vancaillie TG. The Adiana System for permanent contraception: safety and efficacy at 3 years. J Minim Invasive Gynecol 2011;18(5):612–6.

101. Donnez J, Malvaux V, Nisolle M, et al. Hysteroscopic sterilization with the Nd:YAG laser. J Gynecol Surg 1990;6:149–53.

Ovarian Cystic Lesions
A Current Approach to Diagnosis and Management

Susan Ackerman, MD*, Abid Irshad, MBBS,
Madelene Lewis, MD, Munazza Anis, MD

KEYWORDS

- Functional cysts • Nonfunctional cysts • Ovarian tumors

KEY POINTS

- Ultrasonography is the primary imaging modality for the evaluation of cystic ovarian lesions.
- Some lesions are indeterminate, and other modalities such as magnetic resonance imaging or computed tomography can be helpful in further evaluation of the lesion.
- It is important to correlate the patient's clinical signs and symptoms with the imaging features.
- Clinical information such as age, menstrual status, and surgical history are important, as some entities are more common in certain age groups.
- Imaging is used to help guide the management of these patients.

FOLLICLES AND FUNCTIONAL CYSTS

According to the American College of Radiology Appropriateness Criteria, pelvic ultrasonography (US) is the primary and preferred imaging modality for the evaluation of adnexal cysts.[1] In a reproductive-age female, multiple follicles are normally seen within the ovary (**Fig. 1**), and there is a varied appearance throughout the menstrual cycle with developing follicles, 1 or more dominant follicles, and development of a corpus luteum.

A follicle is a thin-walled, anechoic, unilocular, avascular, round to oval space within the ovary (**Fig. 2**). Follicles usually measure 2 to 9 mm, and 1 or more dominant follicles will grow to 20 to 25 mm.[2,3] The dominant follicle will rupture at ovulation, releasing an oocyte. The preovulatory dominant follicle may demonstrate a tiny peripheral curved line representing the ovum surrounded by a cumulus oophorus within the mature follicle (**Fig. 3**). After ovulation, the dominant follicle becomes the corpus luteum. The corpus luteum may demonstrate thickened walls, crenulated inner margins, internal echoes, and a ring of peripheral vascularity, and is usually smaller than 3 cm.[4–6] A functional or follicular cyst results from failure of the follicle to rupture or regress.[7] Follicular cysts are simple unilocular or minimally complicated cysts with thin walls, sharply marginated borders, internal fluid, and no internal vascularity (**Fig. 4**).[4] Folliculogenesis ceases after menopause.

Simple cysts of up to 10 cm in a patient of any age are highly likely to be benign with a malignancy rate of less than 1%.[8,9] In the premenopausal female, follicles or simple cysts up to 3 cm are considered physiologic findings, and no follow-up is recommended. Simple cysts larger

The authors have no disclosures.
Department of Radiology and Radiological Sciences, Medical University of South Carolina, 96 Jonathan Lucas Street, Charleston, SC 29425, USA
* Corresponding author.
E-mail address: ackerman@musc.edu

Radiol Clin N Am 51 (2013) 1067–1085
http://dx.doi.org/10.1016/j.rcl.2013.07.010

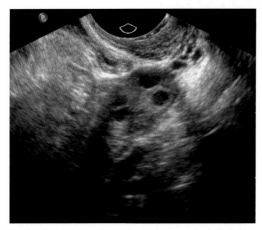

Fig. 1. Normal sonographic appearance of the ovary with multiple follicles.

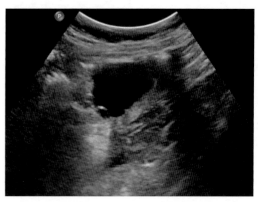

Fig. 3. A preovulatory dominant follicle with an internal peripheral curved line representing the ovum surrounded by a cumulus oophorus within the mature follicle, a physiologic finding for which no follow-up is recommended.

than 3 cm but less than or equal to 5 cm are almost certainly benign and require no follow-up. Simple cysts measuring greater than 5 cm but less than or equal to 7 cm are almost certainly benign, with annual follow-up recommended. Simple cysts larger than 7 cm are difficult to evaluate completely, and for this reason magnetic resonance (MR) imaging or surgical evaluation is recommended.[5] A corpus luteum measuring less than 3 cm is considered normal, and no imaging follow-up is indicated.[4]

In the postmenopausal female, simple cysts up to 1 cm in size may be seen in 21% of patients.[10] These simple cysts are of no clinical significance, are considered benign, and do not require follow-up. Simple cysts between 1 cm and 7 cm in size are almost certainly benign, and yearly follow-up is recommended. For simple cysts larger than 7 cm, MR imaging or surgical evaluation is recommended.[5]

Functional cysts typically resolve in 8 to 12 weeks and are typically asymptomatic.[6] If cysts become large symptoms can result, including pressure effects, pain, or cyst rupture, or the cyst may serve as a lead point for ovarian torsion. There is little evidence to guide when to decrease the frequency or cease follow-up (Box 1).

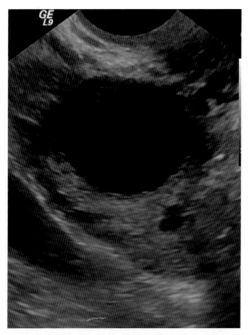

Fig. 2. Unilocular, ovoid, thin-walled, anechoic space within the ovary demonstrating posterior acoustic enhancement measuring less than 3 cm, a dominant follicle; this is a physiologic finding for which no follow-up is recommended.

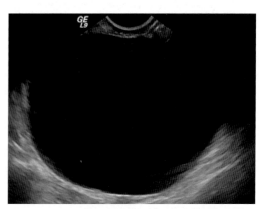

Fig. 4. A 6-cm simple cyst in a premenopausal female, for which yearly follow-up is recommended.

Box 1
Management of functional cysts

Premenopausal Simple Cyst

   5 cm and smaller: Follow-up not needed

   Between 5 and 7 cm: Yearly follow-up

Postmenopausal Simple Cyst

   Between 1 and 7 cm: Yearly follow-up

Any age with cyst larger than 7 cm: MR imaging or surgical evaluation

---

HEMORRHAGIC CYSTS

Hemorrhage into a corpus luteum or other functional cyst frequently occurs in premenopausal women. These patients can present with an abrupt onset of pelvic pain.

The imaging appearance can be variable depending on the age of the blood products. Classic sonographic features have been described, allowing for definitive diagnosis in most cases. These signs include a complex cystic mass with a reticular pattern of internal echoes and/or a solid-appearing area with concave margins that demonstrates no internal flow on color Doppler.[6,11,12] The reticular pattern secondary to fibrin strands has been described in the literature as fishnet, cobweb, spongy, and lacy (**Fig. 5**).[6,11] The cyst wall may be of variable thickness and may demonstrate circumferential blood flow. Hemorrhagic cysts may also demonstrate a fluid-fluid level (**Fig. 6**).[13] The MR appearance of hemorrhagic cysts is variable, with most demonstrating low signal intensity on T1-weighted images and heterogeneous appearance on T2-weighted images.[14]

When not classic in appearance, hemorrhagic cysts can mimic a variety of solid and mixed cystic masses. When present, it is important to recognize the classic appearance to avoid any additional unnecessary testing. The reticular pattern can be distinguished from internal septations, as the reticular lines are very fine and do not completely traverse the cyst. Intracystic clot also needs to be distinguished from mural nodularity. Neoplastic mural nodules typically demonstrate convex contours and internal vascularity. In the setting of cyst rupture, hemoperitoneum may result, and it is important to correlate with the patients' quantitative β subunit of human chorionic gonadotropin (β-hCG) to exclude rupture ectopic pregnancy, as they may present with similar clinical pictures.

Hemorrhagic cysts typically resolve within 8 weeks.[15] In females of reproductive age with a classic-appearing hemorrhagic cyst, no follow-up is indicated for cysts less than or equal to 5 cm. For hemorrhagic cysts larger than 5 cm even with a classic appearance, short-interval follow-up US in 6 to 12 weeks is recommended to ensure resolution.[5] Postmenopausal women should never develop a hemorrhagic cyst, and surgical evaluation in these cases should be considered. Women in early menopause may occasionally ovulate, and cysts with a hemorrhagic appearance are appropriate for short-interval follow-up US in 6 to 12 weeks.[5]

Clinical management is typically conservative and supportive. Occasionally these cysts can rupture, resulting in life-threatening hemoperitoneum and hypotension for which surgery may be indicated (**Boxes 2 and 3, Fig. 7**).

OVARIAN HYPERSTIMULATION SYNDROME

Ovarian hyperstimulation syndrome (OHSS) is an iatrogenic complication following drug therapy for infertility. It occurs during the luteal phase of the menstrual cycle or during early pregnancy. OHSS may persist or worsen if the patient becomes pregnant. The incidence ranges from 6% to 50%.[5,16] Patients' symptoms include pain, abdominal distension, nausea, vomiting, and weight gain.

US is the imaging modality of choice for diagnosis.[17] Both ovaries demonstrate cystic enlargement (**Fig. 8**). The cysts are usually anechoic; however, they occasionally appear complex, secondary to hemorrhage. Signs of third spacing are also present, including ascites and pleural effusions (**Fig. 9**).[18] A "wheel-spoke" pattern of the ovaries has been described on computed tomography (CT) and MR imaging, with peripheral

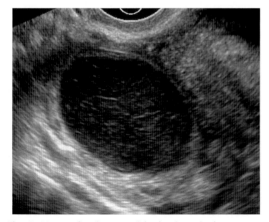

Fig. 5. Hemorrhagic cyst with classic reticular pattern secondary to fibrin strands.

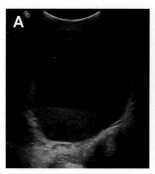 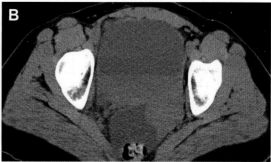

Fig. 6. (A) Transabdominal US and (B) axial CT images demonstrate fluid-fluid level within a hemorrhagic cyst.

location of follicles surrounding a central core of ovarian stroma.[19]

The incorrect diagnosis of ovarian cystic neoplasm can be avoided given the classic imaging appearance and clinical history of drug therapy for infertility. If there remains a question of ovarian cystic neoplasm, MR imaging can be obtained. MR imaging should demonstrate no enhancing abnormal soft tissue in or around the cystic ovarian mass.[19] Moreover, OHSS will demonstrate resolution on follow-up US.[20]

CT may demonstrate slightly higher attenuation ascites if a cyst with internal hemorrhage has ruptured. Frank hemoperitoneum suggests an alternative diagnosis of rupture ectopic pregnancy, especially in patients undergoing assisted reproduction.[21]

OHSS is usually self-limiting, but in severe cases may be life threatening. Treatment is typically supportive and conservative.[5,18] Surgery is indicated if there are signs of ovarian torsion, which has an incidence of 7.5% in the setting of OHSS (**Boxes 4** and **5**).[22]

OVARIAN REMNANT SYNDROME

Ovarian remnant syndrome (ORS) is a condition resulting from incomplete removal of ovarian tissue during an oophorectomy associated with pain and/or a pelvic mass.[23–25] Though uncommon, it presents a diagnostic challenge. Symptoms most frequently occur within the first 5 years after surgery.[23] Aside from the more common presentations of pain and pelvic mass, ORS

can also present with ureteric or intestinal obstruction, dyspareunia, and dysuria.[24–26] The syndrome is more common in young premenopausal women,[23,24] and occurs more commonly on the left side.[23] Risk factors for development include endometriosis, pelvic adhesions, pelvic inflammatory disease, multiple prior surgeries, and inflammatory bowel disease. Other factors that may contribute to inadvertent incomplete ovarian excision are related to intraoperative bleeding, anatomic variations, and poor surgical technique. In the majority of reported cases of ovarian remnant syndrome, the indication for oophorectomy was endometriosis.[23,26]

The residual ovarian tissue may remain viable and functional despite transection of the blood supply during oophorectomy,[24] and this is likely secondary to development of a parasitic blood supply whereby the ovary remains responsive to the hypothalamic pituitary ovarian axis.[25] In addition, malignancy has been described in women with a history of oophorectomies and ORS.[23]

The diagnosis is not easily made. Pelvic imaging is recommended as a supplemental diagnostic tool in combination with patient history, hormonal assays, and provocative testing.[23,24] A cystic or multiseptated pelvic mass in a patient with history

---

Box 2
Classic ultrasonographic features of hemorrhagic cysts

Reticular pattern of internal echoes

Intracystic clot with concave margins

No internal flow

Box 3
Management of classic-appearing hemorrhagic cysts

Premenopausal

- 5 cm and smaller: No follow-up needed
- Larger than 5 cm: 6- to 12-week follow-up

Early Postmenopause

- Any size of cyst: 6- to 12-week follow-up

Postmenopausal

- Consider surgical evaluation

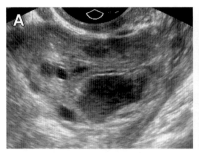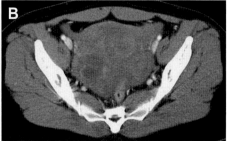

Fig. 7. (A) Transvaginal US and (B) axial CT images demonstrate a ruptured hemorrhagic cyst resulting in hemoperitoneum.

of an ipsilateral oophorectomy suggests the diagnosis of ORS (**Fig. 10**). A definitive diagnosis is obtained at the time of surgical exploration by histologic confirmation of remnant ovarian tissue.

Surgical excision remains the treatment of choice.[23,24] The operation is usually technically challenging and requires a surgeon with knowledge and experience of difficult pelvic dissection. Particularly in patients with risk factors for developing ORS after oophorectomy, prevention is the key, with care taken to completely excise all ovarian tissue and thus reduce the risk of occurrence.

ORS should not be confused with residual ovarian syndrome or supernumerary ovary syndrome. Residual ovarian syndrome occurs when the ovary is intentionally left during gynecologic surgery and subsequently causes pain. Supernumerary ovary syndrome is a rare congenital condition whereby extra ovaries develop embryologically (**Box 6**).

ENDOMETRIOSIS (ENDOMETRIOMA)

Endometriomas are focal cystic fluid collections that are sequelae of endometriosis. Endometriosis is the presence of functional uterine endometrial glands outside the uterine cavity. Women of reproductive age usually present with pelvic pain (usually cyclical) or for the evaluation of infertility. The mean age is 25 to 29 years.[27] About 5% cases may occur in postmenopausal women, in whom hormone replacement therapy is suggested to play a role.[28] Endometriomas typically appear as unilocular or multilocular complex cysts that on US usually show low-level internal echogenicity owing to the presence of homogeneous hemorrhagic fluid content (**Fig. 11**). These cysts can be unilateral or bilateral, and can be seen within the ovaries or be extraovarian. Sometimes, echogenic foci or small nodularity is seen along the wall of an endometrioma (see **Fig. 11**). Color Doppler imaging does not show internal vascularity. A small percentage of endometriomas may have features that are less typical and may show anechoic fluid on US, a fluid-fluid level, or calcifications. When chronic, they may occasionally appear solid on US. On CT, endometriomas usually show slightly higher-density fluid in the cysts compared with simple cysts. MR imaging has greater specificity for diagnosing endometriomas. A T1-weighted fat-suppressed sequence should always be added to eliminate fat-containing lesions from the differential diagnosis. Typical blood products on various

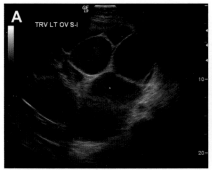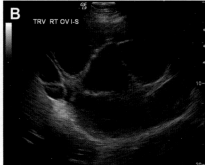

Fig. 8. (A, B) Bilateral cystic ovarian enlargement in a patient undergoing assisted reproduction therapy. The patient's ovaries were greater than 12 cm in size with the presence of ascites and pleural effusions, consistent with severe ovarian hyperstimulation syndrome (OHSS).

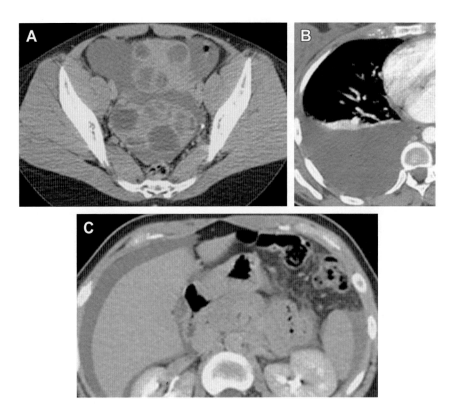

Fig. 9. OHSS. (*A*) Axial CT image of the pelvis shows bilateral cystic enlargement of the ovaries in the presence of ascites. (*B, C*) Axial CT images of the chest and upper abdomen demonstrate pleural effusion and ascites from third spacing, which occurs in OHSS.

sequences are seen with high T1 and variable T2 signals. Gadolinium-enhanced sequences do not particularly help in making a diagnosis because endometriomas may show variable and heterogeneous contrast enhancement. Sometimes loss of signal on T2 sequences, also called "shading," may be seen in endometriomas, reflecting a chronic nature.[29–31] Presence of T2 shading and

presence of multiple T1-hyperintense cystic lesions strongly suggest endometriomas.[29] Treatment can be expectant, medical, or surgical, depending on the severity of symptoms. Medical treatment consists of symptomatic treatment and hormonal manipulation with the menstrual cycle. Conservative surgery retaining the reproductive function can be performed with laparoscopy and laparotomy. Definitive surgery includes hysterectomy and oophorectomy (**Box 7**).

POLYCYSTIC OVARIAN DISEASE/SYNDROME

Polycystic ovarian disease (also known as polycystic ovarian syndrome or PCOS) is a condition of hormonal imbalance. The classic symptomatology of amenorrhea, infertility, obesity, and hirsutism in these patients with enlarged polycystic ovaries was first described by Stein and Leventhal in

---

Box 4
Modified Golan classification for OHSS

Category	Ovarian Size (cm)	Signs and Symptoms
Mild	<6	Abdominal distention, nausea, vomiting
Moderate	6–12	Ascites
Severe	>12	Ascites/hydrothorax, hypovolumia, hemoconcentration, oliguria, coagulation disorder, shock

Data from Ritchie WG. Sonographic evaluation of normal and induced ovulation. Radiology 1986; 161(1):1–10.

Box 5
Hallmark imaging findings in OHSS

Bilateral symmetric cystic ovarian enlargement

Ascites

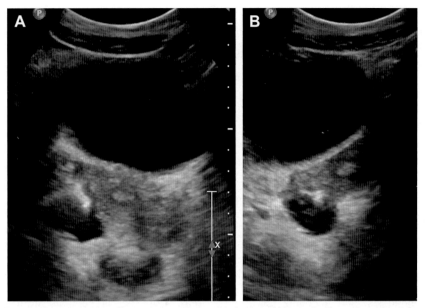

Fig. 10. (A, B) Complex cyst in the adnexa in a patient who had undergone ipsilateral oophorectomy for endometriosis 3 years previously. The patient presented with chronic pelvic pain and dyspareunia.

1935. Polycystic ovaries are not the cause of this disorder but are merely a sign of an underlying anovulatory endocrine disorder, which is usually associated with androgen excess and increased luteinizing hormone/follicle-stimulating hormone ratio. PCOS has a prevalence of 6.6% in women of reproductive age in the United States.[32] Transvaginal US is the standard imaging technique, as up to 30% of cases may not be detected on transabdominal US.[33] Transvaginal US usually shows slightly enlarged ovaries with numerous peripheral subcentimeter (2–9 mm) cysts/follicles without the presence of a dominant follicle (Fig. 12). During the last decade, The US appearance of the polycystic ovaries has been incorporated as 1 of the criteria for the diagnosis of this condition along with other clinical criteria. The US criteria incorporated in the guidelines of the American College of Obstetricians and Gynecologists takes into account 2 US features. Polycystic ovaries are present when (1) one or both ovaries demonstrate 12 or more follicles measuring 2 to 9 mm, or (2) the ovarian volume exceeds 10 mL. Only one ovary meeting one of these criteria is sufficient to establish the presence of polycystic ovaries.[32] Association

with other clinical criteria is important, and presence of polycystic ovaries alone in the absence of other criteria is insufficient for making a diagnosis of this syndrome. Data suggest that about 23% of women of reproductive age will have polycystic ovaries.[34] However, only 5% to 10% of these women will have symptoms of PCOS.[35] MR imaging should be reserved for the patients in whom either transvaginal US cannot be performed or is inconclusive. MR shows hypointense central stroma on T2-weighted images with small

| Box 6 |
| ORS |
| |
| History of oophorectomy with ipsilateral cystic or multiseptated mass |

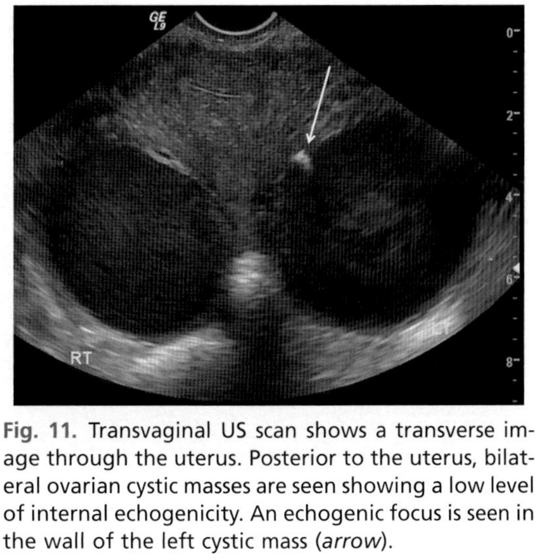

Fig. 11. Transvaginal US scan shows a transverse image through the uterus. Posterior to the uterus, bilateral ovarian cystic masses are seen showing a low level of internal echogenicity. An echogenic focus is seen in the wall of the left cystic mass (arrow).

<table>
<tr><td>

Box 7
Differential diagnosis of cystic mass with internal echoes

Hemorrhagic cyst

Endometrioma

Tubo-ovarian abscess

Ovarian neoplasm

Ectopic pregnancy

</td><td>

Box 8
Differential diagnosis of multiple small cystic lesions in the ovaries

Normal ovaries

Polycystic ovarian syndrome

Ovarian hyperstimulation syndrome

</td></tr>
</table>

peripheral hyperintense cysts. CT is not used for the evaluation of PCOS (**Box 8**).

ECTOPIC PREGNANCY

Ectopic pregnancy is a rare cause of cystic ovarian or adnexal mass. Its incidence is about 2% of all reported pregnancies, and accounts for about 9% of deaths related to pregnancy.[36] These patients usually present with abdominal pain and vaginal bleeding. In the setting of positive β-hCG, the differential diagnosis includes a normal intra-uterine pregnancy (IUP), abnormal IUP, spontaneous abortion, molar pregnancy, or ectopic pregnancy. High-resolution transvaginal US is the best way to evaluate these patients. A large majority of ectopic pregnancies occur in the fallopian tube (90%–95%). Ovarian pregnancies are rare and account for less than 1% of cases of ectopic pregnancy. By the fifth week of gestation in a normal pregnancy, a more clearly defined gestational sac should be observed, with a "double-decidual-sac" sign consisting of 2 hyperechoic

curvilinear lines at the margin of the developing gestational sac separated by hypoechoic material. A gestational pseudosac may be seen in 10% to 20% of ectopic pregnancies.[37] When a pregnancy test is positive and there is no evidence of IUP, any adnexal abnormality should be looked at with suspicion. The findings that have highest specificity include a live extrauterine embryo, adnexal mass with yolk sac or a nonliving embryo, complex or solid adnexal mass, and an echogenic tubal ring (**Fig. 13A**) that is separate from the ovary.[38] Ovarian corpus luteum can mimic the appearance of an ectopic pregnancy. Demonstrating that an adnexal "mass" is within the ovary, or arising from it, in an exophytic manner virtually excludes ectopic pregnancy because intraovarian ectopic pregnancies are extremely rare (<1%). When pressure is applied by the vaginal probe internally and by manual compression externally, the corpus luteum will move with the ovary while the adnexal mass can be observed moving separate from the ovary. Color Doppler may show the so-called ring-of-fire appearance caused by peripheral increased vascularity around the tubal ring (see **Fig. 13B**). However, this finding is also frequently observed in corpus luteum cysts of the ovary. In

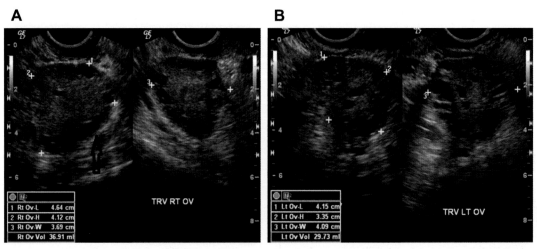

A

1 Rt Ov-L   4.64 cm
2 Rt Ov-H   4.12 cm
3 Rt Ov-W   3.69 cm
Rt Ov Vol 36.91 ml

TRV RT OV

B

1 Lt Ov-L   4.15 cm
2 Lt Ov-H   3.35 cm
3 Lt Ov-W   4.09 cm
Lt Ov Vol 29.73 ml

TRV LT OV

Fig. 12. (*A, B*) Transvaginal US images through right (*A*) and left (*B*) ovaries show enlarged ovaries with increased volumes. Numerous small subcentimeter follicles are present bilaterally with a more peripheral arrangement (*arrow*).

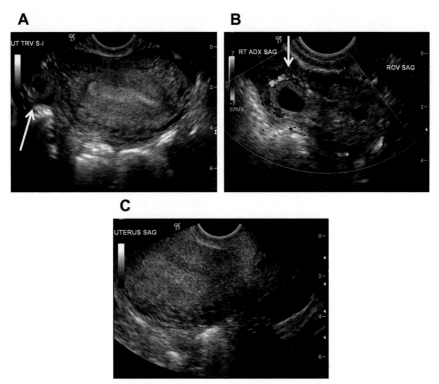

Fig. 13. (*A–C*) Transvaginal US through the uterus and right adnexa. (*A*) A transverse image of the uterus showing normal and empty endometrial stripe. An echogenic ring is seen outside the uterus in the right adnexa (*arrow*). (*B*) A color Doppler image through the right adnexal region shows peripheral hypervascularity or "ring of fire" appearance (*arrow*). (*C*) A sagittal image through the uterus shows slightly thickened endometrial stripe without an intrauterine pregnancy. Fluid/blood is noted posterior to the uterus.

ruptured ectopic, free intraperitoneal blood is seen within the pelvis (see **Fig. 13C**). MR imaging is generally not indicated for diagnosis, as it may show nonspecific features of complex adnexal mass with variable contrast enhancement (**Boxes 9** and **10**).

PARAOVARIAN CYSTS

Paraovarian cysts are benign intraperitoneal mesothelial cysts that consist of about 10% to 20% of all adnexal masses, which usually present in third and fourth decades of life.[39] These cysts usually arise from the broad ligament of uterus and are usually adjacent to the fallopian tubes. Paraovarian cysts can be of various sizes but have an average size of 8 cm,[40] and may be unilateral or bilateral. On US they are usually seen as simple, anechoic, unilocular, round or oval cysts separate from the ipsilateral ovary. If a paraovarian cyst is seen adjacent to the ovary, it may be

Box 9
Differential diagnosis of complex adnexal mass with positive β-hCG
Ectopic pregnancy
Corpus luteal cyst in early IUP
Theca luteal cyst in molar pregnancy
Hormone-secreting ovarian tumor

Box 10
Nonovarian cystic lesions mimicking ovarian lesions
Paraovarian cyst
Peritoneal inclusion cyst
Hydrosalpinx
Lymphocele
Mucocele of the appendix
Lymphangioma
Enteric duplication cyst
Cystic degeneration in exophytic fibroid
Anterior spinal cysts

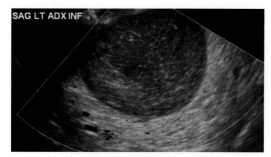

Fig. 14. Color Doppler image of an enlarged, edematous ovary.

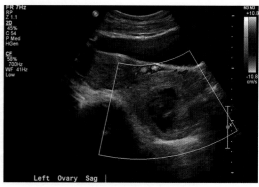

Fig. 16. Color Doppler image of a torsed ovary exhibiting twisted vessels known as the whirlpool sign.

difficult to differentiate it from an ovarian cyst. On real-time US scanning, applying gentle pressure with the transvaginal transducer or with manual pressure at the lower abdomen may help to show the cyst moving separate from the ovary. Their anatomic orientation is better delineated by MR imaging, which shows circumscribed T2 bright-signal and T1 low-signal structure without any significant solid enhancing components or wall thickening. Occasionally they may undergo torsion and show high T1 signal attributable to hemorrhage, along with wall thickening.

PERITONEAL INCLUSION CYSTS

Peritoneal inclusion cysts are also intraperitoneal mesothelial cysts that are almost exclusively seen in premenopausal females with active ovarian function. These cysts are usually seen as an incidental finding; however, some patients may present with pelvic pain. Such cysts form secondarily to previous peritoneal insult such as

surgery, trauma, endometriosis, and infection. The peritoneal fluid starts to accumulate around the ovaries, which may appear entrapped within these cysts. Peritoneal inclusion cysts may be multilocular with thin septations, but usually assume the shape of the adjacent peritoneal cavity. Occasionally the septations may be thickened and may show detectable flow on color Doppler US. Although the ovaries may appear to be entrapped in the cysts on US or MR imaging, the cysts are separate from the ovaries. US may show multiloculated simple anechoic cysts around the ovaries that may be unilateral or bilateral. On MR imaging, these cysts usually show simple fluid content without significant enhancing solid component, which are usually low intensity on T1-weighted images and high intensity on T2-weighted images. Occasionally they may be T1 bright if there is internal hemorrhage,[41] and may show high-density fluid on CT.

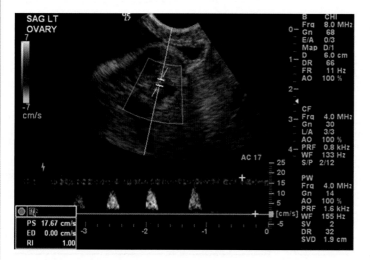

Fig. 15. Spectral Doppler image of a torsed ovary with high-resistance waveform and no diastolic flow.

HYDROSALPINX/CYSTIC DILATATION OF THE FALLOPIAN TUBE

Occasionally, cystic dilatation of the fallopian tube in hydrosalpinx, pyosalpinx, or hematosalpinx may be mistaken for cystic ovarian lesions. Hydrosalpinx occurs as a result of blockage of the fallopian tube, usually secondary to pelvic inflammatory disease or endometriosis.[42] On US, the structure appears tubular and usually can be separated from the adjacent ovary. The helpful signs toward correct diagnosis include the "beads-on-a-string" sign whereby multiple nodular mucosal folds are seen projecting along the wall, and diametrically opposed indentations called the "waist" sign.[43] MR imaging shows similar features but with a better anatomic delineation. Pyosalpinx is usually secondary to pelvic inflammatory disease, and presents with pelvic pain and constitutional symptoms. Hematosalpinx may show internal echoes on US, high-density fluid on CT, and typical MR findings of blood products on various sequences.

LYMPHOCELE

A lymphocele is a lymphatic fluid collection without any epithelial lining, which usually forms after lymphadenectomy for pelvic malignancy. It is usually seen 3 to 8 weeks after surgery, and occurs in 12% to 24% patients after radical lymphadenectomy.[44] On imaging it is usually a unilocular, thin-walled, fluid-filled structure, which many times cannot be differentiated from other cystic lesions. Fluid aspiration and analysis sometimes help in making a differentiation.[45] Lymphoceles are usually seen adjacent to the iliac vessels at the site of pelvic lymphadenectomy. A lymphocele does not show any enhancing solid components, the presence of which should raise the suspicion for recurrent malignancy.

Box 11
Differential diagnosis for ovarian torsion

Hemorrhagic cyst

Ectopic pregnancy

Pelvic inflammatory disease

Massive edema of the ovary

OVARIAN TORSION

Adnexal torsion involves the rotation of the ovary, fallopian tube, or both on its vascular pedicle. Clinically, patients usually present with sudden onset of pelvic pain accompanied by vomiting. In adults, 50% to 80% of adnexal torsion is associated with a cyst or benign ovarian tumor.[46] The risk factors for ovarian torsion include ipsilateral ovarian mass, pregnancy, hypermobility of adnexal structures, and prior tubal ligation.[47] The most common lesions associated with a torsed ovary is a follicular or corpus luteal cyst. Ipsilateral adnexal masses causing ovarian torsion usually measure greater than 5 cm.[47] The most common tumor associated with a torsed ovary is a dermoid, reported in 20% of cases.[48] It is unusual to see ovarian torsion in a cyst smaller than 5 cm.[49] The imaging findings usually depend on the degree and duration of the torsion. Although transvaginal US with Doppler is the initial imaging modality, CT can provide a better evaluation of the abnormal location of the ovary and the torsed pedicle. Occasionally, if the patient's clinical presentation is confusing and other entities such as renal stones or gastrointestinal problems are of concern, the patient may undergo a CT scan first. On gray-scale US, one of the most common imaging findings of ovarian torsion is an enlarged, edematous ovary (**Fig. 14**). The ovary may appear cystic because of necrosis or hemorrhage. The extent of hemorrhage depends on the

---

Box 12
Pearls and pitfalls of ovarian torsion

Interpretative Pearls:

- Enlarged ovary
- Residual ovarian tissue disproportionate to ovarian mass
- Twisted vascular pedicle

Imaging Pitfalls:

- Incorrect Doppler settings
- Underlying complex mass obscuring visualization of normal ovarian architecture

---

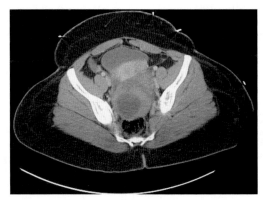

Fig. 17. Axial CT image demonstrating a hemorrhagic cyst in the left ovary and displaced left adnexa.

A   **B**

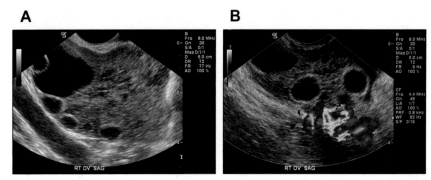

Fig. 18. (*A, B*) Gray-scale and color Doppler images demonstrating an enlarged, edematous ovary with peripheral follicles.

degree and duration of torsion. If there is an ovarian mass, the residual ovarian tissue may be disproportionately enlarged by the mass. Ovarian follicles may be displaced peripherally and may contain debris secondary to hemorrhage. If only the fallopian tube is twisted, it may give the appearance of a beaked structure. The classic color Doppler finding is absence of arterial flow. Color Doppler may show normal adnexal flow, particularly in early or partial torsion. One may also see decreased or absent diastolic flow and no venous flow (**Fig. 15**). The most frequent findings is a decrease or absence of venous flow.[49] No flow is more common in a nonviable ovary. The vascular pedicle can be twisted, with coiled or circular vessels showing the whirlpool sign (**Fig. 16**).[49] There may be an abrupt change in vascularity on color Doppler in the enlarged ovary from present to absent. Pelvic fluid may be simple or hemorrhagic. It is important that Doppler settings be optimized to detect low flow; this includes high spectral/color gain without creating artifact, decrease in pulse-repetition frequency, and color scale and low wall filter.[47] CT findings include a hemorrhagic ovarian cyst, an adnexal mass, a twisted ovarian vascular pedicle, and abnormal location of the adnexa (**Fig. 17**). The uterus may be deviated toward the torsed ovary. MR imaging findings include a T1-hyperintense rim of a subacute hematoma in an enlarged ovary.[50] Treatment of ovarian torsion includes laparoscopic surgical untwisting in noninfarcted ovary or, in the case of ovarian infarction, a laparoscopic salpingo-oophorectomy (**Boxes 11** and **12**).

MASSIVE EDEMA OF THE OVARY

Massive edema of the ovary occurs when there is partial or intermittent torsion leading to venous and lymphatic obstruction. Clinically this occurs in young adult patients who present with a long-term history of intermittent pain localized to one side. Unilateral involvement of the right ovary occurs 75% of the time,[47] and may be secondary to elevated right ovarian pressure relative to the left ovary, thus predisposing the right ovary to partially torse more. US gray-scale findings demonstrate an enlarged, edematous ovary with peripheral follicles (**Fig. 18**). The ovary maintains its usual ovoid shape. When scanning over the affected ovary, patients usually demonstrate focal tenderness. Color Doppler will demonstrate flow; however, venous waveforms may be difficult to obtain with spectral Doppler. The presence of blood flow does not exclude the diagnosis of massive edema of the ovary. Massive edema of the ovary can occur with a preexisting ovarian lesion.[51] MR imaging will show a low signal in ovarian stroma on T1-weighted imaging and a higher signal on T2-weighted imaging. Central enhancement of the ovary is noted.[52,53] Given that it is important to exclude an underlying tumor,

---

Box 13
Differential diagnosis of massive edema of the ovary

Ovarian torsion

Hemorrhagic cyst

Ovarian neoplasm

Box 14
Interpretation pearls for massive edema of the ovary

Enlarged edematous ovary with peripherally located follicles

Presence of blood flow does not exclude this diagnosis

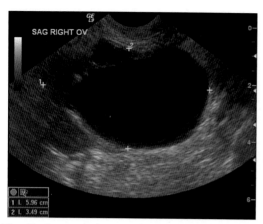

Fig. 19. Gray-scale image of an indeterminate cystic ovarian lesion. Irregular wall thickening with thick septation is noted.

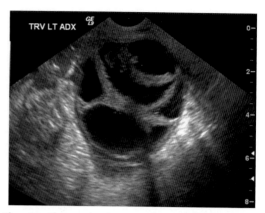

Fig. 20. Gray-scale image of a malignant cystic ovarian lesion (serous cystadenocarcinoma) demonstrating multiple thick, irregular septations and papillary excrescences.

management includes detorsion and frozen section to exclude tumor (**Boxes 13 and 14**).

OVARIAN CYSTIC NEOPLASMS

Ovarian cystic neoplasms can be divided into 2 main categories: benign and malignant. Most ovarian cystic neoplasms are benign. US is considered the primary imaging modality for ovarian cystic lesions. MR imaging is used as a problem-solving tool. Whereas US and MR imaging are highly sensitive for characterizing ovarian cystic lesions, MR imaging is more specific for characterization of fat and blood products. MR imaging can evaluate solid components in lesions that cannot be fully visualized on US.[52] CT or MR imaging can be used in staging to evaluate patients for metastatic disease. Distinguishing benign from potentially malignant lesions is important. Some sonographic features can be seen in both benign and malignant ovarian lesions. The goal of using US to assess an ovarian cystic lesion is to determine if it is likely benign, indeterminate, or malignant. A cyst that is otherwise simple but has a single thin septation (<3 mm) or a calcification in the wall is almost always benign.[5] Sonographic features that classify a lesion as indeterminate are multiple thin septations or a

solid nodule and no detectable Doppler flow (**Fig. 19**).[5] These features suggest a benign etiology. Cysts with irregular wall thickening may be difficult to distinguish from malignancies and are thus indeterminate. MR imaging may be useful to evaluate for contrast enhancement in any solid areas. In a woman of reproductive age, these indeterminate lesions usually require a short-interval follow-up of 6 to 12 weeks with US.[5] A 6- to 12-week period would allow a functional cyst to resolve. If a lesion is persistent then surgical consultation may be warranted. Thick septations or focal areas of wall thickening (>3 mm), papillary projections, and solid components with flow at Doppler US are concerning for a malignant ovarian neoplasm (**Box 15, Fig. 20**).[5,6] These findings are particularly worrisome when peritoneal masses or ascites are noted in the pelvis (**Fig. 21**).

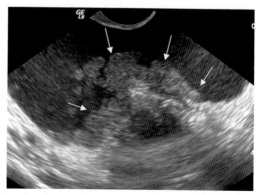

Fig. 21. Gray-scale image of the right lower quadrant demonstrates complex ascites and peritoneal masses (*arrows*) in a patient with mucinous cystadenocarcinoma.

Box 15
Imaging pearls for interpretation of malignant cystic ovarian neoplasms

Thick septations larger than 3 mm

Papillary projections

Solid components with blood flow

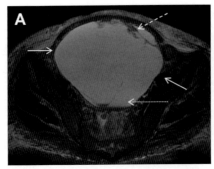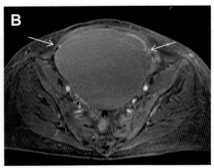

Fig. 22. (A) Axial T2-weighted fat-saturated image demonstrates a large T2-hyperintense cystic lesion (*arrow*) in the mid pelvis with partial septations (*dashed arrow*) and a hematocrit level (*dotted arrow*). (B) Postcontrast axial T1-weighted image demonstrates mild enhancement of the septae (*arrows*); no nodules are present. Findings are compatible with an ovarian serous cystadenoma.

Combining Doppler with gray-scale US is helpful in the assessment of ovarian lesions. Color Doppler US is used to evaluate for the presence or absence of blood flow within any solid areas or septations within the lesion. Spectral Doppler is used to distinguish flow from artifact. Low-resistance Doppler flow is concerning for malignant neovascularity, although this can be seen in benign entities such as a physiologic cyst. There are reports of malignant ovarian lesions with high and low resistance indices.[6] Although there has been much written in the literature about the use of flow parameters to evaluate ovarian cystic lesions and adnexal masses, the sensitivity and specificity are no better than the parameters used in morphologic assessment. The Society of Radiologists in Ultrasound Conference consensus statement affirms that the presence of blood flow in a solid measurement is the most important Doppler feature.[5]

Ovarian tumors are included in the differential of cystic ovarian masses, and are subdivided into 5 main categories according to the World Health Organization classification system[54,55]:

1. Epithelial tumors account for about 75% of all ovarian tumors, and 90% to 95% of ovarian malignancies.
2. Germ-cell tumors account for about 15% to 20% of all ovarian neoplasms.
3. Sex-cord–stromal tumors account for about 5% to 10% of all ovarian neoplasms.
4. Metastatic tumors account for about 1% to 5% of ovarian malignancies, and usually arise from breast, colon, endometrial, stomach, and cervical cancers.

Malignant tumors of the ovaries occur at all ages. Major histologic types can occur in different age groups. Germ-cell tumors constitute the majority of cases in younger females (<20 years),

whereas epithelial ovarian cancers are primarily seen in women older than 50 years. Epithelial ovarian cancer is a relatively common disease in the United States. The lifetime risk of a woman in the United States developing ovarian cancer is approximately 1 in 70.[56] Approximately 23% of gynecologic cancers are ovarian in origin, but is responsible for 47% of all deaths from cancer related to the female genital tract.

Presentation of a cystic adnexal mass in a young female should prompt the physician to obtain diagnostic workup for a germ-cell tumor, whereas in middle aged women epithelial tumors do not usually produce symptoms or signs that would alert the clinician to this diagnosis.[57,58] Approximately two-thirds of all epithelial tumors are Stage III or Stage IV at diagnosis. Symptoms include vague abdominal pain or discomfort, menstrual

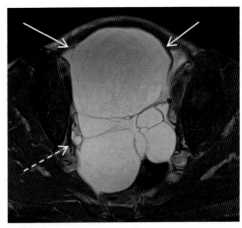

Fig. 23. Axial T2-weighted fat-saturated image demonstrates a septated cystic lesion in the mid pelvis (*arrows*) abutting the right ovary (*dashed arrow*). Findings are concerning for low malignant potential serous cystadenoma.

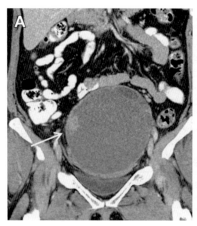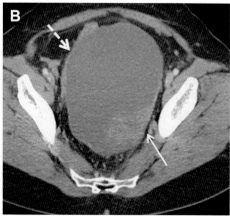

Fig. 24. (A) Coronal CT image demonstrates a complex cystic lesion in the mid abdomen and pelvis with an eccentric nodule along the right lateral (*arrow*), concerning for ovarian cystadenocarcinoma. (B) Axial CT image demonstrates a complex cystic lesion (*dashed arrow*) in the mid abdomen and pelvis with an eccentric nodule along the left posterior wall (*arrow*), concerning for ovarian cystadenocarcinoma.

irregularities, dyspepsia, and other mild digestive issues.

Epithelial Tumors

Epithelial tumors[55,58,59] usually present as unilocular or multilocular cystic adnexal masses. Epithelial ovarian tumors can be subclassified as benign, borderline, or malignant, according to their histologic features and clinical behavior. Tumors of borderline malignancy are characterized by lack of stromal invasion, infrequent and late recurrence, and long survival rates.

Serous tumors are the most common type within both the benign and malignant categories. Serous carcinomas account for 60% to 80% of all epithelial malignancies of the ovary. Approximately 25% of serous tumors are malignant.[58] Benign tumors generally present as unilocular cystic adnexal lesions (**Fig. 22**) and more likely to be bilateral than the mucinous variety. Tumors of low malignant potential may show increased septations and enhancement, although stromal invasion is not present (**Fig. 23**). The malignant lesions tend to have more solid tissue (**Fig. 24**) and areas of hemorrhage or necrosis than benign tumors. These tumors show papillary formations, with up to 30% demonstrating psammomatous calcifications.

Mucinous tumors are typically very large (**Fig. 25**) and multilocular, with numerous smooth, thin-walled cysts. Mucoid material is found within the cysts, sometimes accompanied by hemorrhagic or cellular debris. Ten percent of mucinous ovarian tumors are malignant and tend to have a proportionately greater solid-tissue component. CT and MR imaging may demonstrate high attenuation in some loculi, owing to the high protein content of the mucoid material. At histologic analysis, mucinous carcinomas of the ovary are difficult to differentiate from metastases to the ovary from an intestinal primary tumor.

Endometrioid carcinoma also presents as a cystic adnexal mass, although such tumors are associated with endometrial hyperplasia or carcinoma in 20% to 33% of the cases. Clear-cell carcinomas are identical to the endometrial clear-cell cancers, and also present as unilocular adnexal cysts with 1 or more tumor nodules protruding into the cavity.

Germ-Cell Tumors

Germ-cell tumors are frequently diagnosed by finding a palpable abdominal mass in a young

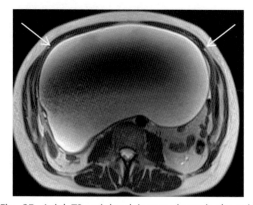

Fig. 25. Axial T2-weighted image through the mid abdomen reveals a large central cystic lesion (*arrows*). Central T2-hypointense signal is artifactually related to the large size of the lesion. Findings are suggestive of mucinous ovarian cystadenoma.

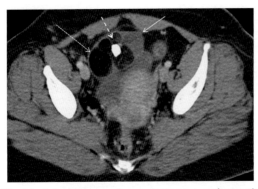

Fig. 26. Axial CT image demonstrates a complex cystic mass in the right adnexa, which demonstrates solid (*arrow*), fat (*dashed arrow*), and osseous components (*dotted arrow*) compatible with a mature teratoma.

woman who complains of abdominal pain. Imaging may reveal a cystic adnexal mass. These ovarian tumors arise from the primitive germ cells of the embryonic gonad. Only a minority of these tumors are malignant at presentation. These tumors can be further divided into dysgerminomas and nondysgerminomas (embryonal cancers), such as teratoma and choriocarcinoma.[56] These tumors are generally associated with abnormalities in serum lactic dehydrogenase, serum α-fetoprotein, or hCG.

The most common germ-cell tumor is a mature teratoma,[60] which can present as a cystic adnexal mass. Mature cystic teratoma (also known as dermoid cyst) typically contains mature tissues of ectodermal (skin, brain), mesodermal (muscle, fat), and endodermal (mucinous or ciliated epithelium) origin (**Fig. 26**). MR imaging aids the diagnosis by demonstrating signal loss on fat-suppressed sequences within a dermoid cyst (**Fig. 27**).

Dysgerminoma is the second most common germ-cell tumor after teratoma, and accounts for only 1% to 2% of all malignant ovarian tumors, with a high association with hypercalcemia. Dysgerminoma occurs mainly in children and young women, and presents as a large solid tumor with areas of hemorrhage and minimal necrosis.

Sex-Cord Tumors

Sex-cord–stromal tumors arise from the gonadal stroma and account for 5% to 10% of ovarian tumors. Sex-cord tumors include granulosa cell tumors, thecomas, fibromas, and Sertoli-Leydig cell tumors.[56] These tumors occur in the fourth to fifth decade of life, although Sertoli-Leydig cell tumor is more common in the third decade. Sex-cord–stromal tumors are usually unilateral and mostly solid, and appear homogeneous. However, granulosa cell tumors can be large and cystic in postmenopausal women. Thecomas mostly present as solid or partially cystic tumors in postmenopausal women with signs of hyperestrogenism, whereas Sertoli-Leydig tumors present as solid/cystic masses in younger females with signs of androgen excess.[61,62]

Some of the sex-cord tumors are associated with clinical syndromes; for example, 30% of patients with sex-cord tumors with annular tubules have Peutz-Jeghers syndrome, an autosomal dominant disorder characterized by multiple gastrointestinal hamartomatous polyps, melanocytic macules of the lips, buccal mucosa, and so forth. Fibromas are associated with Meig syndrome,

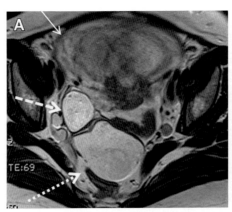
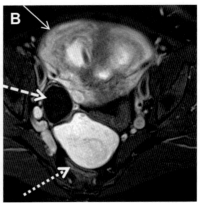

Fig. 27. (*A*) T2-weighted axial image demonstrates a gravid uterus (*arrow*). The posterior midline larger cystic structure (*dashed arrow*) and the right adnexal lesion both demonstrate T2-hyperintense signal (*dotted arrow*). (*B*) T2-weighted axial fat-saturated image demonstrates the posterior midline to retain hyperintense signal compatible with a cyst (*dotted arrow*); however, the right adnexal cyst demonstrates complete loss of signal in keeping with a dermoid cyst (*dashed arrow*). Gravid uterus is noted in the anterior pelvis (*arrow*).

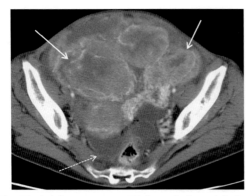

Fig. 28. Axial postcontrast CT through the pelvis demonstrates bilateral large adnexal masses (*arrows*) with free fluid (*dashed arrow*), compatible with Krukenberg tumors.

characterized by a benign ovarian tumor (fibroma) with ascites and pleural effusion.

Metastases to the Ovary

Metastases to the ovary account for 1% of ovarian tumors. However, these are mostly solid masses; central necrosis can lead to a cystic appearance (**Fig. 28**). Krukenberg tumor refers to metastases in the ovary arising mostly from a gastrointestinal primary. Gastric adenocarcinoma is a common primary tumor that metastasizes to the ovary. These tumors are generally bilateral (>80% of cases).

SUMMARY

US is the primary imaging modality for the evaluation of cystic ovarian lesions. Most of these lesions are benign. However, some are indeterminate, and other modalities such as MR imaging or CT can be helpful in further evaluation. It is important to correlate the patient's clinical signs and symptoms with the imaging features. Clinical information such as age, menstrual status, and surgical history are important, as some entities are more common in certain age groups. Imaging is used to help guide the management of these patients.

REFERENCES

1. Harris RD, Javitt MC, Glanc P, et al. American College of Radiology. ACR appropriateness criteria: clinically suspected adnexal masses. Available at: http://www.acr.org/~/media/ACR/Documents/AppCriteria/Diagnostic/ClinicallySuspectedAdnexalMass.pdf. Accessed April 2013.
2. Ritchie WG. Sonographic evaluation of normal and induced ovulation. Radiology 1986;161(1):1–10.
3. Bakos O, Lundkvist O, Wide L, et al. Ultrasonographical and hormonal description of the normal ovulatory and menstrual cycle. Acta Obstet Gynecol Scand 1994;73(10):790–6.
4. Langer JE, Oliver ER, Lev-Toaff AS, et al. Imaging of the female pelvis through the live cycle. Radiographics 2012;32:1575–97.
5. Levine D, Brown DL, Andreotti RF, et al. Management of asymptomatic ovarian and other adnexal cysts imaged at US: Society of Radiologists in Ultrasound consensus conference statement. Radiology 2010;256(30):943–54.
6. Laing FC, Allison S. US of the ovary and adnexa: to worry or not to worry? Radiographics 2012;32: 1621–39.
7. Feong YY, Outwater EK, Kang HK. Imaging evaluation of ovarian masses. Radiographics 2000;20: 1445–70.
8. Ekerhovd E, Wienerroith H, Staudach A, et al. Preoperative assessment of unilocular adnexal cysts by transvaginal ultrasonography: a comparison between ultrasonographic morphologic imaging and histopathologic diagnosis. Am J Obstet Gynecol 2001;184(2):48–54.
9. Modesitt SC, Pavlik EJ, Ueland FR, et al. Risk of malignancy in unilocular ovarian cystic tumors less than 10 centimeters in diameter. Obstet Gynecol 2003;102(3):594–9.
10. Healy DL, Bell R, Roberston DM, et al. Ovarian status in healthy postmenopausal women. Menopause 2008;15(6):1109–14.
11. Patel MD, Feldstein VA, Filly RA. The likelihood ratio of sonographic findings for the diagnosis of hemorrhagic ovarian cysts. J Ultrasound Med 2005;24(5): 607–14.
12. Valentin L. Use of morphology to characterize and manage common adnexal masses. Best Pract Res Clin Obstet Gynaecol 2004;18(1):71–89.
13. Jain KA. Sonographic spectrum of hemorrhagic ovarian cysts. J Ultrasound Med 2002;21:879–86.
14. Kanso HN, Hachem K, Aoun NJ. Variable MR findings in ovarian functional hemorrhagic cysts. J Magn Reson Imaging 2006;24:356–61.
15. Okai T, Kobayashi K, Ryo E, et al. Transvaginal sonographic appearance of hemorrhagic functional ovarian cysts and their spontaneous regression. Int J Gynaecol Obstet 1994;44(1): 47–52.
16. Schenker JG, Weinstein D. Ovarian hyperstimulation syndrome: a current survey. Fertil Steril 1978; 30:255–68.
17. Zivi E, Simon A, Laufer N. Ovarian hyperstimulation syndrome: definition, incidence, and classification. Semin Reprod Med 2010;28(6):441–7.
18. Haning RV Jr, Zweibel WJ. Ultrasound assistance in clinical management of infertility. Semin Ultrasound CT MR 1983;4:226–33.

19. Kim IY, Lee BH. Ovarian hyperstimulation syndrome US and CT appearances. Clin Imaging 1997;21:284–6.

20. Jung BG, Kim H. Severe spontaneous ovarian hyperstimulation syndrome with MR findings. J Comput Assist Tomogr 2001;24(2):215–7.

21. Jung SE, Byun JY, Lee JM, et al. MR imaging of maternal disease in pregnancy. AJR Am J Roentgenol 2001;177(6):1293–300.

22. Baron KT, Babagbemi KT, Arleo EK, et al. Emergent complications of assisted reproduction: expecting the unexpected. Radiographics 2013;33:229–44.

23. Mashiach S, Bider D, Moran O, et al. Adnexal torsion of hyperstimulated ovaries in pregnancies after gonadotropin therapy. Fertil Steril 1990;53(1):76–80.

24. Kho RM, Abrao MS. Ovarian remnant syndrome: etiology, diagnosis, treatment and impact of endometriosis. Curr Opin Obstet Gynecol 2012;42(4):210–4.

25. Magtibay PM, Magrina JF. Ovarian remnant syndrome. Clin Obstet Gynecol 2006;49(3):526–34.

26. Fleischer AC, Tait D, Mayo J, et al. Sonographic features of ovarian remnants. J Ultrasound Med 1998;17(9):551–5.

27. Phillips HE, McGahan JP. Ovarian remnant syndrome. Radiology 1982;142(2):487.

28. Dmowski WP, Lesniewicz R, Rana N, et al. Changing trends in the diagnosis of endometriosis: a comparative study of women with pelvic endometriosis presenting with chronic pelvic pain or infertility. Fertil Steril 1997;67:238–43.

29. Clement PB. Pathology of endometriosis. Pathol Annu 1990;25:245–95.

30. Togashi K, Nishimura K, Kimura I, et al. Endometrial cysts: diagnosis with MR imaging. Radiology 1991;180:73–8.

31. Siegelman ES, Outwater EK. Tissue characterization in the female pelvis by means of MR imaging. Radiology 1999;212:5–18.

32. Rosenfield RL. Clinical review: identifying children at risk for polycystic ovary syndrome. J Clin Endocrinol Metab 2007;92(3):787–96.

33. Azziz R, Woods KS, Reyna R, et al. The prevalence and features of the polycystic ovary syndrome in an unselected population. J Clin Endocrinol Metab 2004;89(6):2745–9.

34. Balen AH, Laven JS, Tan SL, et al. Ultrasound assessment of the polycystic ovary: international consensus definitions. Hum Reprod Update 2003;9(6):505–14.

35. Polson DW, Adams J, Wadsworth J, et al. Polycystic ovaries: a common finding in normal women. Lancet 1988;1(8590):870–2.

36. Lakhani K, Seifalian AM, Atiomo WU, et al. Polycystic ovaries. Br J Radiol 2002;75(889):9–16.

37. Centers for Disease Control. Ectopic pregnancy—United States, 1988–1989. MMWR Morb Mortal Wkly Rep 1992;41:591–4.

38. Levine D. Ectopic pregnancy. Radiology 2007;245:385–97.

39. Brown DL, Doubilet PM. Transvaginal sonography for diagnosing ectopic pregnancy: positivity criteria and performance characteristics. J Ultrasound Med 1994;13:259–66.

40. Kishimoto K, Ito K, Awaya H, et al. Paraovarian cyst: MR imaging features. Abdom Imaging 2002;27(6):685–9.

41. Kim JS, Woo SK, Suh SJ, et al. Sonographic diagnosis of paraovarian cysts: value of detecting a separate ipsilateral ovary. AJR Am J Roentgenol 1995;164(6):1441–4.

42. Levy AD, Arnaiz J, Shaw JC, et al. Primary peritoneal tumors: imaging features with pathologic correlation. Radiographics 2008;28(2):583–607 [quiz: 621–2].

43. Horrow MM. Ultrasound of pelvic inflammatory disease. Ultrasound Q 2004;20:171–9.

44. Patel MD, Acord DL, Young SW. Likelihood ratio of sonographic findings in discriminating hydrosalpinx from other adnexal masses. AJR Am J Roentgenol 2006;186(4):1033–8.

45. Yang DM, Jung DH, Kim H, et al. Retroperitoneal cystic masses: CT, clinical, and pathologic findings and literature review. Radiographics 2004;24(5):1353–65.

46. Kim HY, Kim JW, Kim SH, et al. An analysis of the risk factors and management of lymphocele after pelvic lymphadenectomy in patients with gynecologic malignancies. Cancer Res Treat 2004;36(6):377–83.

47. Atri M, Reinhold C. Diagnostic Imaging: Gynecology. Chapter 7: the ovary. 1st edition. Salt Lake City, Utah: Amirsys; 2007.

48. Cichiello L, Hamper U, Scoutt L. Ultrasound evaluation of gynecologic causes of pelvic pain. Obstet Gynecol Clin North Am 2011;38:86–114.

49. Abayam F, Hamper U. Ovarian and adnexal torsion: spectrum of sonographic findings with pathologic correlation. J Ultrasound Med 2001;20:1063–9.

50. Chang H. Pearls and pitfalls in diagnosis of ovarian torsion. Radiographics 2008;28:1355–68.

51. Duigenen S. Ovarian torsion: magnetic resonance features on CT and MRI with pathologic correlation. AJR Am J Roentgenol 2012;198(2):W122–31.

52. Cepri I. Massive edema of the ovary diagnosed with laparoscopic biopsy and frozen section. J Postgrad Med 2005;51:336–7.

53. Kramer L. Massive edema of the ovary: high resolution MR findings using a phased array pelvic coil. J Magn Reson Imaging 1997;75:758–60.

54. Bell D, Pannu H. Radiologic assessment of gynecologic malignancies. Obstet Gynecol Clin North Am 2011;38:45–68.

55. Scully ER. Classification of human ovarian tumors. Environ Health Perspect 1987;73:15–24.

56. Cotran RS, Kumar V, Robbins SL. Pathologic basis of disease. 4th edition. Philadelphia: Saunders; 1989. p. 1158–9.

57. Denny L, Hacker FN, Gori J, et al. Staging classifications and clinical practice guidelines for gynaecologic cancers. FIGO Committee on Gynecologic Oncology. Int J Gynaecol Obstet 2000;70: 207–312.

58. Bankhead CR, Kehoe ST, Austoker J. Symptoms associated with diagnosis of ovarian cancer. A systematic review. BJOG 2005;112:857–65.

59. Lataifeh I, Marsden DE, Robertson G, et al. Presenting symptoms of epithelial ovarian cancer. Aust N Z J Obstet Gynaecol 2005;45:211–4.

60. Kawamoto S, Urban AB, Fishman E. CT of epithelial ovarian tumors. Radiographics 1999; 19:S85–102.

61. Talerman A. Germ cell tumors of the ovary. In: Kurman RJ, editor. Blaustein's pathology of the female genital tract. 4th edition. New York: Springer-Verlag; 1994. p. 849–914.

62. Lee-Jones L. Ovarian tumors: an overview. Atlas Genet Cytogenet Oncol Haematol 2004;8(2): 245–55.

Current Concepts in the Diagnosis and Management of Endometrial and Cervical Carcinomas

Sree Harsha Tirumani, MD[a],
Alampady K.P. Shanbhogue, MD[b],
Srinivasa R. Prasad, MD[c],*

KEYWORDS

- Endometrial carcinoma • Cervical carcinoma • Magnetic resonance imaging
- International Federation of Gynecologic Oncology (FIGO)

KEY POINTS

- The 2 key magnetic resonance (MR) imaging sequences required for optimal staging of endometrial cancer are high-resolution T2-weighted images, which depict the zonal anatomy of the uterus, and dynamic intravenous contrast-enhanced MR, which identifies viable tumor, enabling accurate assessment of myometrial invasion and nodal disease.
- Diffusion-weighted (DW) imaging has an added value in endometrial cancer by better depiction of the primary tumor, increasing the detection of drop metastases in the cervix and vagina, and diagnosing extrauterine spread to the peritoneum and lymph nodes, particularly in patients with contraindication to intravenous gadolinium contrast.
- MR imaging, by determining the depth of myometrial invasion and detecting cervical stromal invasion, can predict lymphovascular space invasion, a major prognostic risk factor.
- MR imaging plays a key role in the treatment strategies of cervical cancer by determining tumor volume, parametrial invasion, and nodal metastases.
- The presence of an intact stromal ring (with a thickness of >3 mm) in cervical carcinoma has a very high negative predictive value of greater than 96% for parametrial invasion.
- Positron emission tomography combined with computed tomography is highly sensitive and specific for detecting positive pelvic and/or para-aortic lymphadenopathy as well as distant metastases, which necessitates adjuvant radiotherapy and chemotherapy.

INTRODUCTION

Endometrial and cervical cancers, the 2 most common gynecologic malignancies, have distinct epidemiologic patterns, etiologic factors, and management strategies. Recent advances in pathology and genetics have thrown fresh light on the pathogenesis of these cancers. Based on pathogenesis and molecular biology, endometrial cancers have been classified into type 1 and 2 cancers. Type 1 cancers (endometrioid subtype), comprising up to 85% to 90% of all cancers, are

The authors have no conflicts of interest to declare.
[a] Department of Imaging, Dana-Farber Cancer Institute/Brigham and Women's Hospital, Harvard Medical School, 450 Brookline Avenue, Boston, MA 02215, USA; [b] Department of Radiology, Beth Israel Medical Center, 16th Street and 1st Avenue, New York, NY 10003, USA; [c] Department of Radiology, University of Texas MD Anderson Cancer Center, 1400 Pressler Street, Houston, TX 77030, USA
* Corresponding author.
E-mail address: sprasad2@mdanderson.org

Radiol Clin N Am 51 (2013) 1087–1110
http://dx.doi.org/10.1016/j.rcl.2013.07.003

characterized by low-grade, low-stage, estrogen-dependent tumors that are caused by dysregulation of the PI3K/PTEN/AKT pathway.[1] Type 2 cancers (serous/clear-cell carcinomas and carcinosarcomas) are histologically high-grade, biologically aggressive cancers with frequent extrauterine spread of disease that account for 44% of endometrial cancer-related deaths. Type 2 cancers show p53, HER2, and/or p16 mutations.[1] On the other hand, cervical carcinoma comprises squamous cell carcinoma (SCC), the most common subtype that accounts for 80% of all cancers, and mucinous carcinoma, which account for the remainder. SCCs of the cervix are associated with chronic infection by high-risk human papilloma virus (HPV) infection; vaccines against high-risk HPV infection confer protection against development of SCCs.

Recent advances in magnetic resonance (MR) imaging hardware, software, and coil technology permit multiplanar, high-resolution imaging of the uterus and the adnexa. Because of the high-contrast resolution and the multiplanar and tissue-specific imaging capabilities, MR imaging is extremely valuable in the diagnosis, characterization, localization, and accurate locoregional staging of pelvic malignancies, thus enabling optimal triaging and management of patients.

EPIDEMIOLOGY, ETIOPATHOGENESIS, PATHOLOGY, AND GENETICS

Endometrial cancer is the most common gynecologic cancer in the developed countries, and accounts for 6% of all cancers in women. The estimated number of new cases in the United States in the year 2012 was 47,130 and the estimated deaths 8010.[2] The peak age of incidence is the 55- to 65-year group. The risk factors for endometrial cancer include obesity, unopposed estrogen replacement, diabetes, polycystic ovarian syndrome, nulliparity, hypertension, and tamoxifen therapy. The most common presenting symptom is postmenopausal or intermenstrual bleeding, which is responsible for its detection in early stage and consequent longer survival. More than 70% of patients with endometrial cancer present with stages 1 and 2 with resultant excellent prognosis. Histologically, endometrial cancers are divided into 2 types.[3] The most common is the endometrioid adenocarcinoma (type 1). Based on the degree of differentiation, the endometrioid adenocarcinoma is further subdivided into 3 grades: grade 1 (G1) tumors are well differentiated, whereas grade 3 (G3) tumors are poorly differentiated. At a molecular level, type 1 cancers are associated with PTEN, K-RAS, and CTNNB gene mutations. PTEN inactivation is encountered in

up to 80% of endometrioid adenocarcinomas.[1] The other histologic subtypes, namely clear-cell and serous papillary subtypes, constitute type 2 endometrial cancers. In contrast to type 1, type 2 cancers are frequently associated with inactivation of p53 and p16 genes, and gene overexpression of HER-2/neu.[1] From a management and prognosis point of view, high-grade type 1 and all type 2 cancers are associated with poor prognosis.

Cervical cancer is the third most common cancer in women worldwide, but is much more common in the developing countries, which contribute to 85% of new cases.[4] Effective screening strategies with Papanicolaou smear has led to a remarkable decrease in its incidence in the developed countries. In the United States 12,170 new cases and 4220 deaths were reported in the year 2012.[2] The average age at the time of diagnosis is 45 years.[5] Risk factors for cervical cancer, which are often prevalent in the developing countries, include infections with high-risk HPV (types 16, 18), oral contraceptive pills, low socioeconomic status, smoking, and human immunodeficiency virus. Recent studies have shown several molecular mechanisms mediated by the HPV in cervical cancer, including the inactivation of tumor suppressor genes (p53) and retinoblastoma (Rb) genes by the viral oncogenes E6 and E7.[6] SCC is the most common histologic type, accounting for about 75% to 80% cases, and arises from the ectocervix at the squamocolumnar junction.[7] The other less common types that arise from the endocervix include adenocarcinoma, adenosquamous carcinoma, adenocystic carcinoma, small-cell carcinoma, and lymphoma, which constitute up to 20% to 25% of cervical cancers.[8] Cervical cancer is often asymptomatic in the early stages, and the most common presenting symptom is vaginal bleeding.

REVISED INTERNATIONAL FEDERATION OF GYNECOLOGIC ONCOLOGY STAGING OF ENDOMETRIAL AND CERVICAL CANCER (2009)

The International Federation of Gynecologic Oncology (FIGO) revised the 1988 staging of gynecologic malignancies in 2009, consequent to better understanding of the clinical-pathologic characteristics and prognostic factors.[9] According to the 2009 FIGO staging of endometrial cancers (Table 1),[9] stage I tumors are confined to the uterine corpus and are subdivided into stage IA (no or <50% myometrial invasion) and stage IB (≥50% myometrial invasion). Stage II endometrial cancers invade the cervical stroma without parametrial invasion. Stage III endometrial cancers extend

Table 1
Revised FIGO staging, MR imaging features, and management of endometrial cancer

Revised FIGO Stage		MR Imaging Findings	Management	
			Primary	Adjuvant
I	Confined to the corpus uteri			
IA	Confined to the endometrium or invades less than one-half of the myometrium	Hypointense tumor seen within the endometrium or extends less than 50% of the myometrium disrupting the junctional zone	TH + BSO + pelvic and para-aortic node dissection + peritoneal washings for cytology	Observe or vaginal brachytherapy and/or pelvic RT (for G3)
IB	Invades one-half or more of the myometrium	Hypointense tumor extends ≥50% of the myometrium	TH + BSO + pelvic and para-aortic node dissection + peritoneal washings for cytology	Observe (for G1) or vaginal brachytherapy and/or pelvic RT ± chemotherapy (for G3)
II[a]	Invades the cervical stroma but not beyond the serosa	Hypointense cervical stroma disrupted by the tumor	RH + BSO + pelvic and para-aortic node dissection + peritoneal washings for cytology	Vaginal brachytherapy and/or pelvic RT ± chemotherapy (for G3)
III	Extends beyond the uterus or to the regional lymph nodes			
IIIA	Invades the serosa and/or adnexa	Disruption of the hypointense serosa ± adnexal enhancing masses	Resectable: TH + BSO + cytology + surgical debulking ± pelvic and para-aortic node dissection	Chemotherapy ± RT or tumor-directed RT ± pelvic RT ± vaginal brachytherapy
IIIB	Invades the vagina or the parametria	Disruption of the hypointense vaginal wall		Chemotherapy and/or tumor-directed RT
IIIC	Metastasis to the regional nodes		Unresectable: RT + brachytherapy ± chemotherapy ± surgery	Chemotherapy and/or tumor-directed RT
IIIC1	Involvement of pelvic nodes	Enlarged (≥10 mm) pelvic or para-aortic nodes with signal similar to the primary tumor		
IIIC2	Involvement of para-aortic nodes			
IV	Invades urinary bladder and/or rectum, and/or distant metastases			
IVA	Invades urinary bladder and/or rectum	Disruption of the hypointense bladder/rectal muscularis and hyperintense mucosa by abnormal signal tumor	RT ± brachytherapy ± chemotherapy ± surgery	Chemotherapy ± RT
IVB	Distant metastases including inguinal nodes		Palliative TH + BSO ± chemotherapy ± RT ± hormone therapy	Chemotherapy ± RT

Abbreviations: BSO, bilateral salpingo-oophorectomy; FIGO, International Federation of Gynecologic Oncology; G1, grade 1 differentiation at histology; G3, grade 3 differentiation at histology; RH, radical hysterectomy; RT, radiotherapy; TH, total hysterectomy.
[a] Tumor with endocervical glandular involvement is considered stage I.

beyond the uterus, invading the adnexa (IIIA) or vagina/parametria (IIIB), or are associated with pelvic (IIIC1) or para-aortic (IIIC2) nodal involvement. Stage IV endometrial cancers invade the urinary bladder and/or rectum (IVA) or metastasize to distant sites (IVB). Carcinosarcoma (malignant mixed Müllerian tumor), a type of uterine sarcoma, is staged as per the 2009 endometrial cancer staging, whereas new staging systems have been proposed for the remaining uterine sarcomas.[10]

According to the 2009 FIGO staging of cervical cancer (**Table 2**),[9] stage I tumors are confined to the cervix and are subdivided into IA (microscopic tumor with <5 mm deep invasion and <7 mm in largest extent) and IB (clinically visible tumor larger than IA; IB1 <4 cm and IB2 >4 cm). Stage II tumors extend beyond the uterus, invading the upper two-thirds of the vagina (IIA; IIA1 <4 cm and IIA2 >4 cm) or the parametrium (IIB). Stage III tumors invade the lower one-third of the vagina (IIIA) or reach the pelvic side wall, causing hydronephrosis (IIIB). Stage IV tumors invade adjacent organs (IVA) or extend beyond the true pelvis (IVB). The revised FIGO staging allows utilization of computed tomography (CT) and MR imaging for staging purposes where available. The use of cystoscopy and colonoscopy are no longer mandatory.

ENDOMETRIAL AND CERVICAL CANCER: IMAGING MODALITIES
Ultrasonography/Transvaginal Ultrasonography

Ultrasonography (US), especially transvaginal US (TVUS), is the initial and most common imaging test used for the evaluation of postmenopausal bleeding, the most common presentation of endometrial cancer. TVUS can help in the differentiation of benign and malignant causes of bleeding. It is also useful for screening patients with high risk of endometrial cancer, such as those on hormone replacement or tamoxifen therapy. Early endometrial cancer is seen on TVUS as widened endometrial stripe, usually greater than 4 mm (**Fig. 1**). Disruption of the subendometrial halo usually indicates myometrial invasion. Ruangvutilert and colleagues,[11] in a study of 111 patients, found that TVUS had sensitivity of 69.4% and specificity of 70.6% for evaluation of myometrial invasion. The use of saline infusion (ie, sonohysterography) has been shown to increase the accuracy of TVUS. In a study of 53 patients with endometrial cancer evaluated preoperatively with TVUS and saline infusion sonography to assess the depth of myometrial invasion, saline infusion resulted in greater accuracy for predicting deep myometrial invasion (96.4%) than TVUS alone (86%).[12] The major

disadvantage of TVUS is its operator dependence and limited field of view, which makes it difficult to evaluate cervical and extrauterine invasion. TVUS can overestimate myometrial invasion in the presence of large tumors, adenomyosis, and lymphovascular space invasion. Saline infusion can increase the risk of dissemination of malignant cells in up to 7% cases.[13]

US has limited use in cervical cancer for assessing the primary tumor. Transrectal US (TRUS) has been shown to have better accuracy than clinical examination (83% vs 78%), and in some studies than MR imaging (90% vs 81% for detecting tumor and 99% vs 95% for parametrial invasion).[14,15] For detecting bladder invasion based on the intact mobility of bladder over cervix, TRUS has accuracy higher than that of CT or MR imaging.[16] However, the main limitations are inability to assess the pelvic side wall and lymph nodes.[8] TRUS helps in evaluation of hydronephrosis in advanced cervical cancer.

Multidetector-Row Computed Tomography

Multidetector-row CT (MDCT) is used mainly for completing staging of endometrial cancer by detecting nodal and distant metastases (**Fig. 2**). Endometrial thickening incidentally detected on MDCT requires confirmation with TVUS (**Fig. 3**). The major limitation of MDCT lies in local staging of endometrial cancer, as it is less accurate than MR imaging in assessing myometrial and parametrial invasion. The sensitivity and specificity of MDCT for assessing myometrial invasion are 40% to 83% and 42% to 75%, respectively, compared with 90% to 92% and 88% to 90% for MR imaging.[17,18] For detecting cervical invasion, the sensitivity and specificity are 25% and 70%, respectively.[17] MDCT cannot differentiate reactive from metastatic nodes. Similar to endometrial cancer, MDCT mainly helps in the assessment of nodal and distant metastases in cervical cancer (**Fig. 4**). In early cervical cancer MDCT is less useful, as the primary tumor may be isodense to the cervical stroma after intravenous contrast administration. MDCT has an accuracy of 76% to 80% for detecting parametrial invasion, which is seen as eccentric parametrial masses, obliteration of periureteric fat planes, and encasement of parametrial vessels.[19] Because of poor soft-tissue resolution, MDCT can overestimate parametrial invasion.

Magnetic Resonance Imaging

Protocol
High-resolution MR imaging of the pelvis for gynecologic malignancies is performed in the supine position using dedicated surface-array

multichannel coils. Although 3-T scanners offer the advantage of higher signal-to-noise ratio compared with 1.5-T systems, image quality can be degraded owing to artifacts from field inhomogeneity at higher field strength, which can be partially be overcome by using a small field of view (FOV).[20] In young patients with early cervical cancer who are candidates for fertility-preserving surgeries, the use of endovaginal/endorectal coils can provide high-resolution images for treatment planning.[21] Fasting at least 4 hours before the examination, and the use of antiperistaltic agents such as hyoscine butylbromide or glucagon intramuscularly before the examination, can reduce motion artifacts caused by bowel peristalsis. Voiding at least 30 minutes before the start of the examination to achieve a half-filled bladder can also decrease motion and ghosting artifacts. The use of vaginal aqueous gel is recommended by a few investigators to increase the confidence of detecting vaginal invasion, but is not widely practiced.[22]

The standard MR sequences that are applicable to both endometrial and cervical cancers include axial T1-weighted images, axial and sagittal T2-weighted images of the pelvis, and axial T1-weighted or T2-weighted large-FOV images of the abdomen and pelvis to detect metastatic lymph nodes, hydronephrosis, and bone lesions. For detection of the extent of the myometrial invasion in endometrial cancer, high-resolution (512 × 512 matrix) 4-mm sagittal and axial oblique images perpendicular to the endometrial cavity (short axis of the uterine body) with a small FOV (20–25 cm) is recommended.[23] In cervical cancer, similar images at 3 to 6 mm thickness are recommended, but with the short-axis plane perpendicular to the cervical canal.[24] Addition of coronal T2-weighted sequence can improve the depiction of parametrial invasion in cervical cancer.[24] Axial oblique short-axis images through the cervix may be required in endometrial cancer with suspected cervical stromal invasion (**Fig. 5**). Dynamic intravenous contrast-enhanced (DCE) MR imaging with 3-dimensional gradient recalled echo T1-weighted sequences is performed in multiple phases for the staging of endometrial cancer (**Fig. 6**). The acquisition is in the sagittal and axial oblique planes before intravenous contrast administration, in the sagittal plane in the dynamic phase at 1 and 2 minutes, and in the axial oblique plane at 3 minutes, after contrast administration. Dynamic imaging with intravenous contrast is not routinely recommended for cervical cancer. According to the European Society of Urogenital Radiology (ESUR) guidelines, the indications for contrast administration in cervical cancer include small lesions that can be considered for trachelectomy

and detection of tumor recurrence, especially in the setting of postradiation fibrosis.[24] An additional indication for intravenous contrast would be cases of adenocarcinoma on biopsy to determine cervical or endometrial origin of the tumor.

Diffusion-weighted (DW) imaging with low (0–100 s/mm^2) and high (500–1000 s/mm^2) b-values demonstrates endometrial and cervical cancer as areas of high signal intensity, increasing their conspicuity (**Figs. 7** and **8**). DW images are obtained in the sagittal and axial oblique planes. The use of apparent diffusion coefficient (ADC) maps as a quantitative expression of diffusion restriction allows differentiation of high signal, owing to true diffusion restriction from T2 "shine-through" attributable to long T2 relaxation times of some tissues. The tumor with restricted diffusion appears hypointense on ADC maps, whereas T2 shine-through retains the high signal.[25]

MR IMAGING FEATURES OF ENDOMETRIAL AND CERVICAL CANCER: CORRELATION WITH REVISED FIGO (2009) STAGING
Endometrial Cancer

MR imaging features of endometrial cancer as per the FIGO staging are summarized in **Table 1**.

Stage I
Compared to the normal endometrium, endometrial cancer has an isointense signal on T1-weighted images and a hypointense signal on T2-weighted images (**Fig. 9**). After gadolinium administration, dynamic imaging depicts endometrial cancer as a hypovascular mass in comparison with the intensely enhancing myometrium. The maximum contrast between the tumor and myometrium is usually seen at 90 to 150 seconds after intravenous contrast administration (See **Fig. 6**).[23] Stage IA tumors are seen as focal or diffuse intermediate-signal abnormality either within the high-signal endometrial lining or invading less than 50% of the myometrium. Invasion of the myometrium is seen as disruption of the low signal-intensity junctional zone on T2-weighted images and loss of smooth subendometrial enhancement on DCE-MR imaging. Stage IB tumors invade greater than 50% of the myometrial thickness, but do not extend beyond the outer myometrial margin (see **Fig. 9**).

The 2 key MR imaging sequences required for proper staging of endometrial cancer are the high-resolution T2-weighted images, which depict the zonal anatomy of the uterus, and DCE-MR, which identifies viable tumor and enables accurate assessment of myometrial invasion and nodal disease (see **Fig. 9**). Leiomyomas, adenomyosis, and

Table 2
Revised FIGO staging, MR imaging features, and management of cervical cancer

Revised FIGO Stage	MR Imaging Findings	Management	
		Primary	Adjuvant
I	Tumor confined to cervix		
IA	Microscopic tumor with <5 mm deep invasion and <7 mm in largest extent	Primary tumor cannot be seen. MR imaging is not indicated unless trachelectomy is considered	Cone biopsy + pelvic node dissection, extrafascial/ modified RH or radical trachelectomy + pelvic node dissection ± para-aortic node dissection	Observe or pelvic RT + chemotherapy ± vaginal brachytherapy ± para-aortic RT (for positive nodes)
IA1	Invasion <3 mm deep and extent <7 mm			
IA2	Invasion >3 mm deep but <5 mm and extent <7 mm			
IB	Clinically visible tumor larger than IA confined to cervix			Observe or pelvic RT + chemotherapy ± vaginal brachytherapy ± para-aortic RT (for positive nodes)
IB1	Tumor ≤4 cm in greatest dimension	Intermediate/high signal-intensity tumor in the hypointense cervical stroma, subdivided into IB1 and IB2 based on size	RH + pelvic node dissection ± para-aortic node dissection or pelvic RT + brachytherapy ± chemotherapy	
IB2	Tumor >4 cm in greatest dimension		Pelvic RT + brachytherapy ± chemotherapy or RH + pelvic node dissection ± para-aortic node dissection	
II	Tumor extends beyond the uterus, but not to the pelvic wall or the lower third of the vagina			
IIA	Tumor invades the upper two-thirds of vagina with no parametrial invasion	Intermediate signal-intensity tumor disrupts the hypointense vaginal wall, subdivided into IIA1 and IIA2 based on size. No abnormal signal in the parametrium		
IIA1	Tumor ≤4 cm in greatest dimension		Same as IB1	Same as IB1
IIA2	Tumor >4 cm in greatest dimension		Same as IB2	Same as IB2

Stage	Description	Imaging Findings	Treatment	Follow-up
IIB	Tumor with parametrial invasion	Disruption of the hypointense stromal ring with nodular tumor in the parametrium or parametrial vessel encasement	Pelvic RT + chemotherapy + brachytherapy ± para-aortic RT	Surveillance
III	Tumor extends to the pelvic wall and/or lower one-third of vagina or associated with hydronephrosis/nonfunctioning kidney			Surveillance
IIIA	Tumor involves lower one-third of vagina, without pelvic side wall involvement	Disruption of the hypointense wall of the lower one-third of the vagina		
IIIB	Tumor extends to the pelvic side wall or causes hydronephrosis/nonfunctioning kidney	Tumor within 3 mm of the pelvic side wall, hydronephrosis		
IV	Tumor extends beyond true pelvis or invades mucosa of the bladder or rectum			Surveillance
IVA	Invasion of adjacent organs	Disruption of the low signal-intensity muscularis of the bladder/rectum and involvement of the mucosa, loss of perivesical or perirectal fat planes	Pelvic RT + chemotherapy + brachytherapy ± para-aortic RT	
IVB	Distant metastases		Systemic therapy ± individualized RT	

Abbreviations: FIGO, International Federation of Gynecologic Oncology; RH, radical hysterectomy; RT, radiotherapy.

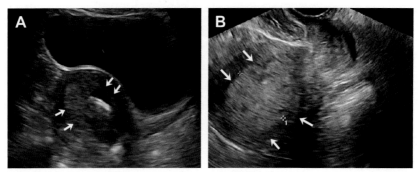

Fig. 1. (*A, B*) A 45-year-old woman with a history of intermenstrual bleeding. Longitudinal transabdominal and transvaginal ultrasonographic images demonstrate diffusely thickened echogenic endometrial stripe (*white arrows*). Endometrial biopsy revealed high-grade endometrial carcinoma.

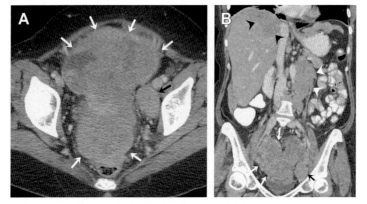

Fig. 2. (*A, B*) A 52-year-old woman with newly diagnosed endometrial carcinoma (serous papillary). Axial and coronal reformatted contrast-enhanced computed tomography (CT) images demonstrate a large heterogeneous mass replacing the uterus (*white arrows*). There are metastatic left external iliac (*black arrow*) and retroperitoneal lymphadenopathy (*white arrowheads*) as well as hepatic metastasis (*black arrowheads*).

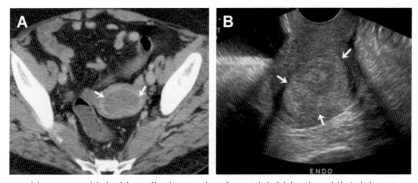

Fig. 3. A 66-year-old woman with incidentally detected endometrial thickening. (*A*) Axial contrast-enhanced CT image demonstrates thick hypodense endometrium (*white arrows*). (*B*) Transverse transvaginal ultrasonographic image confirms diffusely thickened echogenic endometrial stripe (*white arrows*). Surgical histopathology confirmed stage IA endometrial carcinoma.

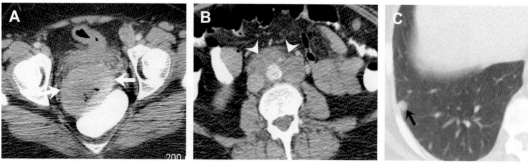

Fig. 4. A 52-year-old woman with cervical carcinoma. (*A, B*) Axial contrast-enhanced CT images of the abdomen and pelvis demonstrate a large heterogeneous cervical mass with central necrosis (*white arrows*) with metastatic retroperitoneal lymphadenopathy (*white arrowheads*). (*C*) Axial CT image of the chest reveals a right pulmonary nodule (*black arrow*) consistent with pulmonary metastasis.

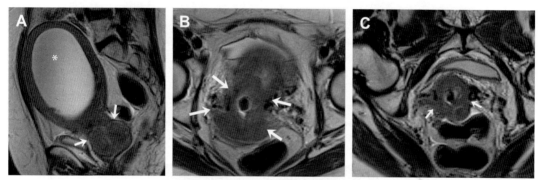

Fig. 5. A 67-year-old woman with endometrial carcinoma. (*A*) Sagittal T2-weighted MR image demonstrates distended endometrial cavity (hydrometra) with enlarged cervix (*arrows*). (*B*) Straight axial and (*C*) oblique axial (perpendicular to the cervix) T2-weighted images demonstrate heterogeneous mass replacing the normal cervical stroma (*arrows*) and causing obstruction to the endocervical canal with resultant hydrometra (*asterisk in A*). Note that the actual extent of the tumor is better depicted on the oblique axial images. The straight axial images overestimate the parametrial extension of the tumor.

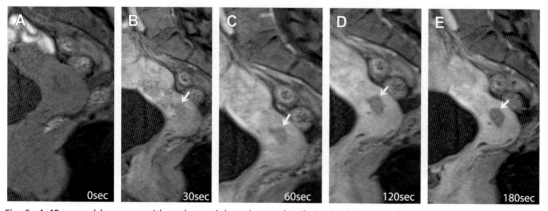

Fig. 6. A 49-year-old woman with endometrial carcinoma (*A–E*). Sagittal dynamic fat-suppressed postgadolinium T1-weighted MR images demonstrate the primary tumor as an isointense mass (*arrows*) on the pregadolinium images, and hypovascular to the normal myometrium on the dynamic imaging. Note that the tumor-myometrium contrast is best seen at 120 to 180 milliseconds.

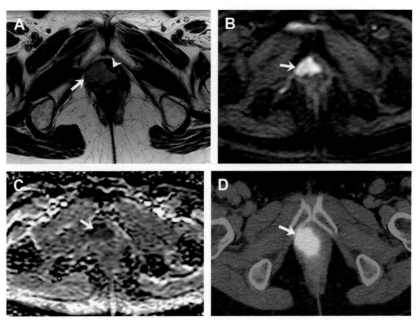

Fig. 7. A 62-year-old woman with cervical carcinoma and drop metastasis to lower vagina. (*A*) Axial T2-weighted MR image of the pelvis demonstrates large intermediate signal intensity mass in the lower vagina (*white arrow*) compressing and displacing the urethra anteriorly (*white arrowhead*). (*B, C*) Axial diffusion-weighted (b-value 500) and corresponding apparent diffusion coefficient (ADC) mapping images reveal significant diffusion restriction in the mass (*white arrow*, 0.9×10^{-3} mm^2/s). (*D*) Axial ^{18F}-fluorodeoxyglucose positron emission tomography (FDG-PET)/CT image demonstrates intense FDG uptake (*white arrow*) in the mass (maximum standardized uptake value [SUV$_{max}$] 11.1). Biopsy of the mass revealed metastasis from cervical carcinoma.

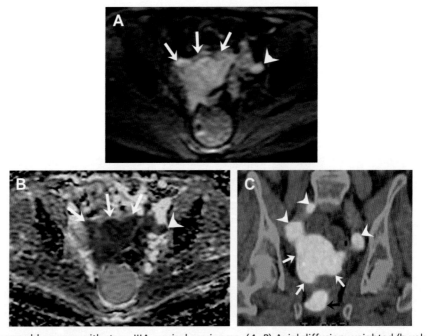

Fig. 8. A 62-year-old woman with stage IIIA cervical carcinoma. (*A, B*) Axial diffusion-weighted (b-value 500) and corresponding ADC mapping images demonstrate large conglomerate pelvic mass involving the uterus (*white arrows*), associated with enlarged left external iliac lymph node (*white arrowhead*). The pelvic mass and the iliac lymph node show marked diffusion restriction with an ADC value of 0.75×10^{-3} mm^2/s. (*C*) Coronal FDG-PET/CT image demonstrates intense FDG uptake in the pelvic mass (*white arrows*), bilateral external and right common iliac lymph nodes (*white arrowheads*), and the lower one-third of the vagina (*black arrow*).

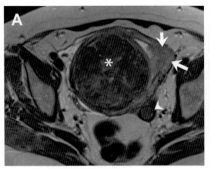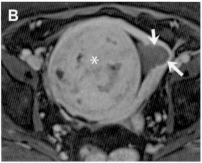

Fig. 9. A 73-year-old woman with stage IB endometrial carcinoma. (*A*) Axial T2-weighted and (*B*) axial fat-suppressed postgadolinium T1-weighted MR images demonstrate intermediate-signal hypovascular tumor in the left uterine cornu invading greater than 50% of the myometrial thickness (*arrows*). Note the incidental large uterine fibroid (*asterisk*) and a left ovarian endometriotic cyst (*arrowhead in A*).

large tumors compressing the myometrium can cause difficulties in assessing myometrial invasion on T2-weighted images. Some studies have found that DCE-MR imaging can increase the accuracy of evaluation of deep myometrial invasion in such cases. Sala and colleagues,[26] in a study of 50 patients with endometrial cancer, found that the accuracy of T2-weighted imaging was increased from 78% to 92% by the addition of DCE-MR imaging.

DW imaging has an added value in endometrial cancer by better depicting the primary tumor, increasing the detection of drop metastases in the cervix and vagina as well as extrauterine spread to the peritoneum and lymph nodes, especially in patients with contraindication to intravenous gadolinium contrast agents.[25] Underestimation of myometrial invasion can occur on DCE-MR imaging in the uterine cornu because of the thin myometrium in this region. Overestimation can occur in the presence of peritumoral enhancement and poor tumor to myometrium contrast.[3] Concurrent evaluation of DCE-MR imaging and DW imaging can increase the accuracy of myometrial invasion in these conditions. Beddy and colleagues,[27] in their study of 48 patients with endometrial cancer, found that the diagnostic accuracy for detecting myometrial invasion was higher in DW images (85%–90%) than with DCE-MR imaging (71%–79%). The pearls and pitfalls in the MR interpretation of endometrial cancer are summarized in **Table 3**.

Stage II

The normal cervical stroma demonstrates low signal intensity on T2-weighted images. In the presence of cervical stromal invasion in stage II tumors, the low signal intensity of the cervical stroma is replaced by the intermediate signal-intensity tumor (**Fig. 10**). The stromal invasion is

best seen on the delayed DCE-MR images (see **Fig. 10**). In some cases, bulky endometrial masses can project in to the endocervical canal, which can mimic cervical stromal invasion. Delayed DCE-MR images in the oblique axial plane (perpendicular to the cervical canal) clearly demonstrate the intact cervical mucosa in these cases. The sensitivity and specificity of MR imaging for detecting cervical invasion can be as high as 80% and 96%, respectively.[28] DCE-MR imaging increases the sensitivity and specificity of cervical invasion from 75% and 88% on T2-weighted images to 100% and 94%, respectively.[29]

Stage III

Stage IIIA endometrial cancer extends beyond the confines of the uterus but not the true pelvis. The tumor disrupts the smooth hypointense outline of the serosa on T2-weighted images, and can cause subtle irregularity of the uterine contour in very early stages. DCE-MR imaging shows discontinuity in the enhancing outer margin of the myometrium and contiguous adnexal or parametrial masses. In the case of grade 3 endometrioid and type 2 endometrial cancers, noncontiguous T2 intermediate signal-intensity foci and enhancing adnexal or parametrial masses can be seen without serosal invasion. DW imaging can be useful in detecting such deposits by increasing their conspicuity.

Stage IIIB endometrial cancer is seen on T2-weighted images as invasion of the hypointense vaginal wall or the parametria (**Fig. 11**). The tumor can be contiguous with the primary tumor or can occur as metastatic disease. Stage IIIC disease is seen as enlarged pelvic (IIIC1) or para-aortic nodes (with or without pelvic nodes) (IIIC2). The MR features of metastatic nodes include size larger than 1 cm, intermediate signal intensity on T2-weighted and hypointense signal intensity

Table 3
Pearls and pitfalls in the interpretation of MR imaging of endometrial and cervical carcinomas

	Endometrial Cancer	Cervical Cancer
Pearls	Concurrent evaluation of T2-weighted and DCE-MR images	Stage IA tumors do not cause signal abnormality
	Knowledge of histology while interpreting MR imaging	Accurate size estimation should be on 2 orthogonal planes
	Use sagittal and axial oblique images for assessing myometrial invasion and cervical invasion	Intact hypointense stromal ring excludes parametrial invasion
	Best time to assess myometrial invasion on DCE-MR: 90–150 s	Intact hypointense signal of the vaginal wall excludes vaginal invasion
	Include DW imaging for better depiction of tumor	Tumors within 3 mm of pelvic side-wall muscles indicate pelvic side-wall invasion
	High index of suspicion for nodal metastases with high-risk tumors	DCE-MR imaging distinguishes endometrial vs cervical origin of biopsy-proven adenocarcinoma
	Intact cervical mucosal enhancement excludes stromal invasion	DCE-MR imaging useful for assessing small tumors
Pitfalls	Adenomyosis, fibroids, large tumors can interfere with evaluation of myometrial invasion: use DCE-MR imaging	Overestimation of parametrial invasion: postbiopsy stranding/hemorrhage, cervical stromal edema, endometriosis, bulky intravaginal tumors
	Poor tumor-myometrial contrast, cornual tumors, peritumoral edema: combined evaluation of DCE-MR and DW imaging	Bullous edema of the bladder wall does not indicate bladder invasion
	Bullous edema of the bladder wall does not indicate bladder invasion	

Abbreviations: DCE-MR, dynamic contrast-enhanced MR; DW, diffusion-weighted.

on T1-weighted images, irregular contour, and multiplicity (**Fig. 12**). The sensitivity and specificity of MR imaging for detecting nodal metastases is 50% and 95% to 96%, respectively.[28,30]

Stage IV

Stage IVA endometrial cancer is seen on T2-weighted images as invasion of the tumor beyond the hypointense muscularis propria of the rectum and/or bladder disrupting the hyperintense mucosa, and as enhancing polypoidal intraluminal tumor in the rectal or bladder lumen on DCE-MR imaging (**Fig. 13**). Bullous edema of the bladder mucosa, which is the result of serosal or muscular layer invasion, does not qualify as stage IVA disease.[3] Stage IVB disease is seen as distant metastases to the para-aortic nodes above the renal vessels, inguinal nodes, and peritoneum, resulting in malignant ascites (see **Fig. 13**). The peritoneal deposits are best seen on delayed contrast-enhanced images of the abdomen and pelvis. High-grade endometrioid endometrial cancer and the type 2 endometrial cancers (serous papillary and clear cell types) have a high propensity to spread to the peritoneal cavity, and behave like ovarian cancers. Distant metastases to the liver,

lung, and bone occur by hematogenous spread, but are rare at initial presentation (see **Fig. 13**).

Cervical Cancer

MR imaging features of cervical cancer as per the FIGO staging are summarized in **Table 2**.

Stage I

Normal cervix has a typical doughnut configuration on oblique axial images. On T2-weighted images, 3 distinct layers are discernible in the cervix: the thin hyperintense mucosa, thick hypointense stroma, and thin outermost intermediate signal-intensity smooth muscle layer. MR imaging is usually not indicated for evaluation of stage IA tumors, as these tumors do not show any signal abnormality. Stage IB tumors have intermediate to high signal intensity compared with the cervical stroma on T2-weighted images, and enhance variably compared with the stroma on DCE-MR imaging (**Fig. 14**). The tumor growth pattern can vary from exophytic, infiltrative, or endocervical.

Stage IB tumors are subdivided into IB1 and IB2, based on size (<4 cm or ≥4 cm, respectively). Tumor size should be measured on

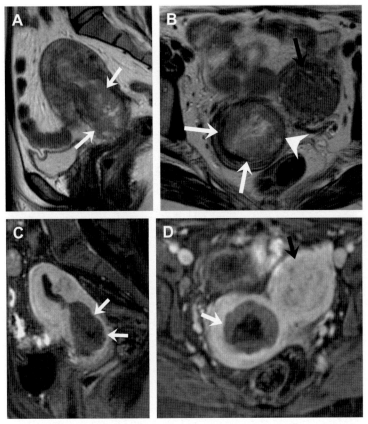

Fig. 10. A 66-year-old woman with stage II endometrial carcinoma. (*A, B*) Axial and sagittal T2-weighted and (*C, D*) axial and sagittal fat-suppressed post-gadolinium T1-weighted MR images demonstrate intermediate signal hypovascular tumor in the lower uterine segment invading the cervical stroma disrupting the normal T2-hypointesne signal (*white arrows*). The peripheral stromal ring is however intact (*arrowhead* in *B*). Note the incidental large uterine fibroid (*black arrows*).

2 orthogonal views and in all 3 dimensions. MR imaging has an accuracy of close to 90% in the assessment of tumor size (see **Fig. 14**). This accuracy is significant, as clinical examination is unreliable for size estimation especially in the case of endocervical lesions. Tumor size also determines the type of treatment; tumors less than 2 cm in size permit fertility-sparing surgery, whereas chemoradiotherapy is offered for tumors larger than 4 cm even in the absence of parametrial invasion. Overestimation can occur in up to 19% cases in comparison with surgical specimens because of postbiopsy hemorrhage and inherent in vivo and in vitro differences.[31] MR imaging helps in the assessment of cervical length and distance from the internal os in patients planned for fertility-sparing surgery.

Stage II

Stage IIA cervical carcinoma involves the upper two-thirds of the vagina without parametrial invasion. Vaginal extension is seen as focal loss of T2-hypointense signal of the vaginal wall. Similarly to stage IB tumors, stage IIA tumors are subdivided into IIA1 and IIA2 based on a tumor size of less than 4 cm and 4 cm or larger, respectively. Bulky exophytic cervical tumors can sometimes mimic apparent vaginal extension; however, the vaginal hypointense ring remains intact in such cases.

Stage IIB cervical cancers invade the parametrium, disrupting the T2-hypointense stromal ring of the cervix without extending to the pelvic side wall (**Fig. 15**). The presence of an intact stromal ring (with a thickness of >3 mm) has a very high negative predictive value of more than 96% for parametrial invasion.[32] The positive predictive value, however, is low (82%–86%).[32] Other reliable MR imaging signs that raise the suspicion of parametrial invasion include distortion of the cervix with displacement to the side of parametrial invasion, irregular interface between the tumor and the parametrium, and enhancing soft tissue in the parametrium encasing the parametrial vessels and/or extending along the uterosacral ligaments

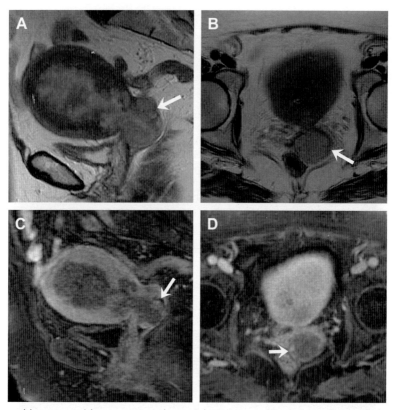

Fig. 11. A 59-year-old woman with stage IIIB endometrial carcinoma. (*A, B*) Sagittal and axial T2-weighted and (*C, D*) sagittal and axial fat-suppressed postgadolinium T1-weighted MR images demonstrate intermediate signal hypovascular tumor in the lower uterine segment invading the cervix and the vagina (*arrows in A, C*), disrupting the normal T2-hypointesne vaginal wall (*arrow in B, D*).

(see **Fig. 15**).[33] Pitfalls in the interpretation of parametrial invasion can occur in the presence of postbiopsy stranding/hemorrhage, peripheral stromal edema that blurs the true tumor-stroma boundary, endometriosis, and bulky intravaginal tumors.[8] When there is full-thickness disruption of the cervical stroma, even in the absence of frank parametrial invasion, microscopic invasion cannot be excluded. Disruption of the stromal ring in the tumors involving the portio vaginalis of the cervix with intact vaginal fornices excludes parametrial invasion. The sensitivity of MR imaging for assessing parametrial invasion can vary from as low as 44% to as high as 100%. Specificity varies between 87% and 93%.[5,34–36] The pearls and pitfalls in the MR interpretation of cervical cancer are summarized in **Table 3**.

Stage III

Direct invasion of the lower one-third of the vagina without pelvic side-wall extension is seen in stage IIIA cervical carcinoma (**Fig. 16**). Stage IIIB cervical carcinomas extend up to the pelvic side wall and are defined as tumor tissue within 3 mm of the pelvic side-wall muscles (**Fig. 17**).[37,38] Presence of hydronephrosis caused by ureteric encasement and encasement of iliac vessels also indicates stage IIIB disease.

Stage IV

Direct invasion of the urinary bladder or the rectal mucosa is seen in stage IVA cervical carcinoma as disruption of the hypointense muscularis propria and invasion of the mucosa by a polypoidal mass, with resultant high signal intensity along the anterior aspect of the posterior bladder wall (**Fig. 18**). Frank vesicovaginal or rectovaginal fistula can be seen in some cases (see **Fig. 18**). Invasion of the bladder is more common than rectal invasion, because of the bare area on the bladder wall posteriorly and the presence of rectovaginal septum separating the posterior fornix from the rectum.[33] Bullous edema can mimic bladder invasion, but can be differentiated by the presence of an intact bladder mucosa and with DCE-MR imaging. The sensitivity of MR imaging for predicting bladder and rectal invasion varies between 83% and 100%, and specificity between 88% and

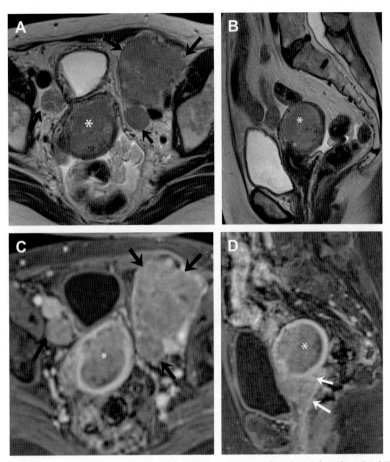

Fig. 12. A 45-year-old woman with stage IIIC1 endometrial carcinoma. (*A, B*) Axial and sagittal T2-weighted and (*C, D*) axial and sagittal fat-suppressed postgadolinium T1-weighted MR images demonstrate large intermediate signal hypovascular tumor in endometrial cavity (*asterisk*) associated with bulky bilateral external iliac lymphadenopathy (*black arrows in A, C*). Note the heterogeneous enhancement of the lateral vaginal fornices concerning for vaginal invasion (*white arrows in D*). Surgical histopathology confirmed vaginal invasion.

100%.[37,39] Stage IVB refers to distant metastases beyond the pelvis to the para-aortic and inguinal nodes, lungs, liver, and bone.

ENDOMETRIAL AND CERVICAL CANCER: RECENT ADVANCES IN IMAGING

DCE-MR imaging can provide information about tumor perfusion and permeability characteristics. Quantitative estimation of these characteristics can be done by plotting curves of the signal intensity after gadolinium administration against time. The various parameters that can be calculated with DCE-MR imaging include signal enhancement ratio, enhancing fraction (E_F), maximum/peak enhancement, K^{trans} (the transfer coefficient between the plasma and extracellular space), k_{ep} (the rate constant), extracellular volume, and IAUGC (the initial area under the gadolinium concentration-time curve).[40,41] The use of these parameters is restricted to research settings for cervical cancer mainly for staging, assessing treatment response, and detecting recurrence. Calculation of ADC values using DW imaging has been shown in some studies to differentiate poorly differentiated tumors from well and moderately differentiated tumors, and to predict response and recurrence.[42] Few studies have shown ADC values as a useful biomarker for assessing treatment response; an increase in responding tumors ADC values occurred earlier than size changes.[43] Proton MR spectroscopy is a metabolic profiling technique that relies on the different resonant frequencies of protons other than those present in the water molecules. These different frequencies can be displayed as different peaks unique to different metabolites. Malignant tumors including cervical and endometrial cancers have high levels of total choline owing to increased cell turnover, which

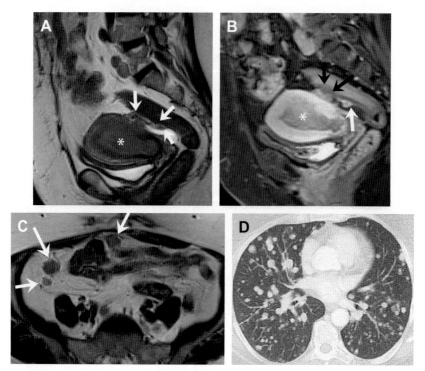

Fig. 13. A 73-year-old woman with stage IV endometrial carcinoma of the serous papillary type. (*A, B*) Sagittal T2-weighted and fat-suppressed postgadolinium T1-weighted MR images demonstrate large intermediate-signal hypovascular tumor replacing the endometrial cavity (*asterisk*) and extending beyond the serosa to involve the anterior surface of the rectum (*white arrows*). There is focal polypoidal thickening of the intraluminal aspect of the rectal wall (*black arrows*), concerning for rectal invasion (confirmed at rectosigmoidoscopy). (*C*) Axial T2-weighted MR image of the lower abdomen demonstrates multiple intermediate-signal peritoneal deposits (*arrows*). (*D*) Axial CT image of the chest demonstrates multiple bilateral pulmonary metastases.

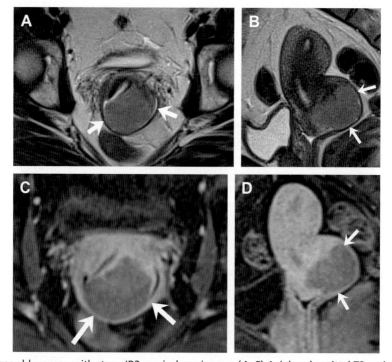

Fig. 14. A 38-year-old woman with stage IB2 cervical carcinoma. (*A, B*) Axial and sagittal T2-weighted and (*C, D*) axial and sagittal fat-suppressed postgadolinium T1-weighted MR images demonstrate a large intermediate-signal hypovascular tumor involving the posterior lip of the uterine cervix (*arrows*). The mass is seen to protrude into the posterior vaginal fornix with intact T2-hypointense vaginal wall.

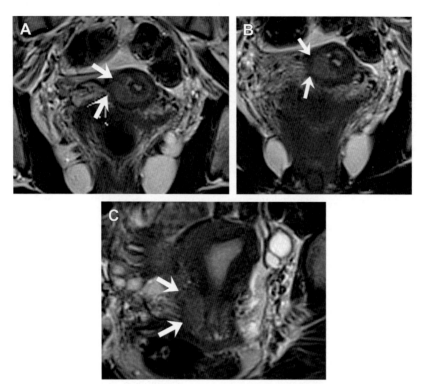

Fig. 15. A 41-year-old woman with stage IIB cervical carcinoma. (*A, B*) Oblique axial and (*C*) straight axial T2-weighted MR images demonstrate an intermediate-signal tumor disrupting the hypointense cervical stromal ring along the right lateral aspect (*arrows*) with irregular interface between the tumor and the parametrium, suggestive of early parametrial invasion.

can be detected with proton MR spectroscopy.[44] MR spectroscopy is still in the research arena. Functional MR imaging techniques such as blood oxygen level–dependent imaging can be used to assess tissue hypoxia, which in turn can help in predicting treatment response in malignant tumors.[45]

[18F]-Fluorodeoxyglucose (FDG) positron emission tomography (PET) combined with CT is a well-established technique finding greater applications in the staging and surveillance of gynecologic malignancies. PET/CT has been shown to increase the accuracy of staging of gynecologic malignancies to the extent of 100% because of

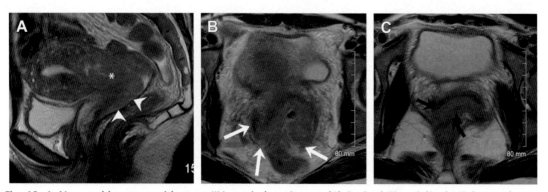

Fig. 16. A 41-year-old woman with stage IIIA cervical carcinoma. (*A*) Sagittal T2-weighted MR image demonstrates a large intermediate signal tumor (*asterisk*) arising from the cervix and invading the lower uterine segment and lower one-third of the vagina (*white arrowheads*). (*B, C*) Axial T2-weighted MR images demonstrate contiguous parametrial invasion (*white arrows in B*) and disruption of the hypointense vaginal wall (*black arrows in C*).

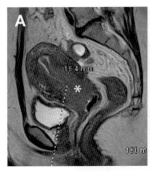
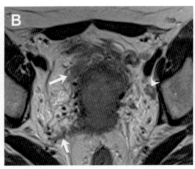
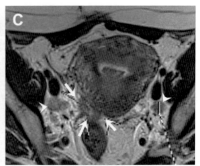

Fig. 17. A 55-year-old woman with stage IIIB cervical carcinoma. (*A–C*) Sagittal and axial T2-weighted MR images of the pelvis demonstrate a large intermediate-signal tumor (*asterisk*) arising from the cervix and invading the lower uterine segment. There is contiguous parametrial invasion with tumor reaching up to the pelvic side wall (*white arrows in B, C*). Note the enlarged bilateral external iliac lymph nodes (*arrowheads in B, C*).

its wider anatomic coverage in a single examination, detecting both locoregional disease and distant metastases (see **Figs. 7** and **8**). In the evaluation of the primary tumor in patients with cervical cancer, the degree of FDG uptake on the preoperative PET/CT has been shown to correlate with the prognosis, as the maximum standardized uptake value was higher in patients with higher-stage tumors, larger tumors, tumors with parametrial invasion, and nodal metastases.[46] PET/CT also predicts disease-specific survival, as patients with metabolically active nodes on PET/CT tend to have worse disease-free survival.[47] Dual-phase PET/CT (imaging at 40 minutes and 3 hours after tracer injection) has been shown to increase the detection rates of para-aortic nodes. In a study of 104 patients with cervical cancer, delayed imaging increased the sensitivity of PET/CT for detecting para-aortic nodes from 81.6% to 100%.[48] PET has been shown to help in modifying treatment

plans and avoiding unnecessary combined-modality treatment by assessing nodal status. PET/CT also aids in delivering intensity-modulated radiation therapy. New tracers for PET, such as [18F]-fluoroazomycin arabinoside, have been shown to help in assessing tumor hypoxia, which predicts response to treatment.[45] The potential of new tracers such as [11C]-choline and [11C]-methionine are being explored in several research studies.[49]

MANAGEMENT OF ENDOMETRIAL AND CERVICAL CANCER: WHAT RADIOLOGISTS SHOULD KNOW AND WHAT GYNECOLOGIC ONCOLOGISTS AND RADIATION ONCOLOGISTS WANT TO KNOW
Endometrial Cancer

Management of endometrial cancer as per the FIGO staging is summarized in **Table 1**. Surgery

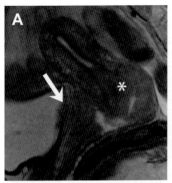
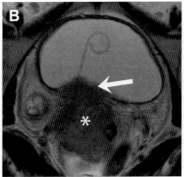
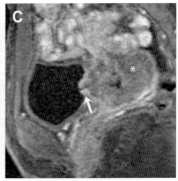

Fig. 18. A 55-year-old woman with stage IVA cervical carcinoma. (*A, B*) Sagittal and axial T2-weighted and (*C*) sagittal fat-suppressed postgadolinium T1-weighted MR images of the pelvis demonstrate a large intermediate-signal tumor (*asterisk*) arising from the cervix and invading the parametrium as well as the urinary bladder (*white arrow in A, B*). There is disruption of the bladder wall with nodular protrusion into the posterior bladder wall (*white arrow in C*). Note the lower end of the right ureteric stent in the bladder lumen (*B*), which was placed to relieve right hydroureteronephrosis.

is the mainstay in the management of endometrial cancer. FIGO endometrial cancer staging is a surgicopathologic staging schemata. Stage I endometrial cancers can be stratified into 3 risk categories based on the histology (grade and type) and depth of myometrial invasion: low, intermediate, and high risk (**Table 4**).[50] The standard surgery for all stage I cancers is total hysterectomy (TH) and bilateral salpingo-oophorectomy (BSO). Considerable controversy exists regarding the role of lymphadenectomy. The National Comprehensive Cancer Network (NCCN) guidelines recommend complete surgical staging in all patients, which includes pelvic and para-aortic node dissection and peritoneal washings for cytology.[51] According to the European Society for Medical Oncology practice guidelines, systemic lymphadenectomy is recommended only for the intermediate-risk and high-risk categories.[50] Stage II endometrial cancers are treated with radical hysterectomy, BSO, cytology, and pelvic/para-aortic lymphadenectomy. Stage III and IV endometrial cancers need extensive debulking in patients with good performance status. In patients who are poor surgical candidates, external radiotherapy with or without tumor-directed brachytherapy has been shown to achieve some degree of local and distant disease control.

The role of adjuvant radiotherapy is contentious in stage I tumors, and depends on the presence of risk factors such as high-grade tumors (G3), deep myometrial invasion, lymphovascular space invasion (LVSI), and serous papillary or clear-cell histology.[51] For stage IA G1 tumors without adverse factors, NCCN recommends observation.[51] For stage IB G3 tumors pelvic radiotherapy

is recommended, with or without vaginal brachytherapy and chemotherapy. For all other stage I tumors, observation or vaginal brachytherapy is recommended depending on adverse factors, with pelvic radiation reserved for high-grade tumors (G3). Combination of pelvic radiotherapy, vaginal brachytherapy, tumor-directed radiotherapy, and chemotherapy are recommended for tumors of stage II to IV. Serous papillary and clear-cell endometrial cancers are managed in the same way as ovarian cancer, with omentectomy and peritoneal biopsies in addition to TH, BSO, and lymphadenectomy.[51]

As endometrial cancer is managed predominantly surgically, the only radiologic investigation recommended by the NCCN guidelines and FIGO staging is chest radiography; MR imaging and CT are optional for advanced cancers.[51] However, preoperative MR imaging provides indispensable information in endometrial cancer and helps in risk stratification, which in turn determines the surgical strategy and need for adjuvant radiotherapy and chemotherapy (see **Table 4**).[50] Although MR imaging cannot directly assess LVSI, by determining the depth of myometrial invasion and detecting cervical stromal invasion it can predict the risk of LVSI. The risk of nodal metastases increases from about 3.5% for grade I tumors with less than 50% myometrial invasion to 17.6% for grade I tumors with greater than 50% is invasion.[52] Similarly, the risk of nodal metastases increased from 9.8% to 32.4% in the presence of cervical stromal invasion.[52] The high accuracy of MR imaging in determining myometrial and cervical stromal invasion make it a dependable proxy for nodal metastases and, hence, LVSI. Because the grade of endometrial cancer also determines LVSI, having knowledge of the histologic type (from endometrial biopsy) before interpreting the MR imaging helps the radiologist to exert caution while interpreting nonenlarged nodes in high-grade cancers. MR imaging can help in planning the surgical approach by providing details about uterine size, adnexal disease, peritoneal deposits (laparoscopic vs open), cervical/parametrial involvement (simple vs radical), and enlarged pelvic and para-aortic nodes (extent of lymphadenectomy). Both CT and PET/CT demonstrate disseminated disease, which can then be targeted with radiotherapy or systemic chemotherapy (see **Fig. 2**).

Cervical Cancer

Management of cervical cancer as per the FIGO staging is summarized in **Table 2**. Cervical cancer is staged clinically according to the FIGO, and

Table 4	
Risk stratification in endometrial carcinoma	
Risk Category	**Type of Endometrial Carcinoma**[a]
Low risk	Stage IA (G1, G2) type 1 histology
Intermediate risk	Stage IA (G3) type 1 histology Stage IB (G1, G2) type 1 histology
High risk	Stage IB (G3) type 1 histology All stages of type 2 histology

Abbreviation: G, grade of differentiation at histology.
[a] Stage as per the revised FIGO staging of endometrial cancer.

includes examination under anesthesia, colposcopy, cystoscopy, sigmoidoscopy, and chest radiography. The revised FIGO staging incorporates MR imaging and CT, where available, in treatment planning. This guideline is based on the premise that clinical staging is much less accurate than surgical or MR imaging staging. Clinical examination is particularly fallacious in detecting parametrial/pelvic side-wall invasion, lymph node metastases, and distant metastases, and in estimating tumor size. When compared with the surgical staging, the clinical staging has a 29% to 33.3% error rate, the maximum errors occurring in stage IIA to IVA (50% to 67%).[36,53] In the assessment of parametrial invasion, the accuracy of clinical staging is 47% to 53%, whereas MR imaging has an accuracy of 86% to 94%[34,54–56] with a specificity of 97% and negative predictive value of 100%.[32] In estimating tumor volume, clinical staging has accuracy of less than 60%, compared with 70% to 93% for MR imaging.[31]

Management of early cervical cancer (stage IA, IB1, IIA1) is mainly radical or modified radical hysterectomy with pelvic lymph node dissection, with or without para-aortic lymph node dissection.[57] For young patients, less aggressive fertility-sparing surgeries such as cone biopsy with or without pelvic lymph node dissection, and radical trachelectomy with or without pelvic lymph node dissection can be considered. Patients with positive pelvic and para-aortic nodes receive adjuvant radiotherapy with or without chemotherapy. For stage IB2, IIA2, and IIB to IV, concurrent chemoradiation is recommended.[57]

MR imaging is not recommended for stage IA cervical cancer. For stage IB and IIA cancers, MR imaging plays a key role in treatment strategies by determining tumor volume and parametrial invasion. In determining the surgical candidates (ie, stage IB1 and IIA1 cancers), MR imaging has an accuracy of 94%.[56] NCCN guidelines recommend MR imaging in stage IB2 and higher to rule out disease high in the endocervix.[57] By estimating the cervical tumor volume in stages IB2 and IIB to IV as well as demonstrating the pelvic and para-aortic nodal disease, MR imaging guides the volume of radiotherapy. Tumor volume as estimated by MR imaging has a significant correlation with 5-year survival.[31] In stage IVA disease, MR imaging has a high negative predictive value in excluding bladder and rectal invasion. Although lymph nodes are not included in the FIGO staging, the presence of positive pelvic and/or para-aortic lymph nodes necessitates adjuvant radiotherapy and chemotherapy. PET/CT is highly sensitive and specific, approaching 90% to 100%, in this context (see **Fig. 8**).[58] PET/CT also helps in the comprehensive evaluation of the whole body for metastatic disease in single session.

ENDOMETRIAL AND CERVICAL CANCER: LYMPH NODE IMAGING

Nodal metastases are a major prognostic factor in patients with endometrial cancer, as the presence of nodal metastases decreases the 5-year survival from 90% to 75% in patients with pelvic nodal metastases and to 38% in patients with para-aortic nodal metastases.[59] The risk of nodal metastases increases with increase in the grade and stage of the tumor, especially with deep myometrial and cervical invasion (see **Fig. 12**).[60] In 17% of patients with endometrial cancer, para-aortic nodal metastases can occur without concurrent pelvic node involvement.[61] Although nodal metastasis is not part of the FIGO staging for cervical cancer, the presence of nodal metastases in cervical cancer decreases 5-year survival from 89% to between 48% and 57% (see **Figs. 8** and **17**).[62] The presence of parametrial invasion increases the risk of nodal metastases by more than 50%.[63] The most common nodes to be involved in cervical cancer are the obturator nodes. The sensitivity and specificity of CT for detecting nodal metastases in endometrial and cervical cancers varies between 50% to 65% and 96% to 97%, respectively.[30,64] For MR imaging they vary between 50% to 71% and 90% to 96%, respectively.[28,64] PET/CT has been shown to have sensitivity and specificity similar to those of MR imaging in endometrial cancer. Kitajima and colleagues,[65] in a study of 40 patients with endometrial cancer, found that PET/CT had a sensitivity and specificity of 50% and 86.7%, respectively. For detecting nodes larger than 10 mm, the sensitivity was 93.3%. Several studies have shown PET/CT to be superior to MR imaging in detecting nodal metastases.[58,66] Choi and colleagues,[66] in a study of 22 patients with cervical cancer, found that sensitivity of PET/CT for detecting metastatic nodes in each of the 7 lymph node groups was higher than that of MR imaging (57.6% vs 30.3%). The use of lymph node–specific contrast agents with US, CT, and MR imaging is under research. MR lymphography with ultrasmall paramagnetic iron oxide particles has been shown to have 90% to 100% sensitivity and greater than 95% specificity for detecting nodal metastases.[67] Sentinel node imaging and biopsy has been used for intraoperative assessment of nodes in cervical and endometrial cancers in some tertiary cancer centers.

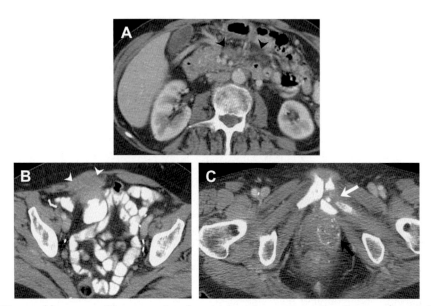

Fig. 19. A 73-year-old woman with recurrent endometrial carcinoma presenting 2 years after total abdominal hysterectomy, bilateral salpingo-oophrectomy, and vaginal brachytherapy for a high-grade stage II endometrial carcinoma. (*A–C*) Axial contrast-enhanced CT images of the abdomen and pelvis demonstrate ill-defined mesenteric soft tissue (*black arrowheads in A*), peritoneal soft-tissue mass (*white arrowheads in B*), a heterogeneous mass with calcification in the vagina (*black arrow in C*), and pathologic fracture of the left inferior pubic mass (*white arrow in C*). Biopsy of the vaginal mass confirmed recurrent endometrial carcinoma.

ENDOMETRIAL AND CERVICAL CANCER: RECURRENCES

The risk of recurrence in endometrial cancer depends on the grade and stage of the tumor, and the degree of LVSI. Most (up to 80%) recurrences occur in the first 3 years of primary treatment, most commonly in the lymph nodes, vaginal vault, peritoneum, and lungs (**Fig. 19**). MR imaging depicts vaginal vault recurrence as a tumor with signal characteristics similar to those of the primary tumor. PET/CT has been shown to have high sensitivity (100%), specificity (83%–94%), and accuracy (93%) in detecting recurrent endometrial cancer (**Fig. 20**).[68,69] Up to 70% of cervical cancers recur in the first 2 years of treatment.[70] Local recurrence in the cervix and vaginal vault is best evaluated with MR imaging, as it can differentiate fibrosis from tumor recurrence because of the high signal of recurrent tumor in contrast to the low signal of fibrotic tissue. PET/CT offers the advantage of detecting distant metastases. The sensitivity and specificity of PET/CT in detecting

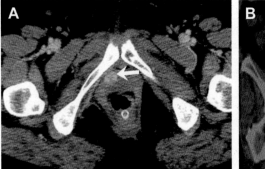
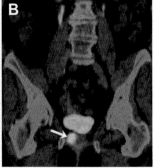

Fig. 20. A 63-year-old woman with recurrent endometrial carcinoma presenting 5 years after total abdominal hysterectomy and bilateral salpingo-oophrectomy for stage I endometrial carcinoma. (*A*) Axial contrast-enhanced CT image of the pelvis demonstrates an enhancing lesion in the right lateral aspect of the vagina (*arrow*). (*B*) Coronal FDG-PET/CT image demonstrates intense FDG uptake in the deposit (*arrow*) (SUV$_{max}$ 7.9) consistent with a metastatic deposit. Biopsy of the vaginal mass confirmed recurrent endometrial carcinoma.

cervical cancer recurrences are 86% and 94%, respectively.[71]

SUMMARY

The revised FIGO staging of endometrial and cervical cancer allows better stratification of patients according to prognostic factors, and achieves better patient care. Though not an integral part of revised staging, cross-sectional imaging is recommended by FIGO where available, as it is increasingly being recognized to have an impact on patient management and outcome. High-resolution MR imaging is the imaging modality of choice for locoregional staging of both endometrial and cervical cancer, and can guide treatment strategies appropriately. Both MDCT and PET/CT play crucial roles in advanced cancers by detecting nodal and distant metastatic disease and aiding treatment planning. Understanding how staging translates to optimal treatment will help radiologists to exercise caution while interpreting imaging studies, making theme an indispensable part of the multidisciplinary gynecologic oncology team.

ACKNOWLEDGMENT

We thank Dr Najla Fasih, Associate Professor of Radiology, The Ottawa Hospital, Ottawa, Canada for contributing to the images in the manuscript.

REFERENCES

1. Hecht JL, Mutter GL. Molecular and pathologic aspects of endometrial carcinogenesis. J Clin Oncol 2006;24(29):4783–91.
2. Siegel R, Naishadham D, Jemal A. Cancer statistics, 2012. CA Cancer J Clin 2012;62(1):10–29.
3. Freeman SJ, Aly AM, Kataoka MY, et al. The revised FIGO staging system for uterine malignancies: implications for MR imaging. Radiographics 2012;32(6):1805–27.
4. Jemal A, Bray F, Center MM, et al. Global cancer statistics. CA Cancer J Clin 2011;61(2):69–90.
5. Nicolet V, Carignan L, Bourdon F, et al. MR imaging of cervical carcinoma: a practical staging approach. Radiographics 2000;20(6):1539–49.
6. Ledwaba T, Dlamini Z, Naicker S, et al. Molecular genetics of human cervical cancer: role of papillomavirus and the apoptotic cascade. Biol Chem 2004;385(8):671–82.
7. Patel S, Liyanage SH, Sahdev A, et al. Imaging of endometrial and cervical cancer. Insights Imaging 2010;1(5–6):309–28.
8. Kaur H, Silverman PM, Iyer RB, et al. Diagnosis, staging, and surveillance of cervical carcinoma. AJR Am J Roentgenol 2003;180(6):1621–31.
9. Pecorelli S. Revised FIGO staging for carcinoma of the vulva, cervix, and endometrium. Int J Gynaecol Obstet 2009;105(2):103–4.
10. Tirumani SH, Ojili V, Shanbhogue AK, et al. Current concepts in the imaging of uterine sarcoma. Abdom Imaging 2013;38(2):397–411.
11. Ruangvutilert P, Sutantawibul A, Sunsaneevithayakul P, et al. Accuracy of transvaginal ultrasound for the evaluation of myometrial invasion in endometrial carcinoma. J Med Assoc Thai 2004;87(1):47–52.
12. Takac I. Transvaginal ultrasonography with and without saline infusion in assessment of myometrial invasion of endometrial cancer. J Ultrasound Med 2007;26(7):949–55 [quiz: 56–7].
13. Alcazar JL, Errasti T, Zornoza A. Saline infusion sonohysterography in endometrial cancer: assessment of malignant cells dissemination risk. Acta Obstet Gynecol Scand 2000;79(4):321–2.
14. Innocenti P, Pulli F, Savino L, et al. Staging of cervical cancer: reliability of transrectal US. Radiology 1992;185(1):201–5.
15. Fischerova D, Cibula D, Stenhova H, et al. Transrectal ultrasound and magnetic resonance imaging in staging of early cervical cancer. Int J Gynecol Cancer 2008;18(4):766–72.
16. Iwamoto K, Kigawa J, Minagawa Y, et al. Transvaginal ultrasonographic diagnosis of bladder-wall invasion in patients with cervical cancer. Obstet Gynecol 1994;83(2):217–9.
17. Hardesty LA, Sumkin JH, Hakim C, et al. The ability of helical CT to preoperatively stage endometrial carcinoma. AJR Am J Roentgenol 2001;176(3):603–6.
18. Kim SH, Kim HD, Song YS, et al. Detection of deep myometrial invasion in endometrial carcinoma: comparison of transvaginal ultrasound, CT, and MRI. J Comput Assist Tomogr 1995;19(5):766–72.
19. Pannu HK, Corl FM, Fishman EK. CT evaluation of cervical cancer: spectrum of disease. Radiographics 2001;21(5):1155–68.
20. Hori M, Kim T, Murakami T, et al. Uterine cervical carcinoma: preoperative staging with 3.0-T MR imaging—comparison with 1.5-T MR imaging. Radiology 2009;251(1):96–104.
21. DeSouza N, Whittle M, Williams A, et al. Magnetic resonance imaging of the primary site in stage I cervical carcinoma: a comparison of endovaginal coil with external phased array coil techniques at 0.5 T. J Magn Reson Imaging 2000;12(6):1020–6.
22. Sala E, Rockall AG, Freeman SJ, et al. The Added role of MR imaging in treatment stratification of patients with gynecologic malignancies: what the radiologist needs to know. Radiology 2013;266(3):717–40.
23. Kinkel K, Forstner R, Danza FM, et al. Staging of endometrial cancer with MRI: guidelines of the

European Society of Urogenital Imaging. Eur Radiol 2009;19(7):1565–74.

24. Balleyguier C, Sala E, Da Cunha T, et al. Staging of uterine cervical cancer with MRI: guidelines of the European Society of Urogenital Radiology. Eur Radiol 2011;21(5):1102–10.

25. Nougaret S, Tirumani SH, Addley H, et al. Pearls and pitfalls in MRI of gynecologic malignancy with diffusion-weighted technique. AJR Am J Roentgenol 2013;200(2):261–76.

26. Sala E, Crawford R, Senior E, et al. Added value of dynamic contrast-enhanced magnetic resonance imaging in predicting advanced stage disease in patients with endometrial carcinoma. Int J Gynecol Cancer 2009;19(1):141–6.

27. Beddy P, Moyle P, Kataoka M, et al. Evaluation of depth of myometrial invasion and overall staging in endometrial cancer: comparison of diffusion-weighted and dynamic contrast-enhanced MR imaging. Radiology 2012;262(2):530–7.

28. Manfredi R, Mirk P, Maresca G, et al. Local-regional staging of endometrial carcinoma: role of MR imaging in surgical planning. Radiology 2004;231(2):372–8.

29. Zandrino F, La Paglia E, Musante F. Magnetic resonance imaging in local staging of endometrial carcinoma: diagnostic performance, pitfalls, and literature review. Tumori 2010;96(4):601–8.

30. Inubashiri E, Hata K, Kanenishi K, et al. Positron emission tomography with the glucose analog [F]-fluoro-2-deoxy-D-glucose for evaluating pelvic lymph node metastasis in uterine corpus cancer: comparison with CT and MRI findings. J Obstet Gynaecol Res 2009;35(1):26–34.

31. Wagenaar HC, Trimbos JB, Postema S, et al. Tumor diameter and volume assessed by magnetic resonance imaging in the prediction of outcome for invasive cervical cancer. Gynecol Oncol 2001;82(3):474–82.

32. Sahdev A, Sohaib SA, Wenaden AE, et al. The performance of magnetic resonance imaging in early cervical carcinoma: a long-term experience. Int J Gynecol Cancer 2007;17(3):629–36.

33. Zand KR, Reinhold C, Abe H, et al. Magnetic resonance imaging of the cervix. Cancer Imaging 2007;7(1):69.

34. Chung HH, Kang SB, Cho JY, et al. Can preoperative MRI accurately evaluate nodal and parametrial invasion in early stage cervical cancer? Jpn J Clin Oncol 2007;37(5):370–5.

35. Shweel MA, Abdel-Gawad EA, Abdel-Gawad EA, et al. Uterine cervical malignancy: diagnostic accuracy of MRI with histopathologic correlation. J Clin Imaging Sci 2012;2:42.

36. Park W, Park YJ, Huh SJ, et al. The usefulness of MRI and PET imaging for the detection of parametrial involvement and lymph node metastasis in

patients with cervical cancer. Jpn J Clin Oncol 2005;35(5):260–4.

37. Hricak H, Yu KK. Radiology in invasive cervical cancer. AJR Am J Roentgenol 1996;167(5):1101–8.

38. Togashi K, Morikawa K, Kataoka ML, et al. Cervical cancer. J Magn Reson Imaging 1998;8(2):391–7.

39. Kim SH, Han MC. Invasion of the urinary bladder by uterine cervical carcinoma: evaluation with MR imaging. AJR Am J Roentgenol 1997;168(2):393–7.

40. Harry VN. Novel imaging techniques as response biomarkers in cervical cancer. Gynecol Oncol 2010;116(2):253–61.

41. Leach MO, Brindle KM, Evelhoch JL, et al. The assessment of antiangiogenic and antivascular therapies in early-stage clinical trials using magnetic resonance imaging: issues and recommendations. Br J Cancer 2005;92(9):1599–610.

42. Payne GS, Schmidt M, Morgan VA, et al. Evaluation of magnetic resonance diffusion and spectroscopy measurements as predictive biomarkers in stage 1 cervical cancer. Gynecol Oncol 2010;116(2):246–52.

43. Liu Y, Bai R, Sun H, et al. Diffusion-weighted imaging in predicting and monitoring the response of uterine cervical cancer to combined chemoradiation. Clin Radiol 2009;64(11):1067–74.

44. Zietkowski D, Davidson R, Eykyn T, et al. Detection of cancer in cervical tissue biopsies using mobile lipid resonances measured with diffusion-weighted 1H magnetic resonance spectroscopy. NMR Biomed 2010;23(4):382–90.

45. Downey K, deSouza NM. Imaging cervical cancer: recent advances and future directions. Curr Opin Oncol 2011;23(5):519–25.

46. Xue F, Lin LL, Dehdashti F, et al. F-18 fluorodeoxyglucose uptake in primary cervical cancer as an indicator of prognosis after radiation therapy. Gynecol Oncol 2006;101(1):147–51.

47. Grigsby PW, Siegel BA, Dehdashti F. Lymph node staging by positron emission tomography in patients with carcinoma of the cervix. J Clin Oncol 2001;19(17):3745–9.

48. Ma SY, See LC, Lai CH, et al. Delayed ^{18}F-FDG PET for detection of paraaortic lymph node metastases in cervical cancer patients. J Nucl Med 2003;44(11):1775–83.

49. Pandit-Taskar N. Oncologic imaging in gynecologic malignancies. J Nucl Med 2005;46(11):1842–50.

50. Colombo N, Preti E, Landoni F, et al. Endometrial cancer: ESMO clinical practice guidelines for diagnosis, treatment and follow-up. Ann Oncol 2011;22(Suppl 6):vi35–9.

51. NCCN clinical practice guidelines in oncology endometrial cancer version 1. 2013. Available at: http://www.nccn.org/professionals/physician_gls/pdf/uterine.pdf. Accessed March 21, 2013.

52. Lee KB, Ki KD, Lee JM, et al. The risk of lymph node metastasis based on myometrial invasion

and tumor grade in endometrioid uterine cancers: a multicenter, retrospective Korean study. Ann Surg Oncol 2009;16(10):2882–7.

53. Reznek RH, Sahdev A. MR imaging in cervical cancer: seeing is believing. The 2004 Mackenzie Davidson Memorial Lecture. Br J Radiol 2005; 78(Spec No 2):S73–85.

54. Sheu MH, Chang CY, Wang JH, et al. Cervical carcinoma: assessment of parametrial invasion and lymph node metastasis with magnetic resonance imaging. Zhonghua Yi Xue Za Zhi (Taipei) 2000; 63(8):634–40.

55. Bipat S, Glas AS, van der Velden J, et al. Computed tomography and magnetic resonance imaging in staging of uterine cervical carcinoma: a systematic review. Gynecol Oncol 2003;91(1):59–66.

56. Subak LL, Hricak H, Powell CB, et al. Cervical carcinoma: computed tomography and magnetic resonance imaging for preoperative staging. Obstet Gynecol 1995;86(1):43–50.

57. NCCN clinical practice guidelines in oncology cervical cancer version 2. 2013. Available at: http://www.nccn.org/professionals/physician_gls/pdf/cervical.pdf. Accessed March 21, 2013.

58. Reinhardt MJ, Ehritt-Braun C, Vogelgesang D, et al. Metastatic lymph nodes in patients with cervical cancer: detection with MR imaging and FDG PET. Radiology 2001;218(3):776–82.

59. Morrow CP, Bundy BN, Kurman RJ, et al. Relationship between surgical-pathological risk factors and outcome in clinical stage I and II carcinoma of the endometrium: a Gynecologic Oncology Group study. Gynecol Oncol 1991;40(1):55–65.

60. Chi D, Barakat R, Palayekar M, et al. The incidence of pelvic lymph node metastasis by FIGO staging for patients with adequately surgically staged endometrial adenocarcinoma of endometrioid histology. Int J Gynecol Cancer 2008;18(2):269–73.

61. McMeekin DS, Lashbrook D, Gold M, et al. Nodal distribution and its significance in FIGO stage IIIc endometrial cancer. Gynecol Oncol 2001;82(2):375–9.

62. Lai G, Rockall AG. Lymph node imaging in gynecologic malignancy. Semin Ultrasound CT MR 2010; 31(5):363.

63. Delgado G, Bundy B, Fowler W, et al. A prospective surgical pathological study of stage I squamous carcinoma of the cervix: a Gynecologic Oncology Group Study. Gynecol Oncol 1989;35(3): 314–20.

64. Yang WT, Lam WW, Yu MY, et al. Comparison of dynamic helical CT and dynamic MR imaging in the evaluation of pelvic lymph nodes in cervical carcinoma. AJR Am J Roentgenol 2000;175(3): 759–66.

65. Kitajima K, Murakami K, Yamasaki E, et al. Accuracy of ^{18}F-FDG PET/CT in detecting pelvic and paraaortic lymph node metastasis in patients with endometrial cancer. AJR Am J Roentgenol 2008; 190(6):1652–8.

66. Choi HJ, Roh JW, Seo SS, et al. Comparison of the accuracy of magnetic resonance imaging and positron emission tomography/computed tomography in the presurgical detection of lymph node metastases in patients with uterine cervical carcinoma. Cancer 2006;106(4):914–22.

67. Rockall AG, Sohaib SA, Harisinghani MG, et al. Diagnostic performance of nanoparticle-enhanced magnetic resonance imaging in the diagnosis of lymph node metastases in patients with endometrial and cervical cancer. J Clin Oncol 2005;23(12):2813–21.

68. Chung HH, Kang WJ, Kim JW, et al. The clinical impact of [18F] FDG PET/CT for the management of recurrent endometrial cancer: correlation with clinical and histological findings. Eur J Nucl Med Mol Imaging 2008;35(6):1081–8.

69. Park JY, Kim EN, Kim DY, et al. Clinical impact of positron emission tomography or positron emission tomography/computed tomography in the post-therapy surveillance of endometrial carcinoma: evaluation of 88 patients. Int J Gynecol Cancer 2008;18(6):1332–8.

70. Rockall AG, Cross S, Flanagan S, et al. The role of FDG-PET/CT in gynaecological cancers. Cancer Imaging 2012;12:49–65.

71. Ryu SY, Kim MH, Choi SC, et al. Detection of early recurrence with ^{18}F-FDG PET in patients with cervical cancer. J Nucl Med 2003;44(3):347–52.

Positron Emission Tomography–Computed Tomography Imaging for Malignancies in Women

Chitra Viswanathan, MD[a],*, Priya R. Bhosale, MD[a],
Shetal N. Shah, MD[b],
Raghunandan Vikram, MBBS, MRCP, FRCR[a]

KEYWORDS

- PET/CT • Cervical cancer • Endometrial cancer • Pitfalls • Gynecologic malignancy

KEY POINTS

- In cervical cancer, survival is correlated with nodal disease, and positron emission tomography (PET)/computed tomography (CT) is superior for nodal staging. Standardized uptake value (SUV) of primary tumor also prognosticates survival at 5 years, and posttreatment SUV predicts survival at 2 years after treatment.
- In ovarian cancer, the value of PET/CT is in detection of disease in symptomatic patients with normal imaging and normal cancer antigen 125 (CA-125) and in patients with normal imaging and increasing CA-125.
- In grade III endometrial cancer and papillary serous tumors, PET/CT is useful in diagnosing nodes above the iliac vessels and detecting distant metastases not included in routine staging surgery, thereby altering treatment.
- PET/CT can help detect the presence of lymph node metastases, the most important prognostic factor, in patients with vulvar carcinoma.
- PET/CT may be helpful in detecting a fallopian tube primary cancer in a patient with widespread metastatic disease of unknown primary tumor.

INTRODUCTION

Gynecologic malignancy is a leading cause of cancer in women worldwide and causes up to 20% of solid tumors in women. In the United States, an estimated 91,730 patients will be diagnosed with gynecologic malignancy and 28,080 will die in 2013.[1] The most common gynecologic malignancy is endometrial cancer in the United States and Western Europe, but ovarian cancer accounts for most of the cancer-related deaths. Ultrasound, computed tomography (CT) and magnetic resonance (MR) imaging are conventionally used for local staging of disease. F-18 fluorodeoxyglucose (FDG) PET/CT has seen increasing acceptance in gynecologic malignancies over the past decade because of its ability to combine physiologic and anatomic information and also to image the whole body in a single examination, helping detect both

The authors have no disclosures.
[a] Diagnostic Radiology, The University of Texas MD Anderson Cancer Center, 1515 Holcombe Boulevard, Unit 1473, Houston, TX 77030, USA; [b] Diagnostic Radiology and PET Imaging, PET-MR, Center for PET and Molecular Imaging, Cleveland Clinic Foundation, Cleveland Clinic Main Campus, Mail Code Hb6, 9500 Euclid Avenue, Cleveland, OH 44195, USA
* Corresponding author.
E-mail address: chitra.viswanathan@mdanderson.org

Radiol Clin N Am 51 (2013) 1111–1125
http://dx.doi.org/10.1016/j.rcl.2013.07.006
0033-8389/13/$ – see front matter © 2013 Elsevier Inc. All rights reserved.

local and distant disease. However, there are several technological and physiologic factors that introduce limitations, artifacts, and pitfalls. Poor spatial resolution limits characterization of sub-centimeter lesions. Misregistration between the CT and PET components may lead to avoidable errors in interpretation. Dependence of standardized uptake value maximum (SUV_{max}) on various factors such as scan time from injection, serum blood glucose, volume averaging from motion, attenuation correction, and difference in scanners can lead to erroneous interpretation of results, particularly when SUV_{max} is used for response assessment.

This article highlights the current status of the role of PET/CT in various gynecologic malignancies in light of current available data, provides imaging examples, and discusses pearls and common pitfalls (**Table 1**).

CERVICAL CANCER

Cervical cancer is the third most common female malignancy worldwide and the second most common cause of cancer-related mortality. An estimated 12,340 cases of invasive cervical cancer are expected to be diagnosed and an estimated 4030 deaths are expected in 2013.[1] However, its incidence in the United States has been decreasing over the past several decades. Since 2004, the rates have decreased by 2.1% per year in women younger than 50 years and 3.1% per year in women 50 years and older. This decrease has been caused by prevention and early detection of cancer as a result of screening with the Papanicolaou (Pap) test. The primary cause of cervical cancer is infection with human papillomavirus (HPV). Long-term use of oral contraceptives is also associated with increased risk of cervical cancer.

The most common type of carcinoma of the cervix is squamous cell cancer (69%), followed by adenocarcinoma (25%) and adenosquamous carcinoma (3%). Other rare tumor types include neuroendocrine tumors, rhabdomyosarcoma, primary lymphoma, and sarcoma. The 2 most common pathologic subtypes of cervical carcinoma are generally FDG avid.

Table 1
Pearls and pitfalls

Malignancy	Pearls	Pitfalls
Cervical cancer	Involvement of lymph nodes provides useful prognostic information Complete metabolic response after chemoradiation is associated with improved survival compared with partial response or progressive disease	PET/CT is poor in defining local extent of cervical cancer in the pelvis Ureteric activity may occasionally mimic pelvic lymphadenopathy
Ovarian cancer	PET/CT is useful in patients with suspected recurrent disease and normal conventional imaging Resolution of metabolic activity on PET/CT, despite the presence of abnormality on conventional CT, is considered response to therapy	Low-grade histologies of ovarian carcinoma may show no or low FDG avidity —
Endometrial cancer	PET/CT is useful in the detection of distant metastatic disease, particularly in the setting of normal conventional imaging	Metabolic activity in the endometrium may be seen during menstruation, and benign conditions such as hyperplasia and polyps can be metabolically FDG avid
Vulvar and vaginal cancers	PET/CT in vulvar and vaginal tumors is highly useful in assessing for lymph node metastatic disease, which affects prognosis and may change management	—
Fallopian tube cancer	In cases of unknown primary tumor, PET/CT may help in distinguishing fallopian tube from ovarian malignancies	Physiologic activity may be seen in the fallopian tubes during menstruation

The National Comprehensive Cancer Network (NCCN) clinical practice guidelines recommend that the use of PET/CT is optional for initial staging of stage 1B tumors or higher, for further evaluation in those patients who have positive para-aortic nodes at surgery, and in surveillance.[2] In both the initial pretreatment evaluation of cervical cancer and in recurrent cervical cancer, the American College of Radiology (ACR) Appropriateness Criteria give PET/CT high ratings.[3,4]

Pretreatment SUV_{max} of the primary lesion at initial staging has been reported as a sensitive marker of overall survival. Analysis of 287 patients treated with curative intent at a single center found that the 5-year survival was greater than 95% when the SUV_{max} of the primary tumor was less than 5.2, decreased to 70% in patients with SUV_{max} values between 5.2 and 13.3, and further decreased to less than 40% when the SUV_{max} was greater than 13.3.[5]

Several early studies showed that judicious use of PET/CT changed management in 24% to 66% of patients with cervical cancer, predominantly because of the ability to detect extrapelvic findings and metastatic disease.[6,7] For example, occult supraclavicular lymph node metastases are seen in up to 8% of patients with advanced cervical cancer; this provides additional information that is valuable in patient management (**Fig. 1**).[8]

PET/CT is useful in detecting lymph node metastases both within the pelvis and in extrapelvic locations. Pelvic nodal involvement almost always precedes para-aortic involvement. Isolated para-aortic lymph node involvement is found in only 1% of patients. Parametrial, obturator, and external iliac nodes are the earliest nodal stations involved in cervical cancer.[9] A meta-analysis reported the pooled sensitivity and specificity for detection of pelvic lymph node involvement with PET as 79% and 99% respectively, and 84% and 95% respectively for para-aortic nodal involvement.[10] The pooled sensitivity and specificity for MR imaging for pelvic lymph node metastases was 72%, 96% and the pooled sensitivity of CT for pelvic lymph node metastases was 47% 50%, and 100% respectively. For entry into three

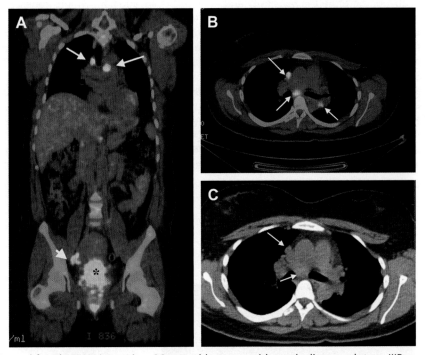

Fig. 1. (A) Coronal fused PET/CT image in a 36-year-old woman with newly diagnosed stage IIIB poorly differentiated squamous cell carcinoma of the cervix. No nodal disease was suspected at presentation. On PET/CT, there is uptake in the cervix (*asterisk*) consistent with the primary tumor. Adjacent pelvic adenopathy was also identified (*short white arrow*). Unexpected uptake was also seen in the nodes of the mediastinum (*long white arrows*). (B) Axial fused PET/CT image through the level of the thorax shows mediastinal and hilar adenopathy with FDG uptake (*long white arrows*). (C) Axial noncontrast CT from the PET/CT shows the same nodes (*white arrows*) are subcentimeter but still have FDG avidity. Biopsy showed poorly differentiated carcinoma from cervical primary. Management was changed from chemoradiation for stage IIIB disease to short-course radiation therapy and extensive chemotherapy for stage IVB disease.

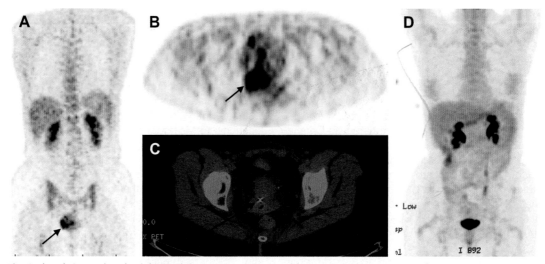

Fig. 2. (*A, B*) Coronal and axial PET/CT images in a 46-year-old woman with carcinoma of the cervix. Pretreatment scan shows marked abnormal FDG uptake in cervix (*black arrow* in *A* and *B*), consistent with tumor. (*C, D*) Axial fused and coronal PET/CT images in a 46-year-old woman with carcinoma of the cervix. Posttreatment scan 5 months later shows significant decrease in abnormal FDG uptake in the cervix, a favorable indicator of survival (*long black arrow* indicates radiation seed).

of the studies in the meta-analysis, negative CT scans were required, therefore the sensitivity and specificity of CT for para-aortic nodes could not be obtained. MR imaging had a sensitivity and specificity of 67% and 100% for para-aortic adenopathy. However, because of resolution limitations, nodes that are less than a centimeter might not be accurately staged on PET/CT.[11–13]

PET/CT is a useful prognostic indicator in patients with cervical carcinoma. Absence or presence of a PET-positive para-aortic node is the most significant prognostic factor for progression-free survival, as shown in a study comparing CT and PET in patients with cervical cancer for nodal staging.[14,15] In addition, lymph nodes above the L5 level are not typically treated with conventional radiation; if FDG-avid nodes are seen above L5, even if they are normal in size, they are included in the radiation portal.

Complete metabolic response, defined as absence of abnormal FDG uptake on postchemoradiation PET scan at sites of abnormal FDG uptake noted on pretreatment scan, has been shown to be a favorable prognostic indicator of survival (**Fig. 2**). Analysis of a mixed retrospective and prospective cohort study at a single center showed

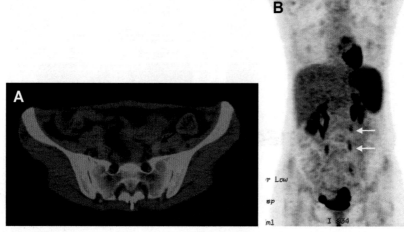

Fig. 3. (*A*) Axial fused PET/CT image shows uptake in the left common iliac region (*black arrow*), which could be mistaken for nodal disease. (*B*) By using the coronal images, this activity is seen to be linear (*white arrows*) and thus represents ureteral activity and not node.

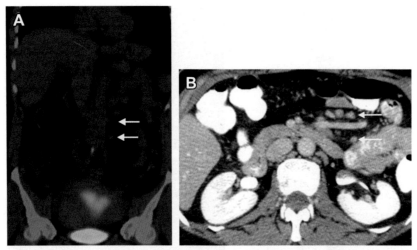

Fig. 4. (A) Coronal fused PET/CT in a 39-year-old woman with treated cervical cancer shows FDG-avid adenopathy in the small bowel mesentery (arrows). (B) Axial contrast-enhanced CT shows better detail of these nodes (arrows). Since the mesenteric lymph nodes are not a usual site of cervical cancer metastases, alternate diagnoses should be considered. Biopsy of these mesenteric nodes showed lymphoma.

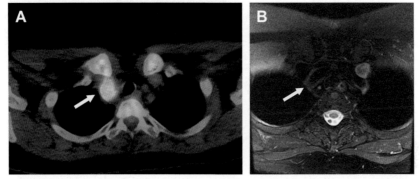

Fig. 5. (A) Axial fused PET/CT in 53-year-old woman with recurrent adenosquamous carcinoma of the cervix treated with radiation and cisplatin-gemcitabine for 1 cycle shows intense increased uptake in the right paratracheal location (arrow), which is concerning for adenopathy. Patient had subsequent head and neck ultrasound, which did not show any nodal disease in this region. (B) Axial T2-weighted MR imaging of the neck shows no adenopathy and thickened and inflamed subclavian artery (arrow). Although angiogram and/or postcontrast images would better evaluate this finding, this patient was unable to have contrast because of an increased creatinine level. Although drug toxicity is rare, this finding is consistent with gemcitabine-induced vasculitis.

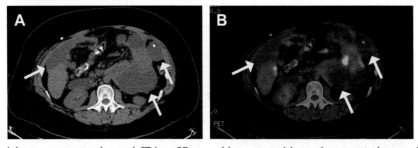

Fig. 6. (A) Axial non–contrast-enhanced CT in a 27-year-old woman with mucinous cystadenocarcinoma shows multiple low-attenuation mucin deposits in the mesentery (white arrows), consistent with metastatic disease. These deposits are difficult to separate from adjacent bowel, and CT with gastrointestinal and intravenous contrast may better evaluate mucinous tumors. There is also a peritoneal catheter in place. (B) Axial fused PET/CT in the same patient shows no FDG avidity in the mucinous portion of the deposits (white arrows) but peripheral activity may represent adjacent bowel. Low-grade tumors may have no or little FDG uptake.

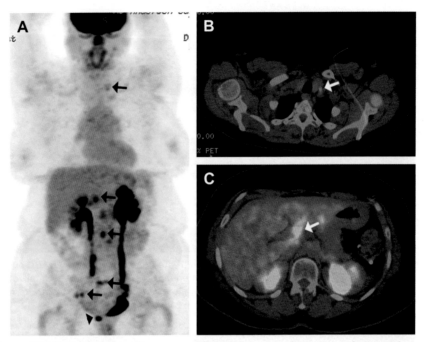

Fig. 7. (*A*) Coronal PET/CT in a 64-year-old woman with ovarian cancer. Six months after completion of therapy, patient had an increasing CA-125. Conventional imaging did not show enlarged nodes, and PET/CT was obtained. There are multiple areas of FDG uptake, corresponding with recurrent disease in the nodes (*arrows*). Recurrent disease is also seen in the pelvis (*arrowhead*). Patient was started on chemotherapy. (*B*) Axial fused PET/CT through the level of the thorax shows normal-sized FDG-avid supraclavicular node (*arrow*), consistent with metastasis. (*C*) Axial fused PET/CT through the abdomen shows FDG-avid porta hepatis node (*arrow*), consistent with metastatic disease.

that the 3-year survival of patients achieving complete metabolic response, partial response, and progressive disease on PET/CT performed 3 months after therapy were 70%, 16%, and 13% respectively.[16]

One of the most common pitfalls is focal activity within the ureter from urinary excretion of FDG, which can mimic a metastatic node (**Fig. 3**). Analyzing the images with normal course of the ureter in mind along with careful search for lymph nodes on the noncontrast CT portion of the PET/CT along the expected pathways of spread often helps in avoiding this misinterpretation. Urinary bladder activity may mask the full extent of disease in the pelvis. Particularly for this reason, the bladder should be emptied before scanning, and the scan should be obtained in a caudal-cranial direction to image the pelvis before bladder filling.

Benign conditions mimicking metastatic disease are a common pitfall encountered in PET-CT scans in patients with nearly all cancer groups. Although discussed here in the context of cervical carcinoma, these may be seen in patients with other malignancies as well. There is an expected pattern of nodal metastases seen in patients with cervical carcinoma. Isolated FDG uptake in distant nodal stations or within the mesenteric lymph nodes is unusual and should alert the radiologist to consider an alternate diagnosis such as lymphoma or sarcoidosis (**Fig. 4**). Unusual activity is sometimes seen as a result of treatment. Hypermetabolism in areas exposed to radiotherapy is common and hence PET/CT is generally contraindicated until 12 weeks after radiotherapy. Although

---

Cervical cancer: pearls and pitfalls

Pearls

- PET/CT is superior to conventional imaging for nodal staging
- Survival correlates with nodal involvement
- High pretreatment SUV_{max} of primary tumor correlates with worse disease-free survival rate

Pitfalls

- Unusual pattern of lymph node uptake should prompt alternate diagnosis
- Ureteral uptake may mimic lymph node

chemotherapy-induced side effects such as vasculitis are seen but are rare,[17] they remain potential pitfalls, particularly in those patients receiving gemcitabine, a common therapeutic agent used in advanced cervical cancer (**Fig. 5**).

OVARIAN CANCER

An estimated 22,240 cases of ovarian cancer are expected to be diagnosed and an estimated 14,030 deaths are expected in 2013.[1] Ovarian cancer accounts for 30% of all gynecologic malignancies but causes more than 50% of deaths in the Western world, because nearly 75% of patients present with advanced-stage disease at the time of diagnosis.[18] However, there has been considerable progress in terms of surgical treatment and chemotherapy, which has improved the median survival of patient with ovarian cancer from 20 months in the 1970s to up to 65 months in recent years.[19,20] Aggressive surgical treatment with total abdominal hysterectomy, bilateral

salpingo-oophorectomy, and optimal tumor debulking that leaves behind no deposits larger than 1 cm followed by chemotherapy is shown to improve overall survival in patients with stage III ovarian carcinoma. Despite these strategies, recurrence rates are high, because more than 50% of patients relapse within 5 years.[21] However, some patients with recurrent disease may benefit from early detection and salvage treatment.[21] Careful monitoring of these patients after optimal treatment to detect recurrent disease is important.

Initial analysis based on a study of 4509 patients with ovarian cancer revealed that use of PET or PET/CT changed intended treatment in 41.4% of patients. When adjusted to the imaging study alone, there was treatment change in 16.2% of patients, highlighting the usefulness of PET and PET/CT in management of ovarian cancer.[22] The NCCN clinical practice guidelines recommend the use of PET/CT for initial staging and in surveillance. PET scan is given a category 2B recommendation (category 2B recommendation is based on

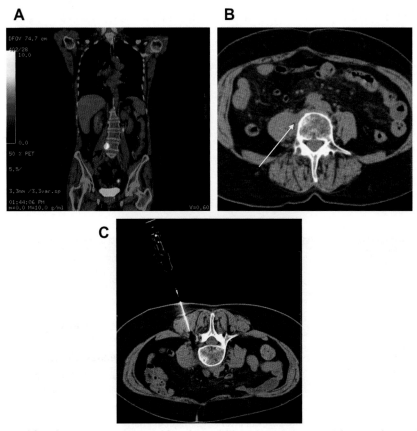

Fig. 8. (A) Coronal fused PET/CT in a 44-year-old patient with ovarian carcinoma with normal CA-125 and normal conventional imaging but with back pain. There is FDG uptake adjacent to and of the right L4 vertebral body (*black arrow*). (B) Corresponding axial noncontrast CT as part of PET/CT shows minimal thickening that is difficult to diagnose prospectively (*long white arrow*). (C) CT guided biopsy obtained of this area showed metastatic ovarian carcinoma.

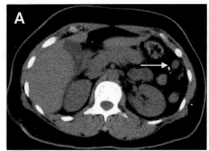
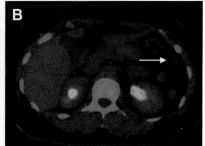

Fig. 9. (*A*) Axial noncontrast CT obtained with PET/CT in a 43-year-old woman with ovarian carcinoma shows a peritoneal nodule in the left upper quadrant (*arrow*). (*B*) Axial fused PET/CT through the same level shows that this peritoneal nodule (*arrow*) does not take up FDG, which is a potential pitfall of PET/CT.

low-level evidence and there is nonuniform consensus but no major disagreement.)[23] The ACR Appropriateness Criteria state that, for the staging of primary ovarian cancer, PET/CT may be useful, but for evaluation of recurrent cancer PET/CT is usually appropriate.[24]

PET/CT is generally not useful in initial diagnosis of ovarian cancer because of a small but significant number of false-positive and false-negative cases.[25] A positive predictive value of 86% and a negative predictive value of 76% was reported by Hubner and colleagues[26] in an early study of the accuracy of PET. Rieber and colleagues[27] reported relative sensitivities of 58%, 92%, and 83%, and specificities of 78%, 59%, and 84%, for PET, transvaginal ultrasound, and MR imaging in diagnosing ovarian malignancy. In contrast, PET/CT could be useful in carefully selected individuals. In a prospective study on 101 patients performed by Risum and colleagues,[28] PET/CT showed a sensitivity of 100% and specificity of 92.5% in identifying primary ovarian cancer in patients with pelvic mass of unknown origin. These patients were selected based on the presence of other risk factors such as cancer antigen 125 (CA-125) levels, ultrasound examination, and postmenopausal state.

In addition, low-grade cystadenocarcinoma or borderline ovarian tumor may show no or low-grade FDG avidity. This avidity seems to be related to low glucose transportase-1 (GLUT-1) expression leading to low accumulation of FDG within the tumor cells. Kurokawa and colleagues[29] reported low GLUT-1 expression in mucinous tumors compared with serous cystadenocarcinomas, and consequently the SUV_{max} of these tumors ranged from 0.7 to 1.9 compared with serous cystadenocarcinomas with SUV_{max} of 2.9 to 8.7 (**Fig. 6**). Potential pitfalls include increased FDG activity seen in normal ovaries of physiologically active young women; inflammatory conditions of the ovary, such as oophoritis, pelvic inflammatory disease, or endometriosis; or dermoid cysts.[30]

PET/CT is perhaps most useful in diagnosis and management of recurrent ovarian cancer, with

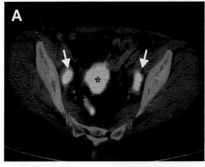
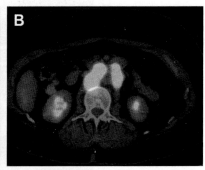

Fig. 10. (*A*) Axial fused PET/CT in 64-year-old woman with newly diagnosed high-grade serous adenocarcinoma of the uterus. PET/CT was ordered before surgical intervention. Axial image through the level of the uterus shows marked FDG uptake in the uterus (*asterisk*; SUV_{max} 14.1) and bilateral external iliac adenopathy (*white arrows*; SUV_{max} 12.6 and 13). (*B*) Axial fused PET/CT through the retroperitoneum shows FDG-avid retroperitoneal para-aortic adenopathy (*black arrows*; SUV_{max} 12.6). This adenopathy was biopsied and found to be metastatic. Although the original plan was to resect these nodes at surgery, the surgeons were unable to resect because of the extensive involvement of the aorta.

some investigators reporting a 25% to 58% change in treatment plan when PET/CT was used.[31–33] The ACR Appropriateness Criteria give a high rating to PET/CT for the evaluation of recurrent ovarian cancer, especially in conjunction with CA-125.[24] PET/CT is also valuable in patients who have an increasing CA-125 but who have had negative CT or MR imaging (**Fig. 7**).[34,35] PET/CT is also useful in identifying disease in symptomatic patients with treated ovarian cancer, with normal conventional imaging, and CA-125 (**Fig. 8**).[34,36]

PET/CT was superior to CA-125, CT, and MR imaging in detecting recurrent disease in a meta-analysis of 34 studies, having the highest pooled sensitivity (0.91).[37] CA-125 had the highest pooled specificity (0.93). Patients do not benefit from treatment if there are no imaging findings to support recurrent disease in the setting of an increased CA-125. PET/CT is particularly helpful in selecting patients for site-specific treatment planning such as biopsy, surgery, or radiotherapy. One potential false-negative finding on PET/CT is small-volume peritoneal disease (carcinomatosis or a subcentimeter peritoneal nodule) that may not be FDG avid (**Fig. 9**).

Ovarian cancer: pearls and pitfalls

Pearls

- PET/CT can help detect the precise location and help guide biopsy in the preoperative setting
- PET/CT is useful for detection of disease in patients with suspected recurrence with normal CA-125 and normal imaging, or increased CA-125 and normal imaging
- PET/CT can be used to assess response to therapy

Pitfalls

- False-positive and false-negative findings may occur

ENDOMETRIAL CANCER

Endometrial cancer is the most common gynecologic malignancy. There are 49,560 projected new cases in 2013, with an estimated 8190 deaths from the disease.[1] The overall 5-year survival rate is 83%. Risk factors for endometrial carcinoma include increase in unopposed estrogen associated with menopause, low parity, obesity, anovulation, and polycystic ovarian syndrome. In addition, hereditary syndromes, such as Lynch syndrome, have an increased risk.

Use of PET and PET/CT changed management in 36.5% of patients with uterine cancer in a study based on analysis of 2869 patients in the National Oncology PET Registry (NOPR).[22,38] The ACR Appropriateness Criteria for endometrial cancer advise use of PET/CT in high-grade tumors and in the posttherapy evaluation of suspected recurrence.[39]

The International Federation of Gynecology and Obstetrics (FIGO) stage and the histologic grade are important determinants of the degree of FDG avidity in the primary tumor. In addition, the SUV_{max} in the primary tumors of patients with metastatic nodal disease is slightly higher than in patients without nodal disease, suggesting that careful evaluation of the lymph node stations in patients with a high tumor grade should be performed. In a series of preoperative patients with endometrial cancer, PET/CT had a sensitivity, specificity, and accuracy of 50%, 86.7%, and 77.5% in detecting lymph node metastases. In grade III endometrial cancer and papillary serous tumors, PET/CT is useful in diagnosing nodes above the iliac vessels and detecting distant metastases not included in routine staging surgery, thereby potentially altering treatment (**Fig. 10**).

PET/CT in endometrial cancer, similar to findings in other gynecologic cancers, has poor sensitivity in detecting micrometastatic disease.[40] It seems that nodal disease is better detected in higher grade tumors. In a study of patients with grade 3 endometrial cancer, Picchio and colleagues[41] found that lymph node detection had

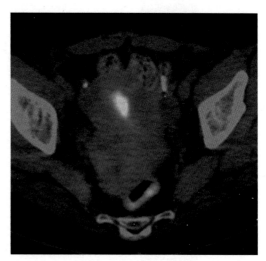

Fig. 11. Axial fused PET/CT in a 48-year-old woman with melanoma shows a linear area of FDG avidity in the uterus corresponding with the endometrial cavity. Endometrial biopsy showed proliferative endometrium.

sensitivity of 57.1%, specificity of 100%, and 88.5% accuracy. In a study of patients with grade II and grade III endometrial carcinoma, the sensitivity, specificity, and accuracy of detecting lymph node metastatic disease were 77.8%, 100%, and 94.4%.

A potential pitfall in the initial diagnosis of endometrial cancer or gynecologic malignancy using PET/CT imaging is endometrial uptake. Endometrial uptake is common in physiologically active women and needs to be distinguished from endometrial carcinoma.[42] Premenopausal women can have endometrial uptake during the menstruating and ovulatory phases (Fig. 11). Increased activity in postmenopausal women is abnormal and must be investigated for possible hyperplasia, polyp, or malignancy. Another possible pitfall is FDG uptake in the endometrium (seen in the evaluation of other gynecologic malignancies such as cervical cancer), which may not represent extension of the primary tumor but may be reactive (Fig. 12).

PET/CT is helpful in determining recurrent disease in endometrial cancer. In patients with suspected recurrent tumor, Kitajima and colleagues[43] found that PET/CT changed management in more patients than CT, having a sensitivity of 91% and a specificity of 94%. In a series of patients analyzed retrospectively by Belhocine and colleagues,[44] PET/CT changed management in approximately 35% of cases by finding recurrence in 88% and asymptomatic recurrence in 12%. The vaginal apex is a common site of recurrence and patients may present with vaginal spotting. Lin and colleagues[45] showed that the use of

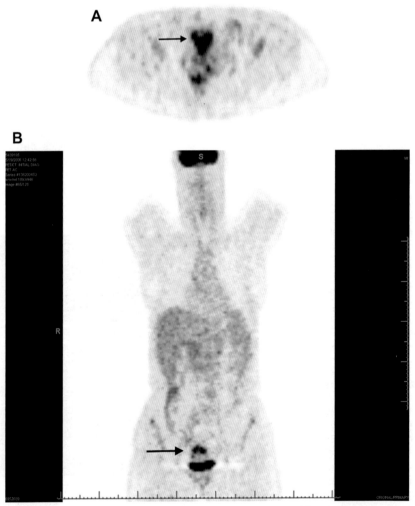

Fig. 12. (A, B) Axial and maximum intensity projection of PET in a 45-year-old patient with cervical cancer shows intense increased FDG avidity in the endometrium of the uterus (*thin arrow*). Endometrial biopsy was negative for malignancy. Patient was having heavy bleeding.

PET/CT in their series of patients with recurrence at the vaginal apex was effective in determining distal metastatic disease and obviating radiotherapy (**Fig. 13**).

Endometrial cancer: pearls and pitfalls

Pearls

- The primary value of PET/CT is in detection of distal metastatic disease.

- PET/CT is useful in patients with recurrence at the vaginal apex to detect distal metastatic disease and prevent unnecessary therapy.

Pitfalls

- Determination of malignancy cannot solely be based on the SUV_{max}. Biopsy may be required.

VULVAR CANCER

Vulvar cancer is a rare cancer, estimated to have 4700 new cases and cause 950 deaths in the United States in the year 2013.[1] Early-stage vulvar carcinoma may have no symptoms, although later-stage disease may present with a vulvar lump, vulvar itching, burning or bleeding, or dysuria. The most common histology of vulvar carcinoma is squamous cell carcinoma.

ACR Appropriateness Criteria advocate the use of PET/CT in the initial work-up and assessment of treatment response, and obtained these guidelines through evaluation of literature and the similarities of vulvar cancers to cervical and anal cancer.

The presence of lymph node metastases is the most important prognostic factor in patients with vulvar carcinoma. PET/CT is perhaps most useful in the evaluation of lymph node status and distal metastatic disease in patients with vulvar cancer

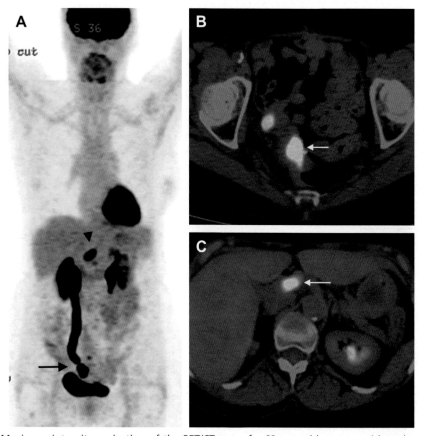

Fig. 13. (*A*) Maximum intensity projection of the PET/CT scan of a 68-year-old woman with endometrial cancer shows a right hydronephrosis (*arrow*) and a focus of uptake in the upper abdomen (*arrowhead*). (*B*) Axial fused PET/CT shows disease at the vaginal apex (*arrow*), which is the cause of the right ureteral obstruction. (*C*) Axial fused PET/CT of the upper abdomen shows FDG-avid periportal adenopathy (*arrow*).

(Fig. 14). Cohn and colleagues[46] reported a sensitivity of 67%, specificity of 95%, positive predictive value of 86%, and negative predictive value of 86% for PET/CT in the detection of nodal disease in patients with vulvar carcinoma. If the vulvar tumor is located in the midline, it is difficult to assess for metastatic lymph nodes even with lymphoscintigraphy because they can drain to bilateral groin lymph nodes. In this situation, PET/CT may be able to assess the FDG-avid metastatic lymph nodes and limit groin dissection to 1 side.

The accuracy of PET/CT is superior to CT and MR imaging in detecting nodal disease and can help plan radiation therapy and surgical management (Fig. 15).

Vulvar cancer: pearls

Pearls

- Similar histology to cervical cancer, and PET/CT indications are similar
- If metastatic pelvic lymph nodes are identified on PET/CT, patients are treated with chemoradiation and do not undergo lymph node dissection

---

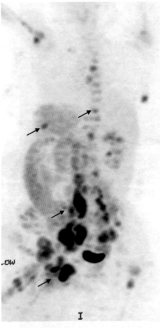

Fig. 14. Maximum intensity projection of a PET scan in a 50-year-old woman with vulvar cancer. Coronal maximum intensity projection PET/CT shows increased FDG avidity in the vulva and widespread metastatic disease in bone, liver, pelvis (examples are marked with *black arrows*).

VAGINAL CANCER

Vaginal carcinoma is also an uncommon cancer, estimated to have 2890 new cases and cause 840 deaths, respectively, in the United States in the year 2013.[1] Squamous cell carcinoma is the most common subtype of primary vaginal carcinoma; however, metastatic disease is more common in the vagina than primary vaginal carcinoma.

Paucity of data in reported literature has made it difficult to recommend generally accepted indications for use of PET/CT in vaginal cancer. Lamoreaux and colleagues[47] reported that the use of PET/CT detected 100% of the primary tumors and twice as many abnormal lymph nodes compared with conventional CT imaging. PET/CT can also be helpful in cases in which recurrence is suspected but other imaging modalities are equivocal.

PRIMARY FALLOPIAN TUBE CANCER

Primary fallopian tube cancer (PFTC) is a rare malignancy of the gynecologic tract. Many cases of PFTC are misdiagnosed as ovarian carcinoma. It accounts for less than 1% of gynecologic malignancies. Risk factors include the hereditary breast and ovarian cancer syndromes and BRCA1.

PET/CT may have a role in detection of metastatic disease and in monitoring treatment. PET/CT may be also useful in diagnosis of fallopian tube carcinoma in metastatic tumors of unknown primary; uptake in the fallopian tube may indicate the primary tumor (Fig. 16). Makhija and colleagues,[48] in their series of 8 patients with ovarian and fallopian tube cancer, showed that PET/CT showed disease in 2 patients with normal CT and increased CA-125. Patel and colleagues[49] also found that PET/CT helped to localize disease in the 2 patients in their study with fallopian tube cancer that was not detectable by CT. PET/CT can also

---

Fallopian tube cancer: pearls and pitfalls

Pearls

- Similar to ovarian cancer, and some cases of presumed ovarian cancer in patients with BRCA may represent fallopian tube malignancy
- PET/CT is useful to localize primary tumor, to distinguish fallopian tube origin from ovarian origin

Pitfalls

- Physiologic uptake may be seen in the fallopian tubes

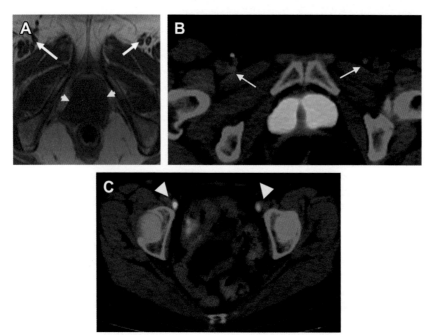

Fig. 15. (A) Axial T1-weighted MR imaging in a 62-year-old woman with history of squamous cell carcinoma of the vulva status post resection and bilateral lymph node dissection in 2005. In 2008, the patient returned with recurrent pelvic tumor (*arrowheads*). The superficial inguinal nodes (*arrows*) appear normal and the initial plan was to irradiate the pelvis and groin to 45 Gy up to L5/S1 and boost to the groin of 50 Gy. (B, C) Axial fused PET/CT shows increased FDG avidity of the superficial inguinal nodes (B, *arrows*) and deep inguinal nodes (C, *arrowheads*). Radiation treatment plan was revised to raise the superior border of the radiation field to L4 to L5 and to increase the dose of the groin boost to 66 Gy to include these FDG-avid deep inguinal lymph nodes.

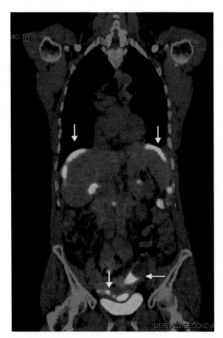

Fig. 16. Coronal fused PET/CT in a 57-year-old woman with bilateral pleural thickening. The patient was initially thought to have mesothelioma. Whole-body PET/CT coronal view shows diffuse FDG-avid disease with bilateral pleural thickening, pelvic implants, and an FDG-avid left adnexal mass and peritoneal carcinomatosis (*arrows*). Pathology was consistent with high-grade serous carcinoma from the fallopian tube.

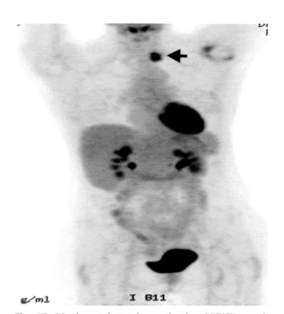

Fig. 17. Maximum intensity projection PET/CT scan in a 51-year-old woman diagnosed with fallopian tube cancer surgically resected 14 years before the study shows no evidence of disease in the pelvis, but there is FDG-avid left supraclavicular lymph node (*arrow*) consistent with metastatic disease.

identify metastatic disease outside the pelvis in cases of suspected recurrence (**Fig. 17**). Presence of a secondary malignancy may be encountered.

Physiologic uptake has been seen in the fallopian tubes on PET/CT. Yun and colleagues[50] found that this occurred in patients of reproductive age in mid–menstrual cycle. The fallopian tubes undergo cyclic changes with ovarian hormones. These changes can be distinguished from ovarian activity by correlation with accompanying noncontrast CT; the fallopian tube activity is typically cylindrical and bilateral.

SUMMARY

PET/CT has been shown to be useful in the management of gynecologic malignancy and is gaining widespread acceptance and roles in standard treatment algorithms, particularly in cervical carcinoma and ovarian carcinoma. The combination of anatomic and functional imaging has improved sensitivity and specificity compared with conventional cross-sectional imaging modalities, although the specificity is often limited by factors such as the size of the lesions and the presence of physiologic visceral uptake, which can mimic malignancy. The particular strengths of PET/CT are the ability to detect disease when conventional imaging modalities fail in suspected recurrences, to scan the whole body, to evaluate treatment response, to use for radiotherapy and surgical treatment planning, and to provide prognostic information. The role of PET/CT in other gynecologic malignancies, including endometrial cancer, cancers of the vagina and vulva, and cancers of the fallopian duct, are yet to be defined adequately.

REFERENCES

1. American Cancer Society. Cancer facts & figures 2013. Atlanta (GA): American Cancer Society; 2013.
2. Koh WJ, Greer BE, Abu-Rustum NR, et al. Cervical Cancer. J Natl Compr Canc Netw 2013;11:320–43.
3. Gaffney DK, Erickson-Wittmann BA, Jhingran A, et al. ACR Appropriateness Criteria® on Advanced Cervical Cancer Expert Panel on Radiation Oncology-Gynecology. Int J Radiat Oncol Biol Phys 2011;81:609–14.
4. Siegel CL, Andreotti RF, Cardenes HR, et al. ACR Appropriateness Criteria® pretreatment planning of invasive cancer of the cervix. J Am Coll Radiol 2012;9:395–402.
5. Kidd EA, Siegel BA, Dehdashti F, et al. The standardized uptake value for F-18 fluorodeoxyglucose is a sensitive predictive biomarker for cervical cancer treatment response and survival. Cancer 2007; 110:1738–44.
6. Yen TC, Lai CH, Ma SY, et al. Comparative benefits and limitations of 18F-FDG PET and CT-MRI in documented or suspected recurrent cervical cancer. Eur J Nucl Med Mol Imaging 2006;33:1399–407.
7. Chung HH, Jo H, Kang WJ, et al. Clinical impact of integrated PET/CT on the management of suspected cervical cancer recurrence. Gynecol Oncol 2007;104:529–34.
8. Tran BN, Grigsby PW, Dehdashti F, et al. Occult supraclavicular lymph node metastasis identified by FDG-PET in patients with carcinoma of the uterine cervix. Gynecol Oncol 2003;90:572–6.
9. Bader AA, Winter R, Haas J, et al. Where to look for the sentinel lymph node in cervical cancer. Am J Obstet Gynecol 2007;197:678.e1–7.
10. Havrilesky LJ, Kulasingam SL, Matchar DB, et al. FDG-PET for management of cervical and ovarian cancer. Gynecol Oncol 2005;97:183–91.
11. Sironi S, Buda A, Picchio M, et al. Lymph node metastasis in patients with clinical early-stage cervical cancer: detection with integrated FDG PET/CT. Radiology 2006;238:272–9.
12. Wright JD, Dehdashti F, Herzog TJ, et al. Preoperative lymph node staging of early-stage cervical carcinoma by [18F]-fluoro-2-deoxy-D-glucose-positron emission tomography. Cancer 2005;104:2484–91.
13. Zand B, Euscher ED, Soliman PT, et al. Rate of para-aortic lymph node micrometastasis in patients with locally advanced cervical cancer. Gynecol Oncol 2010;119:422–5.
14. Grigsby PW, Siegel BA, Dehdashti F. Lymph node staging by positron emission tomography in patients with carcinoma of the cervix. J Clin Oncol 2001;19:3745–9.
15. Singh AK, Grigsby PW, Dehdashti F, et al. FDG-PET lymph node staging and survival of patients with FIGO stage IIIb cervical carcinoma. Int J Radiat Oncol Biol Phys 2003;56:489–93.
16. Schwarz JK, Siegel BA, Dehdashti F, et al. Association of posttherapy positron emission tomography with tumor response and survival in cervical carcinoma. JAMA 2007;298:2289–95.
17. Birlik M, Akar S, Tuzel E, et al. Gemcitabine-induced vasculitis in advanced transitional cell carcinoma of the bladder. J Cancer Res Clin Oncol 2004;130:122–5.
18. Howlader N, Noone AM, Krapcho M, et al. SEER Cancer Statistics Review, 1975–2008. Bethesda (MD): National Cancer Institute; 2011.
19. Harries M, Gore M. Part I: chemotherapy for epithelial ovarian cancer-treatment at first diagnosis. Lancet Oncol 2002;3:529–36.
20. Armstrong DK, Bundy B, Wenzel L, et al. Intraperitoneal cisplatin and paclitaxel in ovarian cancer. N Engl J Med 2006;354:34–43.
21. Sugarbaker PH. Cytoreductive surgery and perioperative intraperitoneal chemotherapy for the treatment

of advanced primary and recurrent ovarian cancer. Curr Opin Obstet Gynecol 2009;21:15–24.

22. Podoloff DA, Ball DW, Ben-Josef E, et al. NCCN task force: clinical utility of PET in a variety of tumor types. J Natl Compr Canc Netw 2009;7(Suppl 2):S1–26.

23. Morgan RJ Jr, Alvarez RD, Armstrong DK, et al. NCCN clinical practice guidelines in oncology: epithelial ovarian cancer. J Natl Compr Canc Netw 2011;9:82–113.

24. Javitt MC. ACR Appropriateness Criteria on staging and follow-up of ovarian cancer. J Am Coll Radiol 2007;4:586–9.

25. Kitajima K, Suzuki K, Senda M, et al. FDG-PET/CT for diagnosis of primary ovarian cancer. Nucl Med Commun 2011;32:549–53.

26. Hubner KF, McDonald TW, Niethammer JG, et al. Assessment of primary and metastatic ovarian cancer by positron emission tomography (PET) using 2-[18F]deoxyglucose (2-[18F]FDG). Gynecol Oncol 1993;51:197–204.

27. Rieber A, Nussle K, Stohr I, et al. Preoperative diagnosis of ovarian tumors with MR imaging: comparison with transvaginal sonography, positron emission tomography, and histologic findings. AJR Am J Roentgenol 2001;177:123–9.

28. Risum S, Hogdall C, Loft A, et al. The diagnostic value of PET/CT for primary ovarian cancer–a prospective study. Gynecol Oncol 2007;105:145–9.

29. Kurokawa T, Yoshida Y, Kawahara K, et al. Expression of GLUT-1 glucose transfer, cellular proliferation activity and grade of tumor correlate with [F-18]-fluorodeoxyglucose uptake by positron emission tomography in epithelial tumors of the ovary. Int J Cancer 2004;109:926–32.

30. Fenchel S, Grab D, Nuessle K, et al. Asymptomatic adnexal masses: correlation of FDG PET and histopathologic findings. Radiology 2002;223:780–8.

31. Simcock B, Neesham D, Quinn M, et al. The impact of PET/CT in the management of recurrent ovarian cancer. Gynecol Oncol 2006;103:271–6.

32. Chung HH, Kang WJ, Kim JW, et al. Role of [18F]FDG PET/CT in the assessment of suspected recurrent ovarian cancer: correlation with clinical or histological findings. Eur J Nucl Med Mol Imaging 2007;34:480–6.

33. Mangili G, Picchio M, Sironi S, et al. Integrated PET/CT as a first-line re-staging modality in patients with suspected recurrence of ovarian cancer. Eur J Nucl Med Mol Imaging 2007;34:658–66.

34. Thrall MM, DeLoia JA, Gallion H, et al. Clinical use of combined positron emission tomography and computed tomography (FDG-PET/CT) in recurrent ovarian cancer. Gynecol Oncol 2007;105:17–22.

35. Salani R, Backes FJ, Fung MF, et al. Posttreatment surveillance and diagnosis of recurrence in women with gynecologic malignancies: Society of Gynecologic Oncologists recommendations. Am J Obstet Gynecol 2011;204:466–78.

36. Bhosale P, Peungjesada S, Wei W, et al. Clinical utility of positron emission tomography/computed tomography in the evaluation of suspected recurrent ovarian cancer in the setting of normal CA-125 levels. Int J Gynecol Cancer 2010;20:936–44.

37. Gu P, Pan LL, Wu SQ, et al. CA 125, PET alone, PET-CT, CT and MRI in diagnosing recurrent ovarian carcinoma: a systematic review and meta-analysis. Eur J Radiol 2009;71:164–74.

38. Hillner BE, Siegel BA, Shields AF, et al. Relationship between cancer type and impact of PET and PET/CT on intended management: findings of the national oncologic PET registry. J Nucl Med 2008;49:1928–35.

39. Lee JH, Dubinsky T, Andreotti RF, et al. ACR Appropriateness Criteria® pretreatment evaluation and follow-up of endometrial cancer of the uterus. Ultrasound Q 2011;27:139–45.

40. Kitajima K, Murakami K, Yamasaki E, et al. Accuracy of 18F-FDG PET/CT in detecting pelvic and paraaortic lymph node metastasis in patients with endometrial cancer. AJR Am J Roentgenol 2008;190:1652–8.

41. Picchio M, Mangili G, Samanes Gajate AM, et al. High-grade endometrial cancer: value of [(18)F]FDG PET/CT in preoperative staging. Nucl Med Commun 2010;31:506–12.

42. Kitajima K, Murakami K, Kaji Y, et al. Spectrum of FDG PET/CT findings of uterine tumors. AJR Am J Roentgenol 2010;195:737–43.

43. Kitajima K, Murakami K, Yamasaki E, et al. Performance of FDG-PET/CT in the diagnosis of recurrent endometrial cancer. Ann Nucl Med 2008;22:103–9.

44. Belhocine T, De Barsy C, Hustinx R, et al. Usefulness of (18)F-FDG PET in the post-therapy surveillance of endometrial carcinoma. Eur J Nucl Med Mol Imaging 2002;29:1132–9.

45. Lin LL, Grigsby PW, Powell MA, et al. Definitive radiotherapy in the management of isolated vaginal recurrences of endometrial cancer. Int J Radiat Oncol Biol Phys 2005;63:500–4.

46. Cohn DE, Dehdashti F, Gibb RK, et al. Prospective evaluation of positron emission tomography for the detection of groin node metastases from vulvar cancer. Gynecol Oncol 2002;85:179–84.

47. Lamoreaux WT, Grigsby PW, Dehdashti F, et al. FDG-PET evaluation of vaginal carcinoma. Int J Radiat Oncol Biol Phys 2005;62:733–7.

48. Makhija S, Howden N, Edwards R, et al. Positron emission tomography/computed tomography imaging for the detection of recurrent ovarian and fallopian tube carcinoma: a retrospective review. Gynecol Oncol 2002;85:53–8.

49. Patel PV, Cohade C, Chin BB. PET-CT localizes previously undetectable metastatic lesions in recurrent fallopian tube carcinoma. Gynecol Oncol 2002;87:323–6.

50. Yun M, Cho A, Lee JH, et al. Physiologic 18F-FDG uptake in the fallopian tubes at mid cycle on PET/CT. J Nucl Med 2010;51:682–5.

Magnetic Resonance Imaging of Pelvic Floor Dysfunction

Neeraj Lalwani, MD[a],*, Mariam Moshiri, MD[b], Jean H. Lee, MD[b],
Puneet Bhargava, MD[c], Manjiri K. Dighe, MD[b]

KEYWORDS

- Pelvic floor dysfunction • MR defecography • Cystocele • Rectocele • Incontinence • Constipation
- Anismus • Descending perineal syndrome

KEY POINTS

- Pelvic floor dysfunction affects roughly 50% of women older than 50 years and can present with nonspecific symptoms, such as urinary or fecal incontinence or chronic constipation, pelvic pain, and organ prolapse.
- A wide array of functional or morphologic pelvic disorders can be responsible for these symptoms, and a precise diagnosis is obligatory before any surgical decision is undertaken.
- Preoperative assessment of pelvic floor dysfunction with dynamic or functional magnetic resonance imaging can change the initial surgical planning in 67% of patients and thus is emerging as one of the most useful tools in complicated cases of pelvic floor dysfunction.

INTRODUCTION

Pelvic floor weakness affects roughly 50% of women older than 50 years.[1] About 10% to 20% of multiparous women seek medical care in gastrointestinal clinics for some sort of evacuation disorder.[2] Almost 11% of these women undergo surgeries, and 30% of these patients may need repeat surgery.[3]

The pelvic floor is a complex anatomic and functional entity that is composed of multiple muscular and fascial sheets. The pelvic floor supports 3 vital anatomic compartments: anterior or urinary (bladder or urethra), middle or genital (vagina, cervix, and uterus), and posterior or anorectal (rectum and anus). Pelvic floor dysfunction can involve any of these compartments and lead to respective symptoms, such as urinary or fecal incontinence or chronic constipation, pelvic pain, and organ prolapse. The underlying functional or morphologic disorders responsible for these symptoms can be cystoceles, urethroceles, urethral hypermobility, rectoceles, rectal prolapse or intussusception, pelvic organ prolapse, abnormal pelvic floor relaxation, enteroceles, peritoneoceles, and dyssynergistic defecation.

Pelvic floor dysfunction is primarily a problem for multiparous and postmenopausal women. However, it may also affect premenopausal women and men in smaller proportions. Multiple vaginal deliveries, prior pelvic surgeries, advancing age, low estrogen levels, connective tissue disorders, smoking, chronic obstructive pulmonary disease, increased body mass index, and excessive Valsalva have been implicated in the pathogenesis of pelvic floor dysfunction. Multiple factors, taken together, contribute to the stretching and widening of the levator ani muscle and subsequent tearing

Disclosures: None.
[a] Department of Radiology, University of Washington, Box 359728, 325 9th Avenue, Seattle, WA 98104-2499, USA; [b] Department of Radiology, University of Washington, 1959 Northeast Pacific Street, Box 357115, Seattle, WA 98195, USA; [c] Department of Radiology, VA Puget Sound Health Care System, Mail Box 358280, S-114/ Radiology, 1660 South Columbian Way, Seattle, WA 98108, USA
* Corresponding author.
E-mail address: neerajl@uw.edu

Radiol Clin N Am 51 (2013) 1127–1139
http://dx.doi.org/10.1016/j.rcl.2013.07.004
0033-8389/13/$ – see front matter © 2013 Elsevier Inc. All rights reserved.

of the supportive fascia. These events lead to pelvic floor dysfunction and descent, which initiates a vicious cycle. Pelvic floor descent of merely 1.35 cm is sufficient to cause stretching of the pudendal nerve by 15%, which is enough to initiate nerve demyelination. Pudendal mononeuropathy caused by such mechanical demyelination is often responsible for organ prolapse.[3] The organ prolapse further worsens the condition and leads to more pelvic floor dysfunction and injury to the muscles and fascia.

Classic physical examination and various clinical staging systems have been used for the assessment of pelvic floor dysfunction. One of the most widely accepted clinical staging systems is Pelvic Organ Prolapse Quantification (POP-Q), proposed by the International Continence Society. However, none of these staging systems or clinical assessments involves a direct assessment of the anatomy. Clinical assessment either underestimates the extent of the dysfunction or misdiagnoses the site of the prolapse (in 45%–90% of cases), and is also less useful for surgical triage and planning.[4] Therefore, other functional investigations, like video urodynamic imaging, evacuation proctography, and dynamic cystoproctography are currently used to evaluate the dynamics of the pelvic floor.

With the recent advent and advances in magnetic resonance (MR) imaging, functional or dynamic MR imaging is emerging as a useful and popular tool for the preoperative planning of patients with pelvic floor dysfunction. MR imaging has been shown to change the initial surgical plan in 67% of patients.[5] Many institutes thus routinely perform dynamic or functional MR imaging to assess pelvic floor dysfunction.

PELVIC FLOOR ANATOMY

The pelvic floor is composed of 3 horizontal layers. Most cranial is the fascia layer, next is the major muscular (or levator ani) layer, and most caudal is the urogenital diaphragm (**Fig. 1**).

The fascia layer of the pelvic floor consists of several ligaments (pubovesicle, uterosacral, and cardinal) and thin layers that cover the parauterine and paravaginal regions. These so-called ligaments are thickened fascia layers or peritoneal reflections that attach the pelvic structures to the pelvic side wall or to the underlying levator ani to provide stability. This layer is mainly responsible for the support of the anterior (urinary bladder and urethra) and the middle (uterus, cervix, and vagina) compartments.

The second layer is composed of the levator ani muscle, which has 3 components: pubococcygeal,

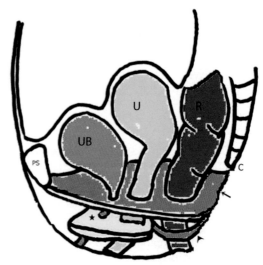

Fig. 1. Anatomy of pelvic floor; the concept of 3 compartments. The anterior compartment is composed of the urinary bladder (UB) and urethra, which is supported by the levator ani muscle (*arrow*) and urogenital diaphragm (*asterisk*). The middle compartment encompasses the vagina, cervix, and uterus (U), whereas the posterior compartment includes the anorectum (R). Both the middle and posterior compartments are mainly supported by the levator ani and fascial ligaments. Arrowhead, puborectalis; C, coccyx; PS, pubic symphysis.

ischiococcygeal, and puborectalis sling. This muscular layer is the major component of the pelvic floor, responsible for providing most of the support for all three compartments. Posterior interlaced fibers of pubococcygeal and puborectalis components of the levator ani muscle are called the levator plate.

The most caudal or inferior layer of the pelvic floor is composed of the urogenital diaphragm, which consists of the transverse perineal muscle, and mainly supports the anterior (urinary bladder and urethra) compartment.

MR IMAGING AND ITS PROTOCOL

Dynamic or functional MR imaging, used to assess pelvic floor dysfunction, should not be confused with functional imaging for metabolic activity (diffusion weighted) or postcontrast T1-weighted (T1W) dynamic inversion recovery sequences. This imaging evaluates the functionality of the pelvic floor and pelvic organs while defecating, hence it is called dynamic or functional MR imaging. It is important to perform a dynamic study because certain abnormalities are revealed only during defecation; for example, rectal prolapse or intussusception.[6]

The imaging is performed using a fast T2-weighted (T2W) sequences (HASTE [Half-Fourier Acquisition Single-Shot Turbo Spin-Echo], single-shot fast field echo), or balanced steady state free precession. The urinary bladder has a natural T2W contrast caused by the presence of urine and is thus highlighted. However, to highlight the rectum and vagina, a contrast medium with high water content is needed that can stay inside the lumen without leaking and does not irritate the mucosa. The literature has mainly described the use of either potato starch or ultrasound gel. However, ultrasound gel has gained practical popularity because of its easy availability, inert nature, high water content, semisolid consistency, and acceptable tolerance among patients. However, short episodes of diarrhea have been reported after ultrasound gel instillation in the rectum, likely caused by mucosal irritation in some patients.[3]

Patient Preparation and Positioning

No rectal preparation is required. The patient may be asked to void the urine at least 30 minutes before the examination. Presence of excessive urine can undermine the precise assessment of the pelvic floor descent and dysfunction. As an alternative, the study can be divided into a cystographic phase, with a filled bladder, and a defecographic phase, with an empty bladder.

Most patients are nervous, apprehensive, or intimidated and may feel awkward about the examination. A lucid preprocedure explanation can play a crucial role in relieving that apprehension and patient concerns. A clear understanding of the instructions given during the study is also important. The imaging is performed at rest, then during squeezing or straining, and then during defecation. The patient should know what these commands mean. For example, squeezing can be better explained as a Kegel exercise.

Approximately 200 mL (120–300 mL) of gel is instilled in the rectum and about 30 to 50 mL instilled in the vagina (**Fig. 2**). The installation can be performed by endocavitary placement of a 30-Fr Foley catheter, which can be performed on the MR table in the lateral decubitus position. The patient is covered with good-quality diapers and pads to avoid leakage, which can lead to electrical hazards or damage to the instrument.[3]

The examination can be performed in a supine position on a closed-configuration magnet or in a sitting position on an open-configuration magnet. In theory, the sitting position seems more physiologic and should be preferred. However, generally both positions are equally effective in diagnosing

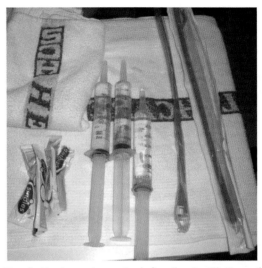

Fig. 2. Equipment required for the instillation of ultrasound gel for MR defecography. Ultrasound gel (*left*), 60-mL syringes filled with ultrasound gel (*middle*), and Foley catheter (*right*). About 180 to 200 mL of ultrasound gel are instilled in the rectum and 30 to 50 mL instilled in the vagina to better delineate the pelvic anatomy using a 30-Fr Foley catheter.

the clinically relevant abnormalities of the pelvic floor.[7] Moreover, open-configuration magnets are not widely available.

A pelvic phased array coil is used for signal transmission and reception, or a cardiac coil can be used, which may provide better resolution (**Fig. 3**).

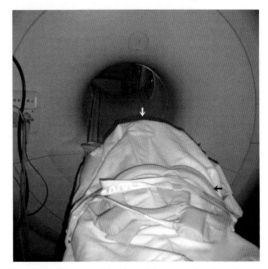

Fig. 3. Patient positioning. The examination is performed with the patient in a supine position with feet first (*white arrow*) on a closed-configuration magnet. A pelvic phased array or cardiac coil is used for signal transmission and reception (*black arrow*). The cardiac coil provides better resolution.

MR Protocol

Pelvic floor imaging is divided into static and dynamic components. The static component includes routine pelvic imaging with T1W and T2W turbo spin echo sequences in 2 or 3 orientations. The static imaging may depict incidental pelvic disorders and provide a morphologic assessment of the pelvis (**Fig. 4**A–C).

The dynamic component includes an ultrafast T2W midsagittal sequence repeated (15–25 times) at the same slice position while the patient is asked to follow the sequential commands of squeezing, straining, and defecation.

Balanced steady state free precession (bSSFP) sequences (TrueFISP [Siemens], FIESTA [GE], and bFFE [Philips]) provide both contrast and speed and are widely used in most institutions. It has been shown that the bSSFP sequence provides a better detection of organ prolapses in all three compartments compared with other sequences like HASTE.[8] The detailed MR protocol is described in **Table 1**.

IMAGING FINDINGS AND IMAGE ANALYSIS

The interpretation of MR imaging is comparable with conventional fluoroscopic study and the visual impression of organ movements remains decisive in most cases. However, certain techniques and aids have been developed to quantify the extent of these observed findings and suspected disorders.

The three compartments of the pelvic floor model remain the mainstay of image analysis.[9]

A quantitative analysis of the disorder is performed by the use of reference lines. However, no general consensus exists about what to measure and how to measure. The most commonly used reference line is the pubococcygeal line (PCL), which is drawn from the inferior border of the symphysis pubis to the last (or second-last)

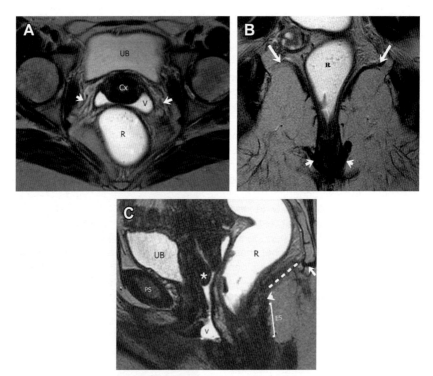

Fig. 4. Static T2W spin echo images. (*A*) Axial images evaluate pelvic anatomy and muscular defects, such as thinning and tears in the muscles. The cardinal or major ligament of the uterus is localized by the presence of uterine vessels (*arrows*). Cx, cervix; R, rectum; V, vagina. (*B*) Coronal images evaluate the levator ani muscle. The ischiococcygeal component of the levator ani shows cephalic convexity on coronal images (*long arrows*). Short arrows, external anal sphincters; R, rectum. (*C*) Sagittal images best delineate the relative position of the UB, cervix (*asterisk*), vagina (V), and rectum (R) at rest. The position of the pelvic organs is determined relative to a line drawn from the PS to the last visible coccygeal joint (*arrow*), which is called the pubococcygeal line (PCL). Posterior interlaced fibers of pubococcygeal and puborectalis components of the levator ani muscle are called the levator plate (*dotted line*). An angle between the levator plate and the PCL that exceeds 10° is an indicator of a loss of pelvic floor support. ES, external anal sphincter. Arrowhead delineates anorectal junction.

Table 1		
Proposed protocol for functional MR imaging to evaluate pelvic floor disorders		
	At Rest	Dynamic Imaging
Sequence	T2W TSE	bSSFP (TrueFISP, bFFE, FIESTA)
Plane	Axial, coronal, sagittal	Midsagittal; single slice repeated 15–25 times at the same slice position
Maneuver	None	Kegel, strain, and defecation[a]
Slice thickness (mm)	4	8
TR (ms)	4230–6940	3.73–4.3
TE (ms)	112	1.87–2.15
Matrix	512 × 205 or 512 × 154	256 × 123 or 128
FOV	275	350–380

Abbreviations: bFFE, balanced fast field echo; FOV, field of view; TE, echo time; TR, recovery time; TSE, turbo spin echo.

[a] Between 180 and 210 mL of ultrasound gel is instilled in the rectal lumen and 30 to 50 mL in the vaginal lumen.

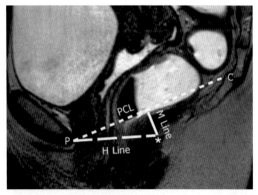

Fig. 5. Useful reference lines. The most widely used reference line is the PCL, which is drawn from the inferior border of the symphysis pubis (P) to the last visible (last or second last) coccygeal joint (C). The anteroposterior diameter of the urogenital or levator hiatus is demarcated by the H line, which is drawn from the inferior border of the pubic symphysis to the posterior wall of the rectum at the level of the anorectal junction (ARJ; *asterisk*). A vertical line drawn at a right angle from the PCL to the most posterior aspect of the H line is called an M Line, which indicates the vertical descent of the levator hiatus.

visible coccygeal joint.[10] The PCL is reproducible, is not influenced by pelvic tilt, and includes the 2 important bony attachments of the pelvic floor (symphysis and coccyx) (Fig. 5).

In addition, the anteroposterior diameter of the urogenital or levator hiatus is demarcated by the H line, which is drawn from the inferior border of the pubic symphysis to the posterior wall of the rectum at the level of the anorectal junction (ARJ; see Fig. 5). The ARJ corresponds with the posterior impression of the transition between the puborectalis and the levator plate.[10] The H line should not exceed 6 cm in normal individuals.[11] The enlargement of the urogenital hiatus can be graded as mild (6–8 cm), moderate (8–10 cm), or severe (>10 cm).[11]

A vertical line drawn at a right angle from the PCL to the most posterior aspect of the H line is called an M Line and signifies the vertical descent of the levator hiatus (see Fig. 5).[10] The M line should not exceed 2 cm in normal individuals.[11] The pelvic floor descent can be graded as mild (2–4 cm), moderate (4–6 cm), or severe (>6 cm).[11]

The HMO (H line, M line, and organ prolapse) classification scheme can be used to quantitate the extent of pelvic organ prolapse and pelvic floor relaxation (Table 2).[12,13]

In addition to these three vital lines, an angle between the central long axis of the anal canal and the posterior border of the rectum is also measured and is called the anorectal angle (ARA; Fig. 6). The ARA measures 94° to 114° at rest.[14,15] However, some authorities have mentioned that normal ARAs can range between 108° and 127°.[10] During squeezing, the pelvic floor elevates and the ARA decreases; whereas during defecation the pelvic floor descends and the ARA increases. The ARA varies by about 15° to 20° between rest and squeezing or rest and defecation.[16,17] There has major debate on the factual relevance and accurate role of the ARA in the assessment of pelvic floor dysfunction, and some authorities do not use ARA for the assessment.

An angle between the levator plate and the PCL that exceeds 10° should be taken as an indicator of a loss of pelvic floor support (see Fig. 4C).[18]

Table 2			
HMO classification: diagnostic criteria			
	Small/ Mild	Moderate	Large/ Severe
H line (cm)	6–8	8–10	>10
M line (cm)	2–4	4–6	>6
Organ descent (rule of 3) (cm)	<3	3–6	>6

H line represents the diameter of levator or urogenital hiatus. M line represents the pelvic floor descent.

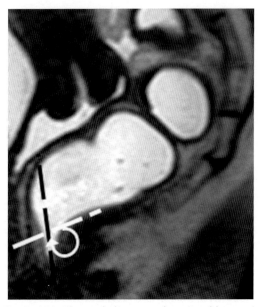

Fig. 6. ARA. The angle between the central long axis of the anal canal (*black dotted line*) and the posterior border of the rectum (*white dotted line*). The ARA measures between 94° and 114° at rest and varies about 15° to 20° between rest and squeezing or rest and defecation.

On the axial images, the vagina shows a typical H shape, which signifies intact paravaginal fascial support. Moreover, the symmetry or thinning of the levator ani can be better assessed on axial or coronal images.[3]

SPECTRUM OF THE PATHOLOGIC FINDINGS AND DIAGNOSTIC CRITERIA

In order to establish the diagnosis of organ descent, the following reference structures from each compartment are assigned together with the reference lines: (1) Anterior compartment: bladder base or most caudal part of the dorsal wall. (2) Middle compartment: posterior cervix or the posterior fornix of the vagina. (3) Posterior compartment: ARJ. The distances from the PCL to the bladder neck, cervix, and ARJ are measured at rest and during defecation and the organ descent is assessed. Most investigators have proposed a grading system of organ prolapse using either 2-cm or 3-cm steps.[7,10,13,19]

ANTERIOR COMPARTMENT DISORDERS
Cystocele

Cystoceles are the most common disorder of the anterior compartment. A cystocele is defined as bulging of the posterior bladder wall or bladder neck below the PCL line (>1 cm) into the anterior

vaginal wall, which signifies a stretched or torn pubocervical fascia (**Fig. 7**). Cystoceles can be graded as small (<3 cm), moderate (3–6 cm), or large (>6 cm).[9]

A bulging bladder base partially occupies the levator (urogenital) hiatus, and as a consequence the H line is elongated (>6 cm). However, a cystocele within the urogenital hiatus could block the prolapse of other pelvic structures (especially the middle compartment) and mask an underlying enterocele, peritoneocele, or rectocele. Repeat imaging with the bladder empty is necessary to reveal disorders that might otherwise be missed.

In addition, a cystocele can displace the uterus and the ARJ posteroinferiorly, causing stretching of the M line (>2 cm).

Recurrent cystocele after retropubic and vaginal operations is confidently diagnosed via functional MR imaging. In this subset of patients, the bladder neck and proximal urethra maintain their normal position above the PCL, but the posterior wall bulges into the anterior vaginal wall.

Urethral Hypermobility

Urethral hypermobility can be an associated finding of cystocele. With increased intra-abdominal pressure, the urethra may rotate horizontally, signifying a loss of intrinsic urethral support and integrity (**Fig. 8**A, B). This finding can be clinically crucial because it needs a pubovaginal sling procedure for repair, whereas retropubic urethropexy is the procedure of choice for uncomplicated stress incontinence.[10]

Kinking of the Urethra-Vesical Junction

Prolapse of the bladder base could also be responsible for kinking of the urethra-vesical junction. This kinking might be a potential cause

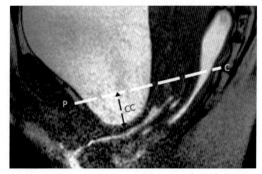

Fig. 7. Cystocele (CC) is the bulging of the posterior bladder wall or bladder neck more than 1 cm below the PCL line. C, last visible coccygeal joint; P, pubic symphysis.

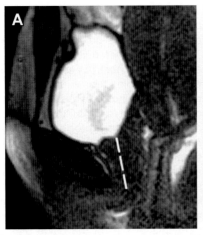

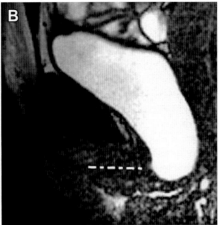

Fig. 8. Urethral hypermobility can be associated with cystocele. (*A*) At rest, the urethra (*dotted line*) is almost vertical. (*B*) With increased intra-abdominal pressure, the urethra (*dotted line*) rotates horizontally.

of urinary retention and can lead to urinary stasis and infection.[10]

MIDDLE COMPARTMENT DISORDERS
Uterovaginal Prolapse

Uterovaginal prolapse is often diagnosed on clinical examination. By definition, movement of the cervix or posterior fornix below the PCL is consistent with uterovaginal prolapse (**Fig. 9A**). The amount of rectal filling can significantly alter the uterovaginal prolapse and is best manifested when the rectum has been emptied. Prolapse can be graded as mild (<3 cm), moderate (3–6 cm), or large (>6 cm).[10] In a case of complete uterine prolapse, the uterus is seen bulging out of the external genitalia, and vaginal walls are everted.

Presence of uterovaginal prolapse signifies injury to the uterosacral ligament, pubocervical fascia, and the rectovaginal fascia. On axial static images, there can be loss of the normal H configuration of the vagina because of the loss of the lateral support provided by the paravaginal fascia (see **Fig. 9B**). On coronal images, the iliococcygeus component of the levator ani can appear as either flat or concave.[3]

Peritoneocele, Enterocele, and Sigmoidocele

Disrupted rectovaginal fascia associated with uteropelvic prolapse can lead to a widening of the pouch of Douglas, yielding potential space for posterior herniation of peritoneal content. The prevalence of this herniation can range from 17% to 37%.[20,21] Women with a history of

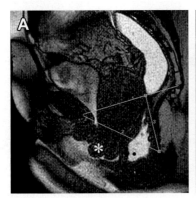

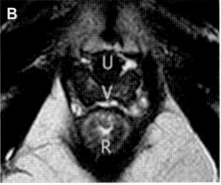

Fig. 9. Uterovaginal prolapse. (*A*) Movement of the cervix below the PCL (1) is consistent with uterovaginal prolapse. In this case the cervix is almost protruding out of the vaginal introitus (*asterisk*). A small anterior rectocele (*black circle*) is also seen. There is a significantly exaggerated M line (3), which indicates severe pelvic descent. Coexisting exaggerated H line (2) signifies enlarged levator hiatus. (*B*) Axial image at the level of the puborectalis sling (or surgical ARJ). The vagina (V) shows a typical H shape, which indicates intact parametrial fascial support.

hysterectomy are predisposed to develop such herniations.[22]

Peritoneocele is the herniation of peritoneal fat without bowel loops, enterocele is herniation of small bowel loops, and sigmoidocele is herniation of the sigmoid colon through the pouch of Douglas below the PCL (**Fig. 10**). They are graded as mild (<3 cm), moderate (3–6 cm), or large (>6 cm).[9,10]

Patients may present with varied symptoms, such as constipation (caused by compression of the anorectum and resulting in outlet obstruction), a feeling of incomplete evacuation, and repeated and unproductive straining or sensation of heaviness in the vagina. These entities are often missed or misdiagnosed in a clinical examination.

Functional MR imaging is most suitable for the diagnosis of these disorders and superior to conventional defecography.[23] MR can confidently diagnose the content of the herniation sac because of an inherent soft tissue contrast without having to fill the bowel lumen with a contrast agent.

These findings are typically picked up in the midsagittal plane at the end of defecation. However, sometimes these herniations are lateral or anterior, so additional dynamic images in the coronal plane can be diagnostic. Large enteroceles can also mask small rectoceles or cystoceles.[20,23]

POSTERIOR COMPARTMENT DISORDERS
Rectoceles

Rectoceles are defined as abnormal bulging of the rectal wall beyond the normal anticipated location, and they indicate inadequate support and laxity of the endopelvic or rectovaginal fascia. Rectoceles

are usually anterior but can be lateral or, rarely, posterior (also termed posterior perineal hernia) and caused by a defect on the levator plate.[24] They are best seen during defecation. Rectoceles do not always obstruct evacuation, but they can be responsible for a sense of incomplete emptying. Their clinical relevance is usually determined by size criteria, extent of retention of contrast, and a need for evacuation maneuvers. Anterior rectoceles measuring more than 2 cm should be considered as abnormal.[25]

Rectoceles are measured as the maximum sagittal depth of a bulge in the rectal wall, which is calculated by measuring the distance between a line drawn parallel to the anal canal and the most inferior part of the bulge (**Fig. 11**).[26] They are graded as small (<2 cm), moderate (2–4 cm), or large (>4 cm).[9] An increased risk of developing rectoceles is associated with a history of vaginal deliveries, hysterectomy, constipation, chronically increased intra-abdominal pressure, and aging.

Rectal Intussusception and Prolapse

Rectal invagination or intussusception can involve mucosa or a full-thickness (mucosa and muscular)

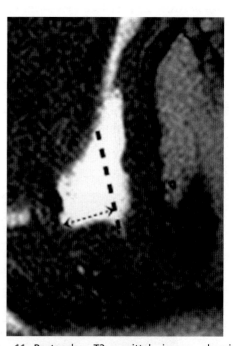

Fig. 11. Rectocele. T2 sagittal image showing abnormal bulging of the rectal wall beyond the normal anticipated location, which is consistent with rectocele. Rectocele is measured as the maximum sagittal depth of a bulge in the rectal wall, which is a distance between a line drawn parallel to the anal canal (*dotted line*) and the most inferior part of the bulge (*dotted double-headed arrow*).

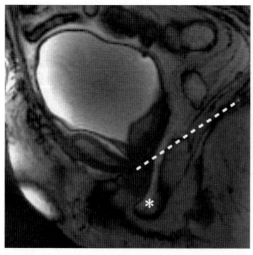

Fig. 10. Peritoneocele. Herniation of peritoneal fat without bowel loops below pubococcygeal line (*dotted line*), which is consistent with peritoneocele (*asterisk*).

wall. It can be located circumferential, anteriorly, or posteriorly, and often is seen as circumferential or focal thickening. Differentiation of mucosal and full-thickness intussusception is possible on functional MR imaging.[27] This differentiation can be of clinical relevance because the mucosal intussusception is treated with transanal excision, whereas full-thickness intussusception requires a rectopexy.[10,28,29]

Invagination could be rectorectal or rectoanal. Rectorectal invagination can be further classified as proximal, middle, or distal rectal. Noticeable internal rectal prolapse is often seen as a V-shaped rectal wall (double rectal wall) on the midsagittal plane (**Fig. 12**). Once the rectoanal prolapse projects outside the anal canal, it is called a rectal prolapse.[9]

Rectal intussusception is associated with coexisting anterior or middle compartment descent in 30% of cases.[27] Functional MR plays a crucial role in diagnosing them.

PELVIC FLOOR RELAXATION (DESCENDING PERINEAL SYNDROME)

Generalized descending of the pelvic floor below the PCL caused by loss of pelvic muscle tone at rest or during defecation is called descending perineal syndrome. This is sometimes confined to the posterior compartment[9] and can present as nonspecific perianal pain and constipation.

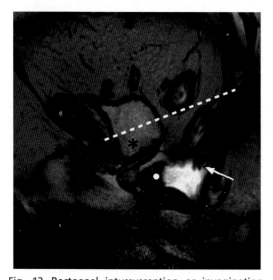

Fig. 12. Rectoanal intussusception or invagination. True full-thickness invagination is seen as a V-shaped rectal wall (double rectal wall) on the midsagittal plane (*arrow*). Once the rectoanal prolapse projects outside the anal canal, it is called a rectal prolapse. Coexisting rectocele (*circle*) and cystocele (*asterisk*) are also noted. Dotted line, PCL.

Incomplete evacuation leads to excessive straining and initiates a cycle of descent, pudendal nerve injury and denervation, and then fecal incontinence.

SPASTIC PELVIC FLOOR SYNDROME (DYSSYNERGIC DEFECATION)

Spastic pelvic floor syndrome is a functional outlet obstruction characterized by prolonged or no defecation that is associated with involuntary, inappropriate, and paradoxic contraction of the striated pelvic floor musculature (puborectalis or anal sphincters). It has also been described as nonrelaxing puborectalis syndrome and anismus.[30,31] However, to clarify that the anismus is not an abnormality of a single muscle, the novel term dyssynergistic defecation was coined, which suggests dyssynergia of the abdominal and pelvic floor muscles involved in defecation.[32]

The exact cause is still unclear, but it has been linked to prior pelvic surgeries, sexual abuse, anxiety, and psychological factors.[33]

The diagnostic findings on functional MR imaging can include a prominent impression of the puborectalis sling, narrow anal canal, upward bulge of the levator plate, failure to increase ARA, and a lack of descent of the pelvic floor.[3,34,35]

PEARLS, PITFALLS, AND VARIANTS

Functional MR (or MR defecography) is a powerful tool to use to evaluate pelvic floor disorders. However, there are certain pearls and pitfalls that can be helpful in performing an ideal or diagnostic study.

As stressed earlier, defecography should be performed with a partially distended bladder. If there is concern about anterior compartment disorders, a repeat study with an empty bladder can be performed to assess the posterior compartment. An overdistended bladder or cystocele may mask findings in the middle compartment, especially enterocele, peritoneocele or sigmoidocele, or underestimate uterovaginal descent (**Fig. 13**A, B).

In addition to midsagittal imaging, dynamic axial imaging at the level of the inferior border of the symphysis can be helpful in evaluating urogenital hiatus, its content, and the puborectalis sling. Moreover, any alteration in the signal intensity and caliber of the femoral vein in this dynamic sequence allows an estimation of the patient's straining effort. This technique can be helpful in differentiating true dyssynergistic defecation from inappropriate or feeble straining effort.

A stack of coronal images during straining may provide a detailed overview of the levator ani and enable a confident diagnosis of the lateral

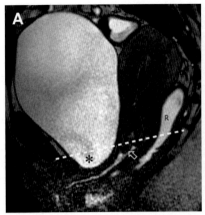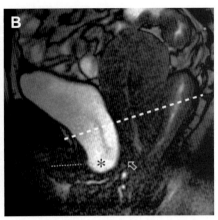

Fig. 13. Effect of an overdistended bladder. (*A*) An overdistended UB or cystocele (*asterisk*) may mask findings in the middle compartment. The cervix (*arrow*) shows a questionable descent below the PCL (*dotted line*). (*B*) Repeat imaging after voiding urine shows a moderate-sized cystocele (*asterisk*), urethral hypermobility (*thin dotted line*), and moderate cervical descent (*arrow*).

rectoceles and rectal intussusceptions. This technique can also differentiate the S-shaped rectal configuration, which can mimic intussusception on sagittal images.

Pelvic organ prolapse is sometimes apparent at a later stage of straining; therefore, it is recommended that the patient continue straining for at least 30 seconds even after the gel is expelled. Sometimes an additional postdefecation sequence may detect an otherwise unrevealed enterocele.

FLUOROSCOPIC VERSUS MR DEFECOGRAPHY

Fluoroscopic defecography has been conventionally used for years. However, introduction of MR defecography in recent years initiated a controversy about the advantages and relevance of MR defecography and its cost-effectiveness compared with the fluoroscopic technique. Studies have shown that functional MR imaging with rectal contrast either has statistically similar frequency of pelvic organ prolapse or is superior to its fluoroscopic counterpart, especially for picking up middle compartment disorders, rectoceles, or diagnosing the degree of bladder descent.[36–38] Disorders like peritoneocele cannot be diagnosed on fluoroscopic examination.

Contrary to the general belief that fluoroscopic examination should yield better results because it is performed in an upright position, it has been shown that no significant difference exists between the results of MR and fluoroscopic examinations despite MR imaging being performed in a supine position.[39] A detailed comparison of the two modalities is provided in **Table 3**.

Table 3
Comparison of functional MR imaging and fluoroscopic examination

	Functional MR Imaging	Fluoroscopy
Diagnostic reliability	Equal or more	Equal or less
Overall sensitivity and specificity	Higher	Lower
Middle compartment disorders	Preferred modality; higher sensitivity	Not sensitive
Identifying content of peritoneal cul-de-sac	No selective opacification of bowel is needed; can differentiate content	Limited; bowel opacification needed
Mucosal vs Full-thickness intussusception	Can diagnose and differentiate both	Can only be inferred
Impact on eventual surgical plan	Significantly altered in 30% of patients	—
Radiation exposure	None	Present
Patient compliance	More	Less
Preparation	None	Oral barium 2 h before
Other pelvic disorders	Can be diagnosed	No

WHAT THE REFERRING PHYSICIAN NEEDS TO KNOW

The patients referred for MR defecography or functional pelvic imaging often present with nonspecific symptoms like fecal incontinence, chronic constipation, perirectal pain, a sense of incomplete evacuation, and organ prolapse. To initiate a patient-specific or tailored management plan, the referring physician needs to know the pertinent findings on each compartment. The principal question is whether or not patients are surgical candidates. If they are, then what procedure is required? An ideal and descriptive report should highlight the disorders in each compartment. A template for an ideal report (**Box 1**) should include the following points:

1. Anterior compartment: presence of cystocele, its size and grade, and mass effect on the vagina; documentation of urethral hypermobility and signs of incontinence.

2. Middle compartment: presence of cervical or vaginal descent and its grading; comment on integrity of paravaginal and rectovaginal fascia and presence of enterocele, peritoneocele, and sigmoidocele.

3. Posterior compartment: presence of rectal intussusception, type of intussusception (full-thickness or mucosal), and its location (intra-rectal, intra-anal, or extra-anal); presence of rectocele and its grade; comment on rectal retention and possible cause.

4. Presence of spastic pelvic floor syndrome.

5. Presence of descending perineal syndrome.

6. Comment on other incidentals or associated findings.

SUMMARY

Functional MR imaging can be a useful tool to use to evaluate patients with suspected pelvic floor dysfunction, and it is emerging as the modality of choice. Because of its inherent soft tissue contrast and multiplanar capabilities, functional MR can provide comprehensive details of pertinent disorders without radiation exposure, and thus can significantly influence the surgical decision.

ACKNOWLEDGMENTS

The authors thank H.K. Pannu, MD, for technical assistance during article preparation.

REFERENCES

1. Law YM, Fielding JR. MRI of pelvic floor dysfunction: review. AJR Am J Roentgenol 2008;191(Suppl 6): S45–53.

2. Drossman DA, Li Z, Andruzzi E, et al. U.S. house-holder survey of functional gastrointestinal disorders. Prevalence, sociodemography, and health impact. Dig Dis Sci 1993;38(9):1569–80.

3. Seynaeve R, Billiet I, Vossaert P, et al. MR imaging of the pelvic floor. JBR-BTR 2006;89(4):182–9.

4. Maglinte DD, Kelvin FM, Fitzgerald K, et al. Association of compartment defects in pelvic floor dysfunction. AJR Am J Roentgenol 1999;172(2):439–44.

5. Hetzer FH, Andreisek G, Tsagari C, et al. MR defecography in patients with fecal incontinence: imaging findings and their effect on surgical management. Radiology 2006;240(2):449–57.

6. Lienemann A, Fischer T. Functional imaging of the pelvic floor. Eur J Radiol 2003;47(2):117–22.

7. Bertschinger KM, Hetzer FH, Roos JE, et al. Dynamic MR imaging of the pelvic floor performed with patient sitting in an open-magnet unit versus with patient supine in a closed-magnet unit. Radiology 2002;223(2):501–8.

8. Hecht EM, Lee VS, Tanpitukpongse TP, et al. MRI of pelvic floor dysfunction: dynamic true fast imaging with steady-state precession versus HASTE. AJR Am J Roentgenol 2008;191(2):352–8.

9. Roos JE, Weishaupt D, Wildermuth S, et al. Experience of 4 years with open MR defecography: pictorial review of anorectal anatomy and disease. Radiographics 2002;22(4):817–32.

10. Colaiacomo MC, Masselli G, Polettini E, et al. Dynamic MR imaging of the pelvic floor: a pictorial review. Radiographics 2009;29(3):e35.

11. Boyadzhyan L, Raman SS, Raz S. Role of static and dynamic MR imaging in surgical pelvic floor dysfunction. Radiographics 2008;28(4):949–67.

12. Barbaric ZL, Marumoto AK, Raz S. Magnetic resonance imaging of the perineum and pelvic floor. Top Magn Reson Imaging 2001;12(2):83–92.

13. Comiter CV, Vasavada SP, Barbaric ZL, et al. Grading pelvic prolapse and pelvic floor relaxation using dynamic magnetic resonance imaging. Urology 1999;54(3):454–7.

14. Bartram CI, Turnbull GK, Lennard-Jones JE. Evacuation proctography: an investigation of rectal expulsion in 20 subjects without defecatory disturbance. Gastrointest Radiol 1988;13(1):72–80.

15. Ekberg O, Nylander G, Fork FT. Defecography. Radiology 1985;155(1):45–8.

16. Healy JC, Halligan S, Reznek RH, et al. Dynamic MR imaging compared with evacuation proctography when evaluating anorectal configuration and pelvic floor movement. AJR Am J Roentgenol 1997;169(3):775–9.

17. Fielding JR, Griffiths DJ, Versi E, et al. MR imaging of pelvic floor continence mechanisms in the supine and sitting positions. AJR Am J Roentgenol 1998;171(6):1607–10.

18. Macura KJ. Magnetic resonance imaging of pelvic floor defects in women. Top Magn Reson Imaging 2006;17(6):417–26.

19. Goh V, Halligan S, Kaplan G, et al. Dynamic MR imaging of the pelvic floor in asymptomatic subjects. AJR Am J Roentgenol 2000;174(3):661–6.

20. Kelvin FM, Maglinte DD, Hale DS, et al. Female pelvic organ prolapse: a comparison of triphasic dynamic MR imaging and triphasic fluoroscopic cystocolpoproctography. AJR Am J Roentgenol 2000;174(1):81–8.

21. Hock D, Lombard R, Jehaes C, et al. Colpocystodefecography. Dis Colon Rectum 1993;36(11):1015–21.

22. Karasick S, Karasick D, Karasick SR. Functional disorders of the anus and rectum: findings on defecography. AJR Am J Roentgenol 1993;160(4):777–82.

23. Lienemann A, Anthuber C, Baron A, et al. Diagnosing enteroceles using dynamic magnetic resonance imaging. Dis Colon Rectum 2000;43(2):205–12 [discussion: 212–3].

24. Mahieu P, Pringot J, Bodart P. Defecography: II. Contribution to the diagnosis of defecation disorders. Gastrointest Radiol 1984;9(3):253–61.

25. Shorvon PJ, McHugh S, Diamant NE, et al. Defecography in normal volunteers: results and implications. Gut 1989;30(12):1737–49.

26. Yoshioka K, Takada H, Hioki K. Rectocele. Nihon Rinsho 1994;(Suppl 6):602–4 [in Japanese].

27. Dvorkin LS, Hetzer F, Scott SM, et al. Open-magnet MR defaecography compared with evacuation proctography in the diagnosis and management of patients with rectal intussusception. Colorectal Dis 2004;6(1):45–53.

28. McCue JL, Thomson JP. Rectopexy for internal rectal intussusception. Br J Surg 1990;77(6):632–4.

29. Tsiaoussis J, Chrysos E, Glynos M, et al. Pathophysiology and treatment of anterior rectal mucosal prolapse syndrome. Br J Surg 1998;85(12):1699–702.

30. Jorge JM, Wexner SD, Ger GC, et al. Cinedefecography and electromyography in the diagnosis of nonrelaxing puborectalis syndrome. Dis Colon Rectum 1993;36(7):668–76.

31. Halligan S, Bartram CI, Park HJ, et al. Proctographic features of anismus. Radiology 1995;197(3):679–82.

32. Bharucha AE, Wald A, Enck P, et al. Functional anorectal disorders. Gastroenterology 2006;130(5):1510–8.

33. Bolog N, Weishaupt D. Dynamic MR imaging of outlet obstruction. Rom J Gastroenterol 2005;14(3):293–302.

34. Karlbom U, Pahlman L, Nilsson S, et al. Relationships between defecographic findings, rectal emptying, and colonic transit time in constipated patients. Gut 1995;36(6):907–12.

35. Kuijpers HC, Bleijenberg G. The spastic pelvic floor syndrome. A cause of constipation. Dis Colon Rectum 1985;28(9):669–72.

36. Lienemann A, Anthuber C, Baron A, et al. Dynamic MR colpocystorectography assessing pelvic-floor descent. Eur Radiol 1997;7(8):1309–17.

37. Pannu HK, Scatarige JC, Eng J. Comparison of supine magnetic resonance imaging with and without rectal contrast to fluoroscopic cystocolpoproctography for the diagnosis of pelvic organ prolapse. J Comput Assist Tomogr 2009;33(1):125–30.

38. Gufler H, Laubenberger J, DeGregorio G, et al. Pelvic floor descent: dynamic MR imaging using a half-Fourier RARE sequence. J Magn Reson Imaging 1999;9(3):378–83.

39. Gufler H, Ohde A, Grau G, et al. Colpocystoproctography in the upright and supine positions correlated with dynamic MRI of the pelvic floor. Eur J Radiol 2004;51(1):41–7.

Index

Note: Page numbers of article titles are in **boldface** type.

Radiol Clin N Am 51 (2013) 1141–1147
http://dx.doi.org/10.1016/S0033-8389(13)00176-0
0033-8389/13/$ – see front matter © 2013 Elsevier Inc. All rights reserved.

United States Postal Service

Statement of Ownership, Management, and Circulation
(All Periodicals Publications Except Requestor Publications)

1. Publication Title
Radiologic Clinics of North America

2. Publication Number
5 9 6 - 5 5 1 0

3. Filing Date
9/14/13

4. Issue Frequency
Jan, Mar, May, Jul, Sep, Nov

5. Number of Issues Published Annually
6

6. Annual Subscription Price
$438.00

7. Complete Mailing Address of Known Office of Publication (Not printer) (Street, city, county, state, and ZIP+4®)

Elsevier Inc.
360 Park Avenue South
New York, NY 10010-1710

Contact Person
Stephen Bushing

Telephone (Include area code)
215-239-3688

8. Complete Mailing Address of Headquarters or General Business Office of Publisher (Not printer)

Elsevier Inc., 360 Park Avenue South, New York, NY 10010-1710

9. Full Names and Complete Mailing Addresses of Publisher, Editor, and Managing Editor (Do not leave blank)

Publisher (Name and complete mailing address)

Linda Belfus, Elsevier, Inc., 1600 John F. Kennedy Blvd. Suite 1800, Philadelphia, PA 19103-2899

Editor (Name and complete mailing address)

Adrianne Brigido, Elsevier, Inc., 1600 John F. Kennedy Blvd. Suite 1800, Philadelphia, PA 19103-2899

Managing Editor (Name and complete mailing address)

Adrianne Brigido, Elsevier, Inc., 1600 John F. Kennedy Blvd. Suite 1800, Philadelphia, PA 19103-2899

10. Owner (Do not leave blank. If the publication is owned by a corporation, give the name and address of the corporation immediately followed by the names and addresses of all stockholders owning or holding 1 percent or more of the total amount of stock. If not owned by a corporation, give the names and addresses of the individual owners. If owned by a partnership or other unincorporated firm, give its name and address as well as those of each individual owner. If the publication is published by a nonprofit organization, give its name and address.)

Full Name	Complete Mailing Address
Wholly owned subsidiary of	1600 John F. Kennedy Blvd., Ste. 1800
Reed/Elsevier, US holdings	Philadelphia, PA 19103-2899

11. Known Bondholders, Mortgagees, and Other Security Holders Owning or Holding 1 Percent or More of Total Amount of Bonds, Mortgages, or Other Securities. If none, check box ☐ None

Full Name	Complete Mailing Address
N/A	

12. Tax Status (For completion by nonprofit organizations authorized to mail at nonprofit rates) (Check one)
The purpose, function, and nonprofit status of this organization and the exempt status for federal income tax purposes:
☐ Has Not Changed During Preceding 12 Months
☐ Has Changed During Preceding 12 Months (Publisher must submit explanation of change with this statement)

PS Form 3526, September 2007 (Page 1 of 3 (Instructions Page 3)) PSN 7530-01-000-9931 PRIVACY NOTICE: See our Privacy policy in www.usps.com

---

13. Publication Title
Radiologic Clinics of North America

14. Issue Date for Circulation Data Below
July 2013

15. Extent and Nature of Circulation

		Average No. Copies Each Issue During Preceding 12 Months	No. Copies of Single Issue Published Nearest to Filing Date
a. Total Number of Copies (Net press run)		3,312	2,640
b. Paid Circulation (By Mail and Outside the Mail)	(1) Mailed Outside-County Paid Subscriptions Stated on PS Form 3541. (Include paid distribution above nominal rate, advertiser's proof copies, and exchange copies)	1,521	1,429
	(2) Mailed In-County Paid Subscriptions Stated on PS Form 3541 (Include paid distribution above nominal rate, advertiser's proof copies, and exchange copies)		
	(3) Paid Distribution Outside the Mails Including Sales Through Dealers and Carriers, Street Vendors, Counter Sales, and Other Paid Distribution Outside USPS®	648	618
	(4) Paid Distribution by Other Classes Mailed Through the USPS (e.g. First-Class Mail®)		
c. Total Paid Distribution (Sum of 15b (1), (2), (3), and (4))	▲	2,169	2,047
d. Free or Nominal Rate Distribution (By Mail and Outside the Mail)	(1) Free or Nominal Rate Outside-County Copies Included on PS Form 3541	69	33
	(2) Free or Nominal Rate In-County Copies Included on PS Form 3541		
	(3) Free or Nominal Rate Copies Mailed at Other Classes Through the USPS (e.g. First-Class Mail)		
	(4) Free or Nominal Rate Distribution Outside the Mail (Carriers or other means)		
e. Total Free or Nominal Rate Distribution (Sum of 15d (1), (2), (3) and (4))	▲	69	33
f. Total Distribution (Sum of 15c and 15e)	▲	2,238	2,080
g. Copies not Distributed (See instructions to publishers #4 (page #3))	▲	1,074	560
h. Total (Sum of 15f and g)	▲	3,312	2,640
i. Percent Paid (15c divided by 15f times 100)		96.92%	98.41%

16. Publication of Statement of Ownership
☐ If the publication is a general publication, publication of this statement is required. Will be printed in the November 2013 issue of this publication. ☐ Publication not required

17. Signature and Title of Editor, Publisher, Business Manager, or Owner

Stephen R. Bushing

Stephen R. Bushing –Inventory Distribution Coordinator

Date
September 14, 2013

I certify that all information furnished on this form is true and complete. I understand that anyone who furnishes false or misleading information on this form or who omits material or information requested on the form may be subject to criminal sanctions (including fines and imprisonment) and/or civil sanctions (including civil penalties).

PS Form 3526, September 2007 (Page 2 of 3)